FIGHT BACK
WITH FOOD

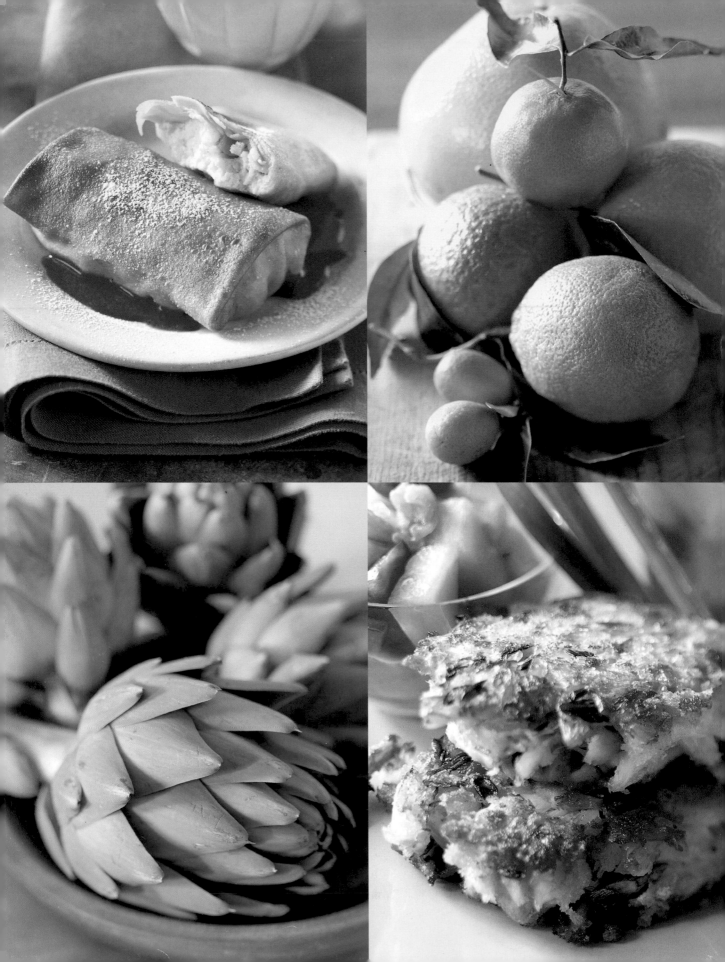

FIGHT BACK
WITH FOOD

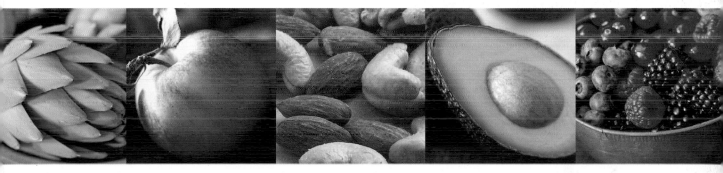

USE NUTRITION TO EASE WHAT AILS YOU

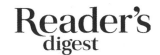

Reader's digest

The Reader's Digest Association, Inc.
New York, NY/Montreal

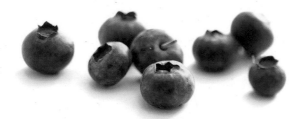

First printing in paperback 2007

Copyright © 2002 The Reader's Digest Association, Inc.

Address any comments about FIGHT BACK WITH FOOD to

The Reader's Digest Association, Inc.

Adult Trade Publishing

44 S. Broadway

White Plains, NY 10601

You can also visit us at www.rd.com

Library of Congress Cataloging in Publication Data

Fight back with food : using nutrition to heal what ails you

p. cm.

Includes index.

ISBN: 0-7621-0342-6 (hardcover)

ISBN: 978-0-7621-0840-4 (paperback)

1. Diet therapy--Popular works. 3. Functional foods--Popular works. I. Reader's Digest Association.

RM216.F527 2002

615.8'54--dc21

2001041621

Printed in China

1 3 5 7 9 10 8 6 4 2 (hardcover)

9 10 (paperback)

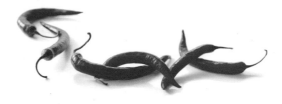

FIGHT BACK WITH FOOD

Reader's Digest Project Staff

EDITORIAL DIRECTOR
Wayne Kalyn

ART DIRECTOR
Joan Mazzeo

ASSOCIATE DESIGNER
Jennifer R. Tokarski

PRODUCTION TECHNOLOGY MANAGER
Douglas A. Croll

EDITORIAL MANAGER
Christine R. Guido

Reader's Digest

PRESIDENT, NORTH AMERICAN BOOKS
AND HOME ENTERTAINMENT
Tom Gardner

VICE PRESIDENT/GENERAL MANAGER
Shirrel Rhoades

MARKETING
James Malloy

Created by Rebus, Inc.

PUBLISHER
Rodney M. Friedman

EXECUTIVE EDITOR
Kate Slate

SENIOR NUTRITION EDITOR
Maureen Mulhern-White

NUTRITION WRITER/RESEARCHER
Patricia Kaupas

TEST KITCHEN DIRECTOR/FOOD EDITOR
Sandra Rose Gluck

ASSISTANT EDITOR
James W. Brown, Jr.

ART DIRECTOR
Timothy Jeffs

DESIGN ASSISTANT
Bree Rock

PHOTOGRAPHER
Alan Richardson

PHOTOGRAPHER'S ASSISTANT
Roy Galaday

FOOD STYLISTS
Anne Disrude, Jee Levin

ASSISTANT FOOD STYLIST
Maggie Ruggiero

PROP STYLIST
Betty Alfenito

CONSULTANTS
Jeanine Barone, M.S.
David M. DeVellis, M.D.
Barbara Levine, Ph.D, R.D.
Hill Nutrition Associates

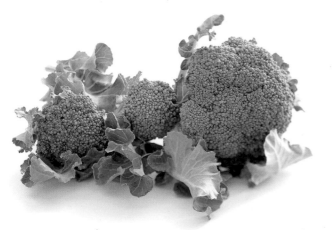

contents

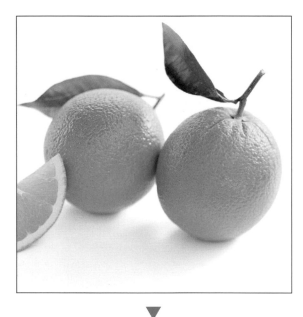

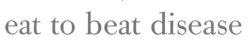

eat to beat disease

An A-to-Z Guide to the Nutrients That
Help Fight Disease

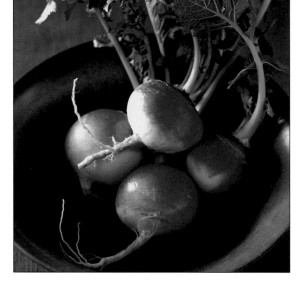

foods that fight back

Super Foods—and the Nutrients in Them—
That Keep You Healthy

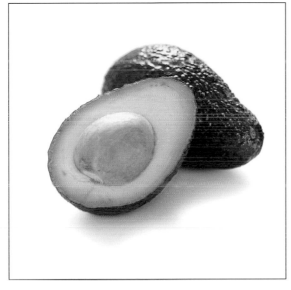

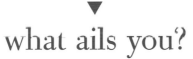

what ails you?

How to Manage or Prevent Common
Ailments Through Diet

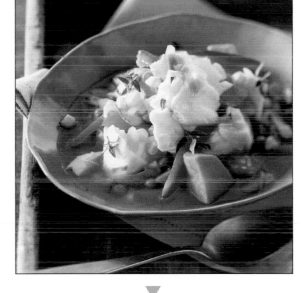

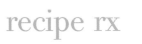

recipe rx

Delicious Dishes That Maximize the
Fighting Power of Food

index

eat to beat disease

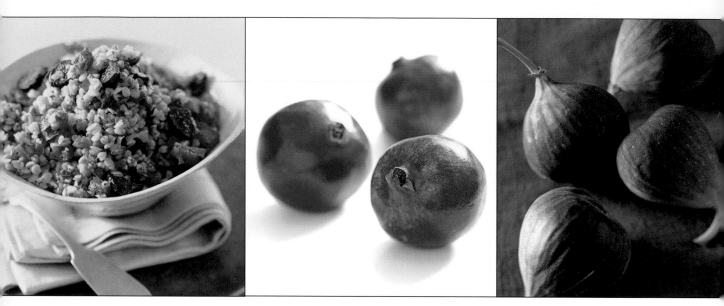

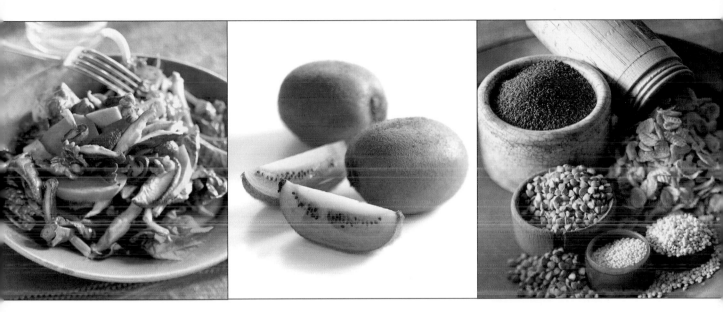

An A-to-Z Guide

to the Nutrients That

Help Fight Disease

eat to beat disease

food as medicine

For thousands of years, people of different cultures have been conscious of the relationship between food and health. Traditional Chinese healers prescribed particular foods to help invigorate the body's vital energy. And the ancient Indians,

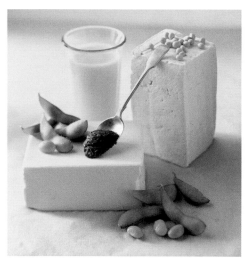

Egyptians, Greeks, and Romans were also keenly aware that medicinal and healing properties of certain foods could play a vital role in human health. This sentiment was put into words over 2,500 years ago when the father of medicine, Hippocrates, wrote "Let medicine be your food, and food your medicine." The idea that food can function as medicine has come full circle. What the people of these ancient cultures believed about the therapeutic value of certain foods, modern nutritional science is now confirming

the foundation

A century ago, scientists discovered the vital food substances—vitamins and minerals—that remedied common debilitating nutritional diseases and maintained good health. They found that if the body doesn't get the proper nutrients, its normal functioning can become impaired. For example, it was discovered that a calcium deficiency could lead to osteoporosis, a lack of iron could cause anemia, and insufficient folate could result in birth defects. Along with this fundamental understanding of the relationship between nutrients and disease prevention came the realization that a broad spectrum of nutrients is also required to energize all the body's cells, foster normal growth and development, and promote longevity.

"Let medicine be your food, and food your medicine."
— Hippocrates

the new nutrition

Today, we are at the forefront of a new and exciting era in nutrition research. Scientists have moved beyond the vitamins and minerals we all know and have begun identifying an army of nutrients that may play an active role in preventing and/or managing disease. Research shows that a single plant food can contain hundreds of disease-fighting nutrients called phytochemicals: compounds that are responsible for the brilliant color and distinct flavor and aroma of fruits, vegetables, and whole grains. Everyday foods—such as green peas or potatoes or apples—contain nutrients that may help ward off cancer, heart disease, depression, obesity, allergies, and other disorders.

Phytochemicals, in their native state, act as protective barriers, shielding plants against insects, bacteria, viruses, UV light, and other environmental threats.

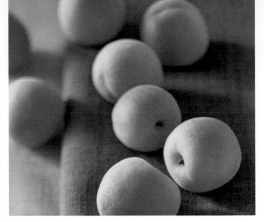

Fortunately, the benefits of phytochemicals extend beyond the botanical world: These potent plant compounds appear to guard the human body from disease in a variety of ways. According to research, many phytochemicals help the body to dispose of potentially hazardous substances, including carcinogens, and may protect DNA in cells from damage that can trigger a disease process. Numerous phytochemicals stimulate the body's immune cells and infection-fighting enzymes. Still other phytochemicals help to balance hormone levels, thus reducing the risk for hormone-related conditions and cancers, such as symptoms of menopause, and breast and prostate cancer. And a vast number of phytochemicals function as antioxidants, which neutralize the harmful free radicals (unstable oxygen molecules) that may play a role in the onset of degenerative diseases.

the importance of whole foods

Because phytochemical research is an emerging science, optimal as well as safe intakes of phytochemicals have not yet been established. The best way to acquire phytochemicals is from consuming a diversity of foods. This is beneficial for several reasons: Just as phytochemicals in a particular food can team up to combat disease and enhance well-being, so do the phytochemicals from a wide range of foods work together to promote good health. It also seems that fiber, vitamins, minerals, and other substances in food may enhance and regulate the actions of phytochemicals.

what the future holds

Current research is now on the road to identifying not only the healthful substances themselves but also their synergies and how the nutrients behave in the human body. For example, scientists are exploring the bioavailability of nutrients in foods (it's in the food, but can our bodies use it?), the mechanism by which these nutrients may fight off environmental toxins, and the effects of processing on the quality of phytonutrients. Researchers are also hoping to discover how certain foods can influence complex aspects of human health, including mood, memory, longevity, and immune responsiveness. We are also witnessing enormously promising innovations resulting from "functional food" research (see *Enhancing Foods for Health, page 18*).

As we enter this new millennium, the science of nutrition will allow us to understand how a food's chemical properties, its nutrient interaction with other foods (as well as medications), its organic compounds, phytochemicals, and micro-

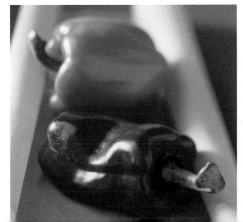

nutrients all work to avoid disease and enhance human health. Each year, researchers discover new interactions and beneficial effects of phytochemicals. Who knows how many healing plant compounds are still to be discovered that will contribute to our arsenal of foods that fight disease?

guide to the new nutrition

The following compendium of nutrition terms and food substances demonstrates the complexity of nutrition today, and the wealth of nutrients that play a part in human health.

For an overview of the most prominent vitamins, minerals, and phytochemicals, see *Top 10 Vitamins and Minerals* (page 14) and *Top 10 Phytochemicals* (page 24).

actinidin An enzyme found in kiwifruit, actinidin is believed to aid digestion. It may also be used as a natural meat tenderizer.

ajoenes These phytochemicals are found in garlic and may reduce LDL ("bad") cholesterol and may possess antithrombotic (anticlotting), anticancer, and antifungal activity. *See also* SULFUR COMPOUNDS.

allicin Responsible for garlic's pungent smell, allicin produces numerous SULFUR COMPOUNDS, possibly with antibacterial properties.

allium compounds See SULFUR COMPOUNDS.

allyl isothiocyanate This ISOTHIOCYANATE compound may battle cancer, and its pungent nature may clear congestion due to colds and flu. Sources: brussels sprouts, cabbage, horseradish, kale, brown mustard seeds.

allyl methyl trisulfide This SULFUR COMPOUND may stimulate the activity of glutathione S-transferase, an enzyme known to assist in the detoxification of carcinogens in the liver and colon. Sources: garlic, onions, leeks.

allyl sulfides These SULFUR COMPOUNDS, found in garlic, onions, leeks, scallions, and other members of the onion family, are under review for their potential to fight cancer.

alpha-carotene Like BETA-CAROTENE, alpha-carotene is an antioxidant carotenoid and a precursor to VITAMIN A. Sources: apricots, carrots, pumpkins, sweet potatoes.

alpha-linolenic acid (ALA) Alpha-linolenic acid (ALA) is an ESSENTIAL FATTY ACID linked to a wide range of health benefits. Vital for many functions, alpha-linolenic acid cannot be made in the body and must therefore be obtained from foods. ALA is important for the maintenance of cell membranes and for creating regulatory substances in the body that protect against inflammatory conditions. ALA converts in the human body into two omega-3 fatty acids: EPA (EICOSAPENTAENOIC ACID) and DHA (DOCOSAHEXAENOIC ACID). Sources: canola oil, soybean oil, flaxseed, purslane, walnuts.

amino acids These are the building blocks of protein. Twenty amino acids are necessary for proper human growth and function. Many amino acids can be synthesized in the body when needed; these are called nonessential. Essential amino acids (such as LYSINE and TRYPTOPHAN to name two) cannot be synthesized in sufficient quantities and must be provided by diet.

anthocyanins Responsible for the red and blue pigments found in certain fruits and vegetables, anthocyanins are FLAVONOIDS under review for their potential to suppress tumor cell growth, to lower LDL ("bad") cholesterol levels, and to prevent blood from forming too many clots. Sources: apples, berries, red cabbage, cherries, red and purple grapes, plums, pomegranates.

antioxidants Found in a wide variety of plant-based foods, antioxidants are compounds that may have the potential to prevent numerous diseases. Serving as internal bodyguards, antioxidants roam through the body and scout out and destroy FREE RADICALS. By scavenging and destroying free radicals, antioxidants may protect against various types of cancer, improve cardiovascular health, enhance immunity, and protect against cataracts and macular degeneration. Some of the most potent disease-fighting powers attributed to certain phytochemicals and vitamins (particularly VITAMIN E, VITAMIN C, CAROTENOIDS, SELENIUM, and FLAVONOIDS) are due to their antioxidant abilities. A natural synergy occurs when some of the antioxidants work together to disarm free radicals and protect cells from damage.

apigenin This compound is a FLAVONOID that may stop tumor growth as well as exert anti-inflammatory action. Sources: celery, parsley.

arginine This cardioprotective nonessential (though it's essential in childhood) amino acid is believed to enhance circulation and strengthen blood flow around the heart. For people who are prone to developing cold sores, however, it may be a good idea to lower your intake

of arginine-rich foods and increase your intake of lysine-rich foods if you are feeling run-down. Food sources: dairy foods, fish, poultry, nuts.

beta-carotene One of the most studied of the CAROTENOIDS, beta-carotene is a potent antioxidant plentiful in red, orange, and yellow plant foods (as well as in dark green vegetables where the orange color is masked by CHLOROPHYLL) and is converted by the body into VITAMIN A. Sources: apricots, carrots, brussels sprouts, dark leafy greens, pumpkin, spinach, sweet potatoes, winter squash.

beta-cryptoxanthin This CAROTENOID may help to prevent colon cancer, and some studies suggest that it may also protect the lungs by offering antioxidant protection. Sources: apricots, oranges, tangerines.

beta-glucan Beta-glucan is a type of soluble dietary FIBER that helps to lower serum cholesterol levels. Sources: barley, brown rice bran, maitake mushrooms, oats, reishi mushrooms, shiitake mushrooms.

beta-sitosterol A PLANT STEROL similar in structure to cholesterol, beta-sitosterol may help to manage benign prostatic hyperplasia (BPH), as well as protect against high choles-

---

The U.S. Diet

The U.S. Dietary Guidelines—established by the U.S. Department of Agriculture (USDA) and the Department of Health and Human Services (HHS)—are designed to help people understand what types of food constitute the foundation of a balanced and sound diet. They also are designed to promote health by helping people meet their nutrient requirements. To meet the Dietary Guidelines, health professionals advocate a low-fat diet with most of the calories coming from nutrient-dense grains, vegetables, and fruits; moderate amounts from low-fat dairy products, lean meats, fish, and poultry; and the fewest calories from fats and sweets.

The U.S. Dietary Guidelines are represented graphically in what is called the "food pyramid": The wide base of the pyramid represents whole grains (bread, cereal, rice, and pasta), vegetables, and fruits. Animal products (dairy, meat, poultry, fish, eggs) are the narrower section, in the center. And sweets, fats, and oils are the smallest part of the pyramid, at the very top.

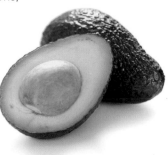

top 10 vitamins & minerals

vitamin/mineral	may be helpful for	where to find it
calcium	osteoporosis, anxiety & stress, high blood pressure, hyperthyroidism, overweight, perimenopause & menopause, PMS, pregnancy	broccoli, dairy products, salmon or sardines with bones, tofu
folate	anemia, cancer, depression, heart disease, infertility & impotence, insomnia, osteoporosis, pregnancy, rheumatoid arthritis	asparagus, avocados, beans, beets, broccoli, cabbage family, citrus fruit, cooking greens, corn, lentils, peas, rice, spinach
iron	anemia, immune deficiency, memory loss, pregnancy	apricots, fatty fish, figs, lentils, meat, peas, poultry, shellfish
magnesium	allergies & asthma, anxiety & stress, chronic fatigue syndrome, constipation, diabetes, high blood pressure, kidney stones, migraine, PMS	avocados, grains, nuts, rice, seeds, shellfish, spinach, winter squash
selenium	allergies & asthma, cancer, hypothyroidism, infertility & impotence, macular degeneration, prostate problems	meats, mushrooms, nuts, poultry, rice, seeds, shellfish, whole grains
vitamin B_6	acne, anemia, anxiety & stress, depression, heart disease, hypothyroidism, insomnia, memory loss, PMS, pregnancy	asparagus, bananas, fatty fish, figs, mushrooms, peas, potatoes, poultry, rice, sweet potatoes, winter squash
vitamin B_{12}	anemia, depression, heart disease, infertility & impotence	dairy products, fatty fish, meat, poultry, shellfish
vitamin C	allergies & asthma, anemia, bronchitis, cancer, cataracts, chronic fatigue syndrome, cold sores, colds & flu, diabetes, eczema, heart disease, hemorrhoids, infertility & impotence, high blood pressure, hyperthyroidism, immune deficiency, macular degeneration, osteoarthritis, osteoporosis, rheumatoid arthritis, sinusitis, sprains & strains	berries, cabbage family, citrus fruits, kiwifruit, melons, peas, peppers, pineapple, potatoes, salad greens, spinach, sweet potatoes, tomatoes, turnips, winter squash
vitamin E	bronchitis, cancer, cataracts, eczema, hyperthyroidism, immune deficiency, infertility & impotence, memory loss, macular degeneration, osteoarthritis, prostate problems, rheumatoid arthritis	avocados, grains, nuts, olive oil, salad greens, seeds
zinc	acne, bronchitis, chronic fatigue syndrome, colds & flu, cold sores, eczema, hemorrhoids, hypothyroidism, immunity, infertility & impotence, macular degeneration, rosacea, sinusitis	beans, grains, meat, poultry, seeds, shellfish

terol and cancer. Sources: avocados, corn oil, rice bran, seeds, soy foods, wheat germ.

betacyanin A type of plant pigment, betacyanin gives beets their rich crimson color and is also linked with antioxidant activity in the body.

betaine This phytochemical may be helpful in lowering HOMOCYSTEINE levels. Source: beets.

biotin This B vitamin is required for the metabolism of fatty acids, amino acids, and carbohydrates from food. Biotin also assists the body in the utilization of blood sugar (glucose), a major source of energy. Sources: barley, legumes, cauliflower, corn, egg yolks, mushrooms, oats, peanut butter, rice, soy foods.

boron This bone-nourishing mineral is thought to enhance the body's ability to use CALCIUM, MAGNESIUM, and VITAMIN D. Sources: beans, nuts.

bromelain An enzyme derived from pineapples, bromelain is believed to have anti-inflammatory and pain-reducing properties.

caffeic acid This widely available PHENOLIC COMPOUND may have antioxidant capabilities and may block carcinogenic substances generated from seared or charred meat and seafood. Sources: apples, carrots, celery, coffee beans, grapes, onions, potatoes, soy foods, tomatoes, spinach.

calcium The most abundant and important mineral in the body, calcium is vital for maintaining the integrity of bones and teeth. Dairy foods are the best dietary sources of calcium. Other sources: broccoli, salmon with bones, sardines with bones.

calcium pectate Responsible for the characteristic crunch of certain fruits and vegetables, calcium pectate is a PECTIN FIBER that may lower LDL ("bad") choles-

terol levels. Sources: apples, cabbage, carrots, onions.

campesterol A PLANT STEROL, campesterol may be helpful in managing symptoms of benign prostatic hyperplasia (BPH) and high cholesterol. Sources: nuts, olive oil, peanuts, seeds, soybeans.

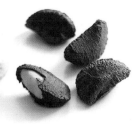

capsaicin This phytochemical gives hot peppers their fiery taste. Along with easing congestion, capsaicin is currently being investigated for its antioxidant and disease-protective effects. Food sources: chili peppers, cayenne pepper.

carbohydrates These energy-yielding nutrients are the most efficient fuel source for the body (PROTEIN and FATS also provide energy to the body). Carbohydrates are readily broken down into glucose, a simple sugar that rapidly and effectively feeds the body's tissues. Though there are many types of carbohydrates (including so-called simple carbohydrates, sometimes also called simple sugars), the type with most nutritional importance is COMPLEX CARBOHYDRATES.

carnosol A substance that has antioxidant potential, carnosol may fight tumors by detoxifying cancerous chemicals. Sources: rosemary, sage.

carotenoids These pigments give certain produce their characteristic orange, yellow, and red colors. They may possess potent antioxidant power to fight heart disease, certain types of cancer, as well as degenerative eye diseases such as cataracts and macular degeneration. To date, more than 600 carotenoids have been identified, but only six are known to provide us with significant health benefits: ALPHA-CAROTENE, BETA-CAROTENE, BETA-CRYPTOXANTHIN, LYCOPENE, LUTEIN, and ZEAXANTHIN.

catechins This class of FLAVONOIDS appears predominantly in green tea and exhibits cardioprotective, chemoprotective, and antimicrobial properties. Sources: dark chocolate, red grapes, red wine, pomegranates, tea. *See also* EGCG (EPIGALLOCATECHIN GALLATE).

chlorogenic acid This PHENOLIC COMPOUND may prevent nitrates from forming into cancer-causing nitrosamines. Sources: artichokes, berries, cherries, potatoes, soybeans, sweet potatoes, tomatoes.

chlorophyll The green pigment of leaves and plants, chlorophyll not only helps to freshen breath but it may also help to prevent DNA damage to cells. Sources: dark leafy greens, kiwifruit, parsley, peas, peppers.

cholesterol This is a type of fat present only in animal foods and is also synthesized by the body. Cholesterol is an important element of all cell membranes and serves as a precursor to VITAMIN D, hormones, and bile (for digestion). Excessive cholesterol circulating in the blood can build up on artery walls, leading to heart disease and stroke.

choline A vitamin-like substance required for cell membrane integrity, choline is also important for normal brain and liver function. Sources: cabbage, cauliflower, dairy foods, eggs, navy beans, soybeans, wheat germ.

Balancing Fats

Health professionals speculate that some chronic diseases in the United States may be due to an imbalance in the types of fats consumed in the average American diet. Over the past 100 years or so, due in part to advances in technology and the prevalence of processed foods, Americans are consuming disproportionately lower levels of the beneficial fats, such as MONOUNSATURATED FATS and OMEGA-3 FATTY ACIDS, and higher levels of SATURATED FATS, TRANS FATTY ACIDS, and OMEGA-6 FATTY ACIDS. For optimal health, it's best to try to shift this balance toward foods rich in omega-3 and monounsaturated fatty acids, since these healthful fats have been linked to the prevention of numerous diseases.

chromium This essential trace mineral is necessary for the manufacture of insulin and for the breakdown of MACRONUTRIENTS. Sources: nuts, potatoes, prunes, seafood, whole grains.

complex carbohydrates FIBER and starch in legumes, vegetables, and grains are complex carbohydrates. A diet that emphasizes complex carbohydrates can help protect against cardiovascular disease, improve blood sugar levels, relieve diarrhea, and ease insomnia. Sources: fruits, grains, legumes, potatoes, rice.

copper This trace mineral is instrumental in bone formation, blood clotting, normal immune function, and skeletal mineralization. Sources: amaranth, avocados, mushrooms, potatoes, shellfish, sunflower seeds.

cruciferous vegetables A family of phytochemical-rich vegetables named for their cross-shaped flowers, cruciferous vegetables are touted for their powerful healing compounds that exhibit cancer-fighting activity in laboratory studies. Cruciferous vegetables include bok choy, broccoli, brussels sprouts, cabbage, cauliflower, kale, mustard greens, radishes, rutabaga, turnips, watercress.

curcumin A phytochemical compound that lends yellow color to turmeric, curcumin is currently under review for its antioxidant abilities. Sources: turmeric, curry powder, certain types of mustard with turmeric.

cyanidin A type of ANTHOCYANIN, cyanidin may reduce pain by blocking inflammatory enzymes in the body. Sources: berries, cherries.

cynarin Found in artichokes, cynarin may support liver health, lower harmful cholesterol, and possibly combat environmental carcinogens. Cynarin also appears to lend a sweet aftertaste to other foods and drinks.

daidzein An ISOFLAVONE found in soy foods, daidzein is thought to inhibit the growth of cancer cells and the onset of osteoporosis, and may improve heart health. Daidzein's mild estrogenic attributes may relieve menopausal symptoms as well. *See also* PHYTOESTROGENS.

DHA An OMEGA-3 FATTY ACID, DHA (docosahexaenoic acid) is important for all phases of the human life cycle. A major building block of human brain tissue and the primary structural fatty acid in the gray matter of the brain and the retina, DHA is vital for brain and eye health. Studies indicate that DHA may have cardiovascular benefits as well as neurological benefits. Although the body can convert ALPHA-LINOLENIC ACID into DHA, the amount produced is minimal so you are better off getting DHA directly from food. Sources: fatty fish, shellfish.

diallyl sulfide A powerful SULFUR COMPOUND, diallyl sulfide may help to prevent stomach cancer and may also have significant cholesterol-lowering properties. Sources: chives, garlic, leeks, onions, scallions, shallots.

diosmin A FLAVONOID found in citrus fruit, diosmin is thought to bolster blood vessels and help prevent certain types of cancer. Sources: citrus fruit, rosemary.

dithiolthiones These phytochemicals are thought to activate enzymes in the body that detoxify carcinogens. Laboratory studies suggest that dithiolthiones may inhibit the development of tumors of the lung, colon, breast, and bladder. Sources: bok choy, broccoli, cabbage, cauliflower.

EGCG A CATECHIN in green tea, EGCG (epigallocatechin gallate) is part of the POLYPHENOL family. As an antioxidant, EGCG appears to destroy harmful free radicals, and may possess cardioprotective and anticancer attributes.

ellagic acid A PHENOLIC COMPOUND with potent antioxidant capabilities, ellagic acid is thought to fight cancer by inducing cancer cell death as well as by inhibiting carcinogens such as tobacco smoke or air pollution. Sources: apples, apricots, berries, grapes, pomegranates, walnuts.

EPA An OMEGA-3 FATTY ACID, eicosapentaenoic acid (EPA) is linked to cardiovascular and anticancer benefits, and may help improve inflammatory conditions such as rheumatoid arthritis. Although the body can convert ALPHA-LINOLENIC ACID into EPA, the amount produced is minimal so you are better off getting EPA directly from food. Sources: mackerel, sardines, salmon, herring, shellfish.

ergosterol Found in mushrooms, ergosterol is converted in the body into VITAMIN D.

eritadenine Preliminary laboratory studies suggest that eritadenine may reduce LDL ("bad") cholesterol. Source: shiitake mushrooms.

essential fatty acids (EFAs) The building blocks of necessary fats, EFAs must be obtained through food. They are involved in the manufacture of anti-inflammatory compounds, the transmission of nerve impulses, energy metabolism, and the promotion of cardiovascular and immune system health. Sources: canola oil, fatty fish, flaxseed oil, sunflower seeds, walnuts, wheat germ.

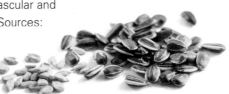

fats An important energy reserve for the body, fat also cushions organs, provides insulation, transports fat-soluble nutrients, and lends structure to cell membranes. The major type of fat in food and in the body is triglycerides. CHOLESTEROL

enhancing foods for health

Research, technology, and widespread interest in nutrition have sparked an explosion of health-promoting foods. Supermarket shelves are filled with foods created to boost health and longevity: calcium-fortified orange juice, folate-fortified cereal, cholesterol-lowering margarine spreads, and many more. Through processing, growing methods, animal feed, or biotechnology, a broad spectrum of foods is supplemented with ingredients designed to ward off disease.

The idea of adding ingredients to food is not new, of course: For example, early last century iodine was first added to salt to help guard against goiter. But with current research, many products and foods are now being enhanced with more esoteric ingredients, such as phytonutrients and cardioprotective fats. To categorize an ever-evolving genre of health-promoting foods, a number of terms have been coined by academia and the food industry.

▶ **enriched foods** Many grain-based foods, such as bread, flour, and cereal, are commonly "enriched" with certain nutrients—riboflavin, thiamin, folate, and iron. These essential nutrients are lost during processing and are added back into the food in varying amounts after it has been processed. Note that whole-grain products possess superior nutrition to processed grains since enrichment does not replace all the nutrients, fiber, and phytochemicals lost during processing. One cup of whole-wheat flour, for example, contains higher levels of nutrients than 1 cup of "enriched" white flour. Another category of enriched foods is omega-3-enriched eggs. Hens are given a feed supplemented with omega-3s to produce a heart-healthy version of the traditional egg.

▶ **fortified foods** To boost protection against chronic disease or to help prevent a nutrient deficiency, certain foods are fortified with nutrients not present in the original food. Vitamin D-fortified milk, iodized salt, folate-fortified wheat products, calcium-fortified orange juice, and cereal fortified with vitamin B_{12} are well-known fortified foods that help to prevent nutrient deficiencies.

▶ **functional food** A loosely defined umbrella term, "functional food" refers to any food that promotes health beyond satisfying basic nutrition needs. The term reflects the growing number of enhanced foods available to us and does not carry scientific or legal meaning. Falling into the category of functional foods are "nutraceuticals," "pharmafoods," and "designer foods," all of which are promoted as imparting a particular health or medicinal benefit, including the prevention and treatment of disease. Genetically modified foods (see below) fall into the category of designer foods. Unenhanced foods with natural disease-fighting properties (such as garlic or tomatoes), as well as enriched and fortified foods, are also considered functional foods.

▶ **genetically modified foods** These are foods whose genetic make-up is altered in an effort to produce a new plant with more desirable characteristics, such as increased resistance to spoilage or improved nutritional content. Considerable controversy surrounds genetically modified foods, as long-term health and environmental effects and ethical issues are not resolved.

▶ **organic foods** Organic foods are grown and/or processed without the use of such synthetic chemicals as pesticides, herbicides, preservatives, growth hormones, and antibiotics. The benefits of organic foods are not clear-cut. Although organic fruits and vegetables may be more flavorful and colorful, their nutritional value has not been established as superior to nonorganic fruits and vegetables. Also, many organic foods tend to spoil faster and organically grown fruits and vegetables may harbor harmful microbes, such as *E. coli*, due to organic methods of fertilization. On the other hand, some experts maintain that certain organic meats have a healthier fatty acid content compared with conventional meat.

is a fatlike substance present in the blood and in food. Fatty acids are the building blocks of triglycerides, and the so-called ESSENTIAL FATTY ACIDS (such as OMEGA-3S and OMEGA-6S) must be obtained from the diet, because they cannot be manufactured by the body. As the most dense source of food energy, fat serves up more than twice the amount of calories per gram as carbohydrate or protein. For optimal health, experts advise a low-fat diet rich in nourishing MONOUNSATURATED FAT and omega-3 fatty acids in place of SATURATED FAT and TRANS FATS.

ferulic acid Research suggests that this phytochemical may inhibit cancer-causing substances, such as nitrosamines. Sources: apples, pineapple.

fiber, insoluble Composed of indigestible plant parts, insoluble fiber adds bulk to stools, which eases elimination. Insoluble fiber may promote satiety as well. Sources: broccoli, cabbage, celery, flaxseed, salad greens, sweet potatoes.

fiber, soluble Soluble fiber forms a gel-like mass around food particles, preventing cholesterol from being absorbed and promoting its excretion. PECTIN and BETA-GLUCAN are two types of soluble fiber that are particularly beneficial for lowering cholesterol levels. Soluble fiber also helps to manage diarrhea and may regulate levels of blood glucose as well. Sources: apples, apricots, beans, berries, figs, oats, plums, prunes, pumpkin.

ficin Found in figs, ficin is an enzyme with mild laxative properties.

flavonoids Powerful antioxidants, flavonoids are phytochemicals linked to a reduced risk of cardiovascular disease and may impede the development of cancer. The free-radical scavenging properties of flavonoids are thought to reduce inflammation associated with rheumatoid arthritis, slow age-related decline in memory function, bolster blood vessels, and improve the potency of immune cells. Some important flavonoid compounds include CATECHINS, ELLAGIC ACID, KAEMPFEROL, QUERCETIN, and RUTIN. Sources: fruits, vegetables, grains, tea, wine.

fluoride Known as a mineral that protects teeth against dental decay, fluoride is also involved in the maintenance of bone structure and is found primarily in bone tissue. Sources: fluoridated water, seafood.

folate This B vitamin is present mostly in green leafy vegetables. The synthetic form is called folic acid, which is found in most fortified cereal. Folate helps to prevent neural tube defects in newborns and may lower levels of the amino acid HOMOCYSTEINE. Sources: asparagus, avocado, beans, beets, broccoli, chicory, lentils, oranges, peas, salad greens, spinach.

free radicals Unstable, highly reactive oxygen molecules, free radicals are the products of metabolism and are also found in the environment: UV radiation from sunlight, smoke, and other forms of pollution. Free radicals contribute to "oxidative stress," which is implicated in premature aging as well as the onset of many diseases.

fructooligosaccharides (FOS) Indigestible carbohydrate compounds, fructooligosaccharides (FOS) are thought to encourage the growth of friendly bacteria in the body and may reduce the amount of toxins produced by unfriendly flora in the colon. Sources: bananas, chicory, onion family.

genistein A potent ISOFLAVONE with estrogenlike activity, genistein may help balance hormones and may reduce the risk for hormone-related cancer, such as prostate cancer, as well as help prevent

Eating the Rainbow

Have you ever wondered what gives a carrot its rich orange color (beta-carotene)? Or why blueberries are a deep bluish purple (anthocyanins)?

Plant pigments such as carotenoids and anthocyanins are responsible for giving color to certain plant foods, and science has discovered that often the most vibrantly colorful fruits and vegetables tend to contain the most potent disease-fighting compounds. For example, a salad that includes slices of orange peppers provides an impressive amount of carotenoids such as alpha-carotene and beta-carotene. Toss in some kernels of corn and you will benefit from a carotenoid called lutein. Add some red tomatoes and you will receive a variety of benefits from lycopene, the carotenoid that gives tomatoes their distinctive red color. Toss with some deep-green lettuce for more beta-carotene.

These vibrant pigments may help to prevent cancer and cardiovascular disease by acting as antioxidants that protect cells from damage by disabling harmful free radicals.

---

fibrocystic breasts and premenstrual syndrome. Sources: soy foods. *See also* PHYTOESTROGENS.

gingerol A phytochemical in ginger, gingerol is believed to reduce swelling and tenderness of the joints. Ginger may help with nausea and vomiting as well.

glucosinolates A class of anticancer phytochemicals present in CRUCIFEROUS VEGETABLES, glucosinolates when ingested are metabolized into various beneficial compounds such as INDOLES, ISOTHIO-CYANATES, and SULFORAPHANE.

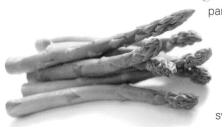

glutathione An essential part of several antioxidant enzymes that naturally occur in the body, glutathione may detoxify carcinogenic compounds and enhance the immune system. Sources: apples, asparagus, avocados.

gluten Gluten is a protein in barley, buckwheat, oats, rye, and wheat. Certain people, particularly those with celiac disease, have an intolerance to gluten; they experience an adverse gastrointestinal reaction to gluten, so they must avoid foods made with these grains.

goitrogens When eaten in large quantities, goitrogens in uncooked foods have the potential to interfere with the absorption of IODINE and slow thyroid function. Goitrogens are primarily found in cabbage, turnips, mustard greens, and radishes, but are present in relatively small quantities.

hesperidin A FLAVONOID found in the zest (or outer, colored portion of the peel) of citrus fruits, hesperidin may improve the integrity of capillary linings.

homocysteine A compound that results from the breakdown of methionine, an essential amino acid, homocysteine, at high levels in the blood, increases the risk for atherosclerosis, and possibly other conditions. An estimated 20% to 40% of people with clogged arteries, or those who have suffered strokes or heart attacks, have abnormally high levels of homocysteine. The good news is that researchers have discovered that several B vitamins, FOLATE, VITAMIN B$_6$ and VITAMIN B$_{12}$, can help lower homocysteine levels.

hydroxytyrosol A PHENOLIC COMPOUND that contributes to the characteristic flavor and aroma of olives and olive oil, hydroxytyrosol may protect against breast cancer, high blood pressure, heart disease, and stroke.

indole-3-carbinol A well-studied INDOLE compound and a member of the GLUCOSINOLATE phytochemical family, indole-3-carbinol is particularly abundant in broccoli. Indole-3-carbinol may offer protection against hormone-dependent cancers, such as breast cancer. Sources: CRUCIFEROUS VEGETABLES.

indoles Partially responsible for the strong taste of broccoli and brussels sprouts, indoles are a class of GLUCOSINOLATE phytochemicals present in CRUCIFEROUS VEGETABLES and may stimulate cancer-fighting enzymes.

inulin An indigestible carbohydrate compound, inulin may help stabilize blood glucose levels, activate immune cells, reduce inflammation, and promote friendly intestinal bacteria. Sources: chicory, jerusalem artichokes.

iodine Tiny amounts of this trace mineral are required for normal cell metabolism and thyroid function. Sources: fish, iodized salt, seaweed, shellfish.

iron This mineral is an essential component of hemoglobin, the oxygen-carrying pigment in red blood cells. Iron is present in food in two forms: Heme iron is found in meat, fish, and poultry and is better absorbed than iron derived from plants or dairy foods (nonheme iron). Sources: amaranth, dried apricots, figs, fish, lentils, meat, poultry, quinoa, shellfish, tofu.

isoflavones Found primarily in soy foods, isoflavones are a major class of PHYTOESTROGENS, which are plant chemicals with mild estrogen activity. GENISTEIN and DAIDZEIN are the most prominent isoflavones. Soy isoflavones are under investigation for their potential to ease menopause symptoms and to protect against osteoporosis-related fractures, Alzheimer's disease, high cholesterol, and hormone-dependent cancers, such as breast and prostate cancer.

isothiocyanates Providing pungency to numerous CRUCIFEROUS VEGETABLES, isothiocyanates are potent cancer fighters. SULFORAPHANE in broccoli and phenethyliocyanate (PEITC) in watercress are two powerful isothiocyanates that may short-circuit enzymes that activate carcinogens as well as stimulate the production of natural anticancer enzymes.

kaempferol A FLAVONOID compound, kaempferol is converted in the liver into QUERCETIN. Kaempferol may lower the risk of mortality from heart disease and enhance the immune system. Sources: berries, cabbage, chives, green beans, horseradish, leeks, onions, radishes.

lecithin Plentiful in egg yolks, lecithin is a fatty substance present in all cells and is involved with fat digestion in the intestines.

lentinan A polysaccharide (carbohydrate compound) extracted from shiitake mushrooms, lentinan may have the potential to enhance immunity, as well as to protect against cancer, high blood pressure, and high cholesterol.

lentinula edodes mycelium (LEM) Present in shiitake mushrooms, LEM is a polysaccharide compound under review for antiviral and cardiovascular benefits.

lignans These compounds are PHYTOESTROGENS with mild estrogenlike activity. They may have antitumor effects, antimicrobial benefits, and provide relief from PMS and protection against osteoporosis. Sources: beans, flaxseeds (ground up), flaxseed oil, olive oil, soy foods, grains.

lignins Similar in chemical make up to LIGNANS, lignins are a type of insoluble fiber that may be useful for relieving constipation. Sources: brown rice, fruits, legumes, seeds, vegetables, grains.

limonene This phytochemical is under review for its ability to inhibit tumors and protect lungs from disease. Sources: zest of lemons, limes, oranges, tangerines.

lutein & zeaxanthin Found in foods that are bright yellow, orange, and green, lutein and zeaxanthin are pigments in the CAROTENOID family that are linked to a reduced risk for macular degeneration and cataracts. Lutein is under investigation for its potential to inhibit atherosclerosis and to prevent lung and colon cancer. Collard greens, spinach, and kale are especially high in lutein. Other sources: broccoli, corn, egg yolks, kiwifruit, mustard greens, oranges, peas, romaine lettuce, turnip greens, zucchini.

luteolin A FLAVONOID present in artichokes, luteolin is under review for its anticancer activity, potential to reduce heart disease risk, and its ability to block the release of histamine, a substance that triggers congestion.

lycopene An antioxidant CAROTENOID that lends red color to numerous foods, lycopene is particularly abundant in red tomatoes. Lycopene may defend immune cells against oxidative damage and protect against macular degeneration, cardiovascular disease, prostate cancer, and possibly male infertility. Sources: apricots, pink and red grapefruit, tomatoes, watermelon.

lysine This essential AMINO ACID must be obtained from dietary sources. Some experts advocate lysine to help prevent or reduce the severity of cold sores. Sources: amaranth, beans, dairy products, chicken, eggs, fish, potatoes.

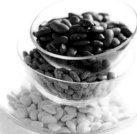

macronutrients The food we eat provides two types of essential building blocks, or nutrients, known as macronutrients and MICRONUTRIENTS. Most food is primarily made up of water, a macronutrient. The remaining macronutrients—CARBOHYDRATE, PROTEIN, and FAT—are vital energy-yielding nutrients that work in harmony with micronutrients to keep the body fit and functioning well.

magnesium Required for hundreds of biochemical reactions, this mineral assists in maintaining normal enzyme, muscle, and nerve function. It also keeps bones and teeth strong and helps to regulate heart rhythm. Sources: amaranth, avoca-

dos, quinoa, brown rice, sunflower seeds, wheat bran, wheat germ.

manganese This trace mineral is important for bone and connective tissue formation, as well as for the actions of enzymes involved in carbohydrate metabolism. Sources: amaranth, blackberries, pineapples.

micronutrients Required in small amounts from the diet, VITAMINS and MINERALS are noncaloric essential nutrients known as micronutrients. They are critical for normal growth, development, and good health. Micronutrients promote and regulate chemical reactions vital for life and participate in all body processes, such as deriving energy from MACRONUTRIENTS, transmitting nerve impulses, and battling infections.

minerals Naturally occurring inorganic nutrients in food, minerals are involved in a variety of specialized roles, such as maintaining skin health and building bone. Minerals also serve as cofactors—assistants to the body's many enzymes. Nutritional requirement for minerals is relatively small but exceedingly important. Minerals are classified as major or trace, according to the body's daily requirements. Major minerals are needed in higher quantities than trace minerals and include POTASSIUM, CALCIUM, and MAGNESIUM. Examples of trace minerals include IRON, ZINC, SELENIUM, and MANGANESE.

molybdenum Essential for normal growth and development, this trace mineral assists several enzymes and is also needed to manufacture red blood cells. Sources: beans, lentils, milk, nuts, peas, whole grains.

monoterpenes A family of phytochemicals that includes LIMONENE, PERILLYL ALCOHOL, and carvone, monoterpenes are under review for their ability to detoxify carcinogens, hinder cancer cell growth, and improve cholesterol levels. Food source: cherries, citrus fruits, caraway, dill, spearmint.

monounsaturated fat Plentiful in many high-fat plant foods, heart-healthy monounsaturated fat is not easily damaged by oxidation, so is less likely than unhealthy SATURATED FAT and TRANS FATS to clog arteries. When consumed in place of saturated and trans fats, monounsaturated fat may protect against high blood pressure, high cholesterol, heart disease, and possibly high blood glucose levels. Researchers believe monounsaturated fat may also lower the risk of breast and colon cancer, though the mechanism is unclear. Sources: avocados, nuts, olives, olive oil.

naringin A FLAVONOID that gives white grapefruit its characteristic bitter flavor, naringin may suppress cancer-causing compounds, bolster blood vessels, and shield delicate lung tissue from environmental toxins. Naringin interferes with the metabolism of certain drugs, causing elevated blood levels of the drug.

niacin An indispensable B vitamin, niacin is required for energy metabolism, as well as healthy skin and proper functioning of the digestive and nervous systems. Sources: eggs, fish, meat, milk, nuts, poultry, whole grains.

nobiletin A FLAVONOID found in the flesh of oranges, nobiletin may possess anti-inflammatory activity, according to preliminary research.

oleic acid When consumed in place of saturated fat, this MONOUNSATURATED FAT is linked to healthier cholesterol levels. Sources: avocados, canola oil, olive oil.

oleuropein A POLYPHENOL with significant antioxidant power, oleuropein may team up with HYDROXYTYROSOL, a phytochemical, to help protect against heart disease, high blood pressure, infertility, and infection-causing bacteria. Source: olive oil.

omega-3 fatty acids Omega-3s are ESSENTIAL FATTY ACIDS. Linolenic acid is the precursor to omega-3s and must be obtained from the diet. The body converts linolenic acid into EPA (EPICOAPENTAENOIC ACID) and DHA (DOCOSAHEXAENOIC ACID). Omega-3s are under review for their potential to improve cardiovascular health, suppress inflammatory compounds, as well as relieve depression. Sources: fatty fish, purslane, and shellfish.

omega-6 fatty acids Omega-6s are ESSENTIAL FATTY ACIDS. They are important for cell membrane structure and are converted by the body into anti-inflammatory compounds, as well as some potentially harmful compounds, some of which are associated with cancer. Most experts advocate an increased intake of OMEGA-3s for better balance, since the U.S. diet is typically excessive in omega-6 fatty acids. Sources: nuts, seeds, whole grains, vegetable oils.

oryzanol Also known as gamma oryzanol, oryzanol is a natural compound found in grains and isolated from rice bran oil. Oryzanol is being studied for its potential to prevent symptoms of menopause and to improve

The Mediterranean Diet

Traditional diets in certain Mediterranean regions such as Crete and other parts of Greece, Spain, southern Italy, southern France, Turkey, and North Africa have been studied for their compelling health benefits. Many people from these regions enjoy an increased life expectancy, and compared with Americans, they suffer from fewer chronic illnesses such as cancer, inflammatory conditions, diabetes, and cardiovascular diseases.

While there is no one typical "Mediterranean" diet (cuisines vary considerably even among different regions within a country), there is, however, one overarching theme: They eat very little meat, very few high-fat dairy foods, little or no prepared products, and there is a primary focus on local, fresh foods such as whole grains, legumes, yogurt, fruit, vegetables, nuts, seeds, fish, olives, olive oil, and red wine.

top 10 phytochemicals

phytochemical	may be helpful for	where to find it
anthocyanins	cancer	apples, beets, berries, cherries, grapes, plums & prunes, pomegranates, potatoes
carotenoids: **beta-carotene** **lutein & zeaxanthin** **lycopene**	anemia, cancer, hyperthyroidism, immune deficiency, memory loss, eye diseases, skin conditions, prostate problems, heart disease, high cholesterol, infertility & impotence	**beta-carotene:** apricots, broccoli, carrots, melons, peppers, spinach, sweet potatoes **lutein & zeaxanthin:** cooking greens, corn, kiwifruit, peas, winter squash **lycopene:** apricots, red & pink grapefruit, tomatoes
catechins	cancer	green tea, pomegranates
flavonoids: **kaempferol** **luteolin** **quercetin** **citrus flavonoids**	cancer, hemorrhoids, high cholesterol, infertility & impotence, memory loss, rheumatoid arthritis	apples, berries, citrus fruit, leeks, onions
glucosinolates: **indoles** **isothiocyanates** **sulforaphane**	cancer	broccoli, brussels sprouts, cabbage, kale
phenolic compounds: **caffeic acid** **ellagic acid** **ferulic acid** **curcumin**	cancer	apples, berries, green tea, pomegranates
phytoestrogens: **soy isoflavones** **(genistein & daidzein)** **lignans**	cancer, osteoporosis, hyperthyroidism	**soy isoflavones:** soy foods **lignans:** flaxseeds, grains, legumes, olive oil
resveratrol	cancer, stroke	red and purple grapes, peanuts, red wine
sulfur compounds **ajoenes** **allicin** **allyl sulfides** **diallyl sulfide**	cancer, high cholesterol	chives, garlic, leeks, onions, shallots
terpenes **limonene** **perillyl alcohol**	cancer	**limonene:** caraway, cardamom, citrus zest (colored portion of peel), coriander, mint, thyme **perillyl alcohol:** cherries

cholesterol levels. Sources: rice bran oil, whole grains.

oxalates Found in the greatest quantities in green vegetables, oxalates are compounds that bind CALCIUM, IRON, and ZINC, blocking their absorption in the body. In addition, people prone to kidney stones should avoid foods high in oxalates since these compounds may fuel the formation of certain types of kidney stones. Sources: beet greens, chocolate, chard, cranberries, dandelion greens, nuts, parsley, rhubarb, spinach, strawberries, tea, wheat bran.

pantothenic acid This bountiful B vitamin is involved in many of the body's processes, including the release of energy from macronutrients, the transmission of nerve impulses, and the synthesis of cell membranes. Sources: avocados, broccoli, chicken, duck, egg yolks, fish, legumes, mushrooms, yogurt.

pectin Pectin is a SOLUBLE FIBER that helps to lower artery-damaging LDL cholesterol. Pectin may also be useful for managing diarrhea and diabetes. Sources: apples, apricots, bananas, carrots, figs, kiwifruit, sweet potatoes.

perillyl alcohol This phytochemical is thought to trigger cell death in tumor cells without harming healthy cells. Sources: cherries, caraway.

phenolic compounds Numerous types of phenolic compounds—CAFFEIC, CHLOROGENIC, ELLAGIC, and FERULIC ACIDS— may battle cancer by destroying free radicals and activating cancer-fighting enzymes that suppress tumors in early stages. Sources: apples, berries, green tea, pomegranates, turmeric.

phosphorus A constituent of every cell, this mineral is involved in almost all metabolic reactions and helps to build strong bones, teeth, and muscles. Sources: almonds, dairy products, fish, legumes, meat, poultry.

phthalides (3-n-butyl phthalide) Present in celery, phthalide phytochemicals are thought to contribute to reduced blood pressure.

phytic acid Also known as inositol hexaphosphate, phytic acid binds to minerals (particularly IRON). This can be beneficial because excessive levels of iron generate harmful free radicals that can contribute to cancer. Phytic acids may also slow starch digestion and help to stabilize blood sugar levels. Sources: grains, soy foods.

phytoestrogens These compounds exhibit estrogenlike activity and may lower the risk of hormone-related cancers, as well as relieve fibrocystic breasts, osteoarthritis, and symptoms of perimenopause and menopause. The two major classes of phytoestrogens are ISOFLAVONES and LIGNANS. Sources: beans, flaxseed, pomegranates, soy foods.

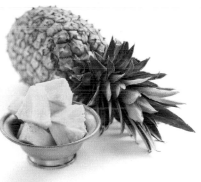

plant sterols Structurally similar to cholesterol, plant sterols may protect against heart disease, cancer, and benign prostatic hyperplasia (BPH). Sources: figs, grains, lentils, nuts, pineapple, seeds, sweet potatoes.

polyphenols A class of ANTIOXIDANTS, polyphenol phytochemicals are under review for their potential to suppress tumor growth, detoxify carcinogens, interfere with the damaging effects of high estrogen levels, lower the risk of stroke, and prevent plaque buildup in the arteries. Sources: apples, berries, citrus fruits, figs, olives, wheat.

polysaccharides Polysaccharides are carbohydrate compounds (starch and glycogen) that may possess disease-fighting properties. LENTINAN in shiitake mushrooms is a type of polysaccharide. Sources: fruits, grains, vegetables.

potassium We need this mineral for the regulation of blood pressure, muscle contraction, heartbeats, and insulin secretion. Potassium functions as an electrolyte and, as such, helps to maintain proper fluid balance in the body. Sources: apricots, avocados, bananas, citrus fruits, dairy, potatoes, quinoa.

probiotics These are a group of beneficial bacteria in the body and are also present in yogurt and fermented milk products with live bacterial cultures. Consuming probiotics may improve immune responses against viruses and cancer cells and may also help to restore the normal balance of bacteria in the colon after a bout of diarrhea.

protease inhibitors Powerful anti-cancer compounds, protease inhibitors appear to short-circuit enzyme production in cancer cells, block the binding of hormones to cells, and inhibit malignant changes in healthy cells. Soy foods are rich in a unique cancer-fighting protease inhibitor known as the Bowman-Birk Inhibitor. Sources: broccoli sprouts, legumes, potatoes, soy foods.

protein Protein is important for health, since AMINO ACIDS—the building blocks of protein—form muscles, hormones, genes, immune cells, brain chemicals, and countless other substances that we rely on daily. While dietary protein from animal sources is generally more digestible and more readily absorbed by the body than plant protein, many animal sources tend to be high in saturated fat. Fish and low-fat dairy products are excel-

lent sources of protein with little to no SATURATED FAT. Among plant sources, protein from soy foods is most bioavailable. Grains high in protein include amaranth and quinoa.

quercetin Red onions are the richest source of quercetin, a potent FLAVONOID linked to a reduced risk of cancer, cardiovascular disease, and cataracts. Quercetin may also prevent the release of histamine, an action essential for managing respiratory and inflammatory conditions. Sources: apples, berries, cherries, grapes, red onions, plums, tea, wine.

resveratrol A phytochemical particularly abundant in the skin of red grapes, resveratrol is under review for its potential to improve cholesterol levels, prevent atherosclerosis, and reduce the risks for stroke and cancer. Sources: peanuts, red and purple grape juice, red wine.

riboflavin Important for the release of energy from carbohydrates, riboflavin is a B vitamin that is important to metabolism. Riboflavin is instrumental in protecting the nervous system, building immunity, and maintaining normal metabolism. Sources: dairy foods, eggs, fish, mushrooms, poultry, quinoa.

rutin Preliminary research suggests that this FLAVONOID may inhibit the formation of cancer cells, improve osteoarthritis symptoms, as well as reduce blood pressure and levels of LDL ("bad") cholesterol. Buckwheat is a particularly good food source of this phytochemical. Other sources: apples, cherries.

saponins Present in many vegetables and grains, saponins are phytochemicals that appear to bind cholesterol and chemical toxins in the digestive tract. Saponins may also inhibit cancer cell replication and increase levels of immune cells. Sources: asparagus, legumes (particularly soybeans), oats, and potatoes.

saturated fat This type of fat is found in animal foods such as meat, poultry, and full-fat dairy products, including butter and whole milk. Tropical cooking oils, such as palm and coconut, are sources of saturated fat as well. High intakes of saturated fat are the primary food factor linked to cardiovascular disease.

selenium This essential trace mineral acts as an antioxidant by promoting the activity of an enzyme that neutralizes free-radical molecules. Selenium also works along with VITAMIN E to reduce free-radical damage linked to chronic diseases such as cancer, heart disease, and some eye diseases. Selenium is required for optimal immunity and thyroid function as well. Sources: Brazil nuts, fish, mushrooms, sunflower seeds, shellfish, turkey, whole grains.

sesaminol compounds Found in sesame seeds, sesaminol compounds—sesaminol, sesamolinol, and pinoresinol—are converted into LIGNANS and appear to possess cardioprotective and anticancer properties.

shogaols Present in ginger, these phytochemicals may help fight cancer and heart disease, as well as improve pain and reduce swelling of inflamed joints.

sodium The major constituent of table salt, sodium is a mineral that is required in small amounts by the body in order to regulate water balance, blood pressure, and blood volume. Most processed foods and fast foods contain excessive sodium, which is linked to high blood pressure. Many experts recommend a maximum sodium intake of 2400mg each day.

sorbitol A natural sugar that has mild laxative properties, sorbitol may help relieve constipation. Note that excess sorbitol can cause diarrhea. Source: prunes.

soy protein Protein derived from soy is high in quality and provides all of the essential amino acids. Eating 25g of soy protein each day as part of a low-fat diet can significantly improve cholesterol levels in people with high cholesterol. Sources: soybeans, soy foods.

sulforaphane A notable SULFUR COMPOUND classified as a GLUCOSINOLATE, sulforaphane may increase the activity of cancer-fighting enzymes in the body, reduce tumor growth, block carcinogens from initiating cancer, and fight hormone-related cancer. Sources: broccoli, cabbage, cooking greens.

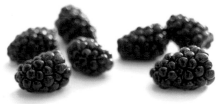

sulfur compounds Sulfur-containing phytochemicals abundant in garlic and the onion family are collectively called sulfur compounds and include ALLYL SULFIDE and AJOENES. Certain sulfur compounds may stimulate cancer-fighting enzymes. Sources: chives, garlic, leeks, onions, scallions, shallots.

syringic acid A phytochemical found in sesame seeds, syringic acid may fight UV sun damage in skin cells, according to experimental research.

tangeretin A FLAVONOID present in tangerines, tangeretin may hinder the growth of tumor cells, according to laboratory studies.

tannins Also called proanthocyanidins, tannins may detoxify carcinogens and scavenge harmful free radicals. Tannins in cranberries may protect against urinary tract infections. Note also that tannins reduce IRON bioavailability. Sources: blackberries, blueberries, cranberries, grapes, lentils, tea, wine.

terpenes Terpenes are a class of phytochemicals that include PERILLYL ALCOHOL in cherries, LIMONENE in the zest of citrus fruit, SAPONINS in grains and vegetables, and eugenol in cloves and nutmeg. Terpene phytochemicals may block cancer, as well as improve immunity and help to fight heart disease.

thiamin Essential for normal development and growth, this B vitamin assists in energy metabolism and ensures proper functioning of the nervous and cardio-vascular systems. Sources: corn, fish, poultry, rice.

thioproline A phytochemical in fresh shiitake mushrooms, thioproline is currently under investigation for its cancer-fighting properties.

trans fatty acids These types of fats in foods are formed when vegetable oils are processed (hydrogenated) to improve their stability and to make them more solid. A food that lists "hydrogenated vegetable oil" on its ingredient list contains trans fatty acids. Growing concern about trans fatty acids is based on research that suggests high intakes of trans fatty acids may contribute to heart disease by elevating LDL ("bad") cholesterol and reducing HDL ("good") cholesterol. Some margarines (especially stick margarines), solid shortenings, certain types of peanut butter, commercial frying fats (used in fast-food establishments), and baked goods are the major sources of trans fats.

tryptophan An essential AMINO ACID, tryptophan is converted by the body into the B vitamin NIACIN. Tryptophan stimulates production of serotonin, a neurotransmitter that supports mental health. COMPLEX CARBOHYDRATES enhance the absorption and use of tryptophan in the brain. Sources: bananas, dairy products, fish, peas, poultry, turnips.

tyrosine A nonessential AMINO ACID, tyrosine is a precursor to numerous chemical messengers (neurotransmitters) in the brain and serves as a protein building block throughout the body. Sources: fatty fish, soy foods.

tyrosine kinase inhibitors These potent compounds in lentils and beans appear to team up with SOLUBLE FIBER to stabilize levels of blood sugar.

vitamins, fat-soluble Fat-soluble vitamins—A, D, E, and K—dissolve in fat before they are absorbed in the bloodstream to carry out their functions. These vitamins are stored in our bodies. Because they are stored in fatty tissues, a buildup from supplement forms of these vitamins may result in toxic levels.

vitamins, water-soluble Water-soluble vitamins—C and the B vitamins—dissolve in water and are not stored in the body long term (with the exception of vitamin B_{12}, which is not readily excreted). Instead, they are eliminated in sweat and urine. Because they are not stored, we need to eat foods rich in these fragile vitamins each day.

vitamin A Known for its vision-enhancing properties, vitamin A is also vital for normal cell growth and maintaining immunity and healthy skin. This fat-soluble vitamin is acquired from animal fats and is also synthesized in the intestines from BETA-CAROTENE and other CAROTENOIDS. Because high levels of vitamin A in supplement form may be toxic, it is best to obtain vitamin A from food. Sources: dried apricots, carrots, pumpkins, sweet potatoes.

vitamin B_6 Also known as pyridoxine, vitamin B_6 is vital for the regulation of mental processes. Vitamin B_6 also helps maintain glucose (blood sugar) levels, healthy nervous and immune systems, and hemoglobin production. Along with

VITAMIN B12 and FOLATE, vitamin B6 is thought to lower levels of HOMOCYSTEINE (a risk factor for heart disease). Sources: avocado, bananas, fish, peas, potatoes, poultry, prune juice.

vitamin B12 Also called cobalamin, vitamin B12 is found only in animal products and some fortified foods. Vitamin B12 is required to produce DNA, the genetic material in all cells. Adequate amounts of vitamin B12 may help to prevent anemia, chronic fatigue syndrome, depression, heart disease, and infertility, and it is vital for healthy nerve cells and red blood cells. Sources: eggs, dairy products, fish, meat, poultry, shellfish.

vitamin C This vitamin, also known as ascorbic acid, has considerable ANTIOXIDANT power. Vitamin C may strengthen the immune system, support connective tissues, prevent nasal congestion, and enhance healing of wounds. Sources: berries, broccoli, citrus fruits, kiwifruit, peppers, pineapple, melons, tomatoes.

vitamin D Important for the absorption of CALCIUM and PHOSPHORUS, vitamin D is a fat-soluble vitamin that is often referred to as the "sunshine vitamin," because the body creates it when the sun's ultraviolet rays strike the skin for about 10 to 15 minutes a day. Sources: fortified milk, fatty fish.

vitamin E A fat-soluble vitamin that is found in foods and supplements in eight different forms, vitamin E is a potent antioxidant. The most biologically active form of vitamin E for our bodies is alpha-tocopherol. Vitamin E may provide antioxidant protection against many ailments, including cancer, vision disorders, eczema, memory loss, and osteoarthritis. Note that large doses of vitamin E may adversely affect people on blood thinners or aspirin therapy. Sources: avocados, nuts, olive oil, sunflower seeds, vegetable oils, wheat germ.

vitamin K This fat-soluble vitamin is critical for blood clotting as well as bone formation. Among various forms of vitamin K, phylloquinone is the form available in foods (vitamin K is also made in the gastrointestinal tract). Note that people who are on blood-thinning medications should not take vitamin K supplements and should avoid foods high in vitamin K. Sources: broccoli, cabbage, cauliflower, soybeans, green leafy vegetables.

water Indispensable for life and comprising about 60 percent of body weight, water regulates temperature, provides lubrication, and serves as a fluid medium for metabolic processes throughout the body. Routinely drinking about eight glasses of water throughout each day is important, as water is constantly lost from the body and must be replaced through regular consumption.

zinc This essential trace mineral is instrumental in maintaining normal skin, hair, immunity, protein metabolism, and numerous enzyme systems. Sources: beans, dairy, meat, nuts, poultry, seeds, shellfish, tofu, wheat germ, whole grains.

When to Take a Supplement

While reaping the multiple benefits of whole foods is the optimal way to prevent and/or manage symptoms of illness, there are situations in which the use of supplements is appropriate. For example, most foods that contain VITAMIN E (a fat-soluble vitamin) tend to be high in fat. So in order to get enough vitamin E, it may be helpful to take a supplement. And taking a general multivitamin every day can be beneficial—though a multivitamin is *not* a substitute for eating nutritious foods.

There are also specific medical conditions that warrant the use of supplements. Women of childbearing age should take supplemental folic acid (the synthetic form of the B vitamin FOLATE) to prevent possible birth defects in an unborn child. In addition, people at risk for osteoporosis should take a CALCIUM supplement. This is particularly important for postmenopausal women who are most at risk for this debilitating bone-thinning disease, though older men are certainly also at risk.

foods that fight back

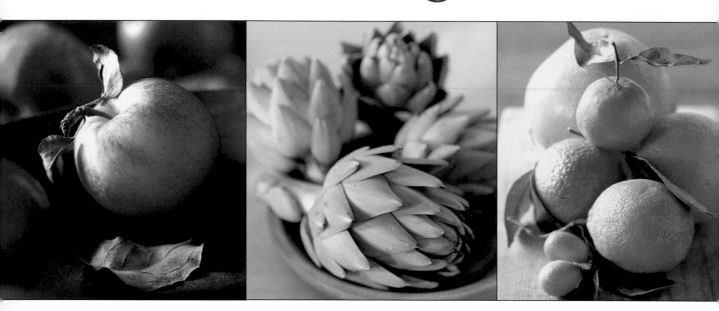

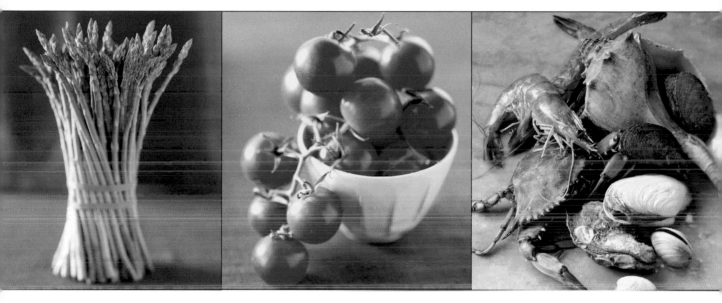

Super Foods—and the
Nutrients in Them—That
Keep You Healthy

apples

Apples are packed with bushels of beneficial substances, such as pectin, vitamin C, and numerous phytochemicals that may help prevent heart disease and certain cancers, and also alleviate symptoms of allergies and asthma.

add more to your diet

▶ Top pancakes, waffles, or even ice cream with applesauce instead of syrup.

▶ Stir diced apples into your breakfast oatmeal or other cereal.

▶ Applesauce makes a surprisingly creamy sorbet. Just freeze your favorite applesauce in an ice-cream maker.

▶ Substitute chopped dried apples for raisins in baked goods.

▶ Core apples and thinly slice them crosswise. Use these fresh, crunchy slices in sandwiches.

▶ Sprinkle diced apples on top of a homemade cheese pizza.

▶ Homemade applesauce is incredibly easy and quick to make: Cook chunks of apple with just a little bit of water or juice over a low flame and in about 15 minutes you'll have applesauce. Certain apples will collapse to a puree by themselves; other types are sturdier and will have to be mashed a bit with a potato masher or fork.

what's in it

anthocyanins Natural food pigments, anthocyanins have antioxidant activity that may defend against carcinogens. They may also lower LDL ("bad") cholesterol and prevent blood clots.

glutathione This antioxidant may have anticancer actions and improve the immune system's ability to fight off infections.

pectin A type of soluble fiber that helps to lower artery-damaging LDL cholesterol, pectin in applesauce is also helpful in managing diarrhea. (A single unpeeled apple provides nearly 4g of dietary fiber, almost half of which is heart-healthy pectin.)

phenolic acids Apples contain caffeic, chlorogenic, ellagic, and ferulic acids, as well as other types of phenolic compounds that may help to fight cancer.

quercetin A flavonoid linked to a reduced risk for cancer development, quercetin may also help to prevent cataracts and reduce symptoms associated with respiratory ailments.

rutin Rutin is a flavonoid that teams up with vitamin C to maintain blood-vessel health.

maximizing the benefits

For **vitamin C** and **glutathione**, eat apples uncooked, as these nutrients are diminished by heat. For **pectin**, it's best to cook the apples, as the pectin is released when the apples' cell walls soften as they cook. For **insoluble fiber** and **anthocyanins**, which are found in the apple skin, use unpeeled apples (buy organic apples if you are concerned about pesticides).

health bites

You may breathe easier if you eat a lot of apples. A recent study linked apple consumption with a reduced risk for lung cancer. Researchers isolated quercetin, a powerful flavonoid, as the possible source of the anticancer effect—although the phenolic acids and vitamin C found in apples may also protect the lungs.

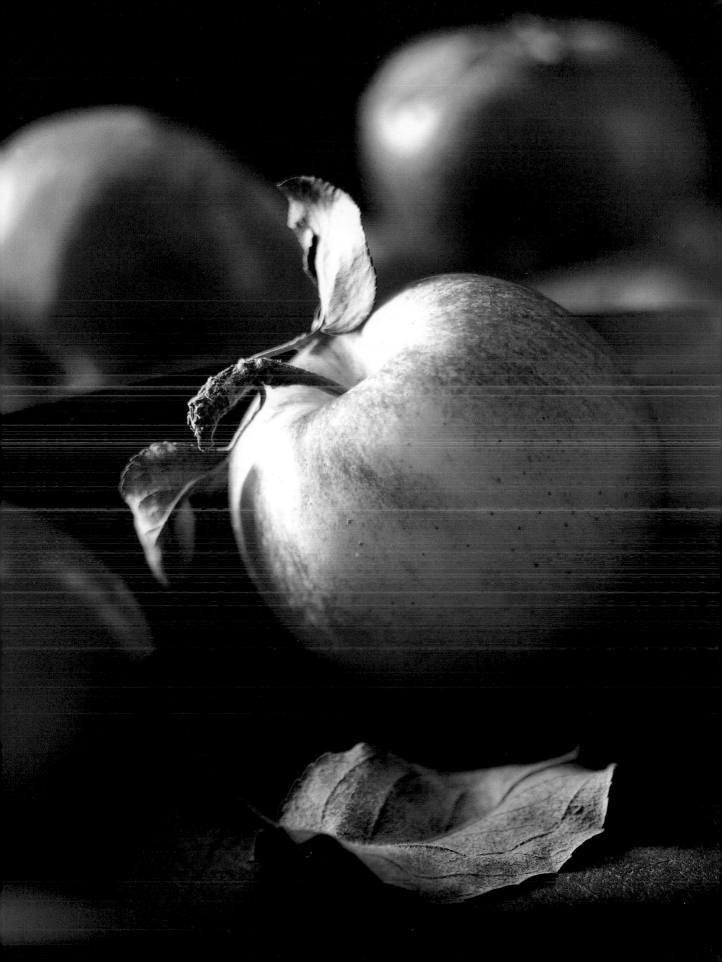

apricots

Apricots' deep golden color indicates the presence of carotenoids, specifically beta-carotene, an important antioxidant. Although fresh apricots are good for you, nutrient-dense dried apricots are even better.

add more to your diet

▶ Cook dried apricots in apple juice or white grape juice until very soft, and then puree to make your own homemade, no-sugar-added fruit spread.

▶ Use diced dried apricots instead of raisins in cakes, cookies, and tea breads.

▶ For a savory fruit accompaniment to grilled meat or poultry, pit and quarter fresh apricots, and gently sauté in olive oil with a touch of minced garlic.

▶ Add chopped dried apricots to poultry stuffings, rice pilafs, or other grain dishes.

▶ Add halved fresh apricots or diced dried apricots to meat or poultry stews.

▶ Make your own trail mix by combining diced dried apricots with an assortment of nuts and seeds such as almonds, walnuts, and pumpkin seeds.

what's in it

beta-carotene A carotenoid whose antioxidant power is linked with cancer prevention, beta-carotene is believed to combat free-radical damage, and is also thought to reinforce the immune system.

ellagic acid A compound that may reduce damage caused by carcinogens such as environmental toxins, ellagic acid is also being studied for its potential to inhibit the growth of cancer cells.

iron Dried apricots are a good source of iron (¼ cup provides 1.5mg, or 8% of the Daily Value for this mineral). Adequate amounts of iron are important for everyone, particularly for pregnant women and children. Iron-deficient anemia can lead to fatigue and vulnerability to infections due to reduced immune response.

lycopene Apricots contain small amounts of this powerful antioxidant, which is believed to reduce LDL ("bad") cholesterol and protect the prostate against cancer.

pectin Pectin is a soluble fiber that lowers LDL cholesterol levels, which are linked to dangerous hardening of the arteries.

potassium This important mineral helps to prevent high blood pressure and is required for healthy nerves and muscles.

maximizing the benefits

Although eating fresh apricots is a way to get the most **vitamin C** (which is depleted by heat and exposure to air when apricots are dried), other substances—such as **beta-carotene, lycopene,** and **pectin**—are actually made more available to the body when the apricots (fresh or dried) are cooked.

health bites

If you are sensitive to the sulfites (sulfur dioxide) that are used to prevent dried apricots from turning brown, look for sulfite-free apricots in health-food stores and the health-food section of some supermarkets.

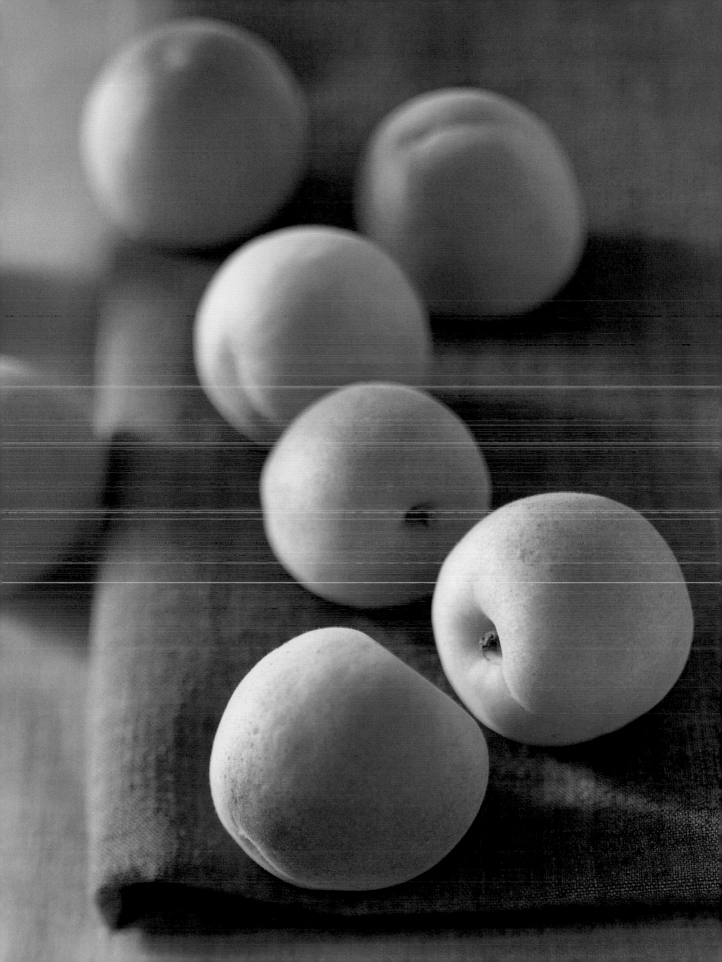

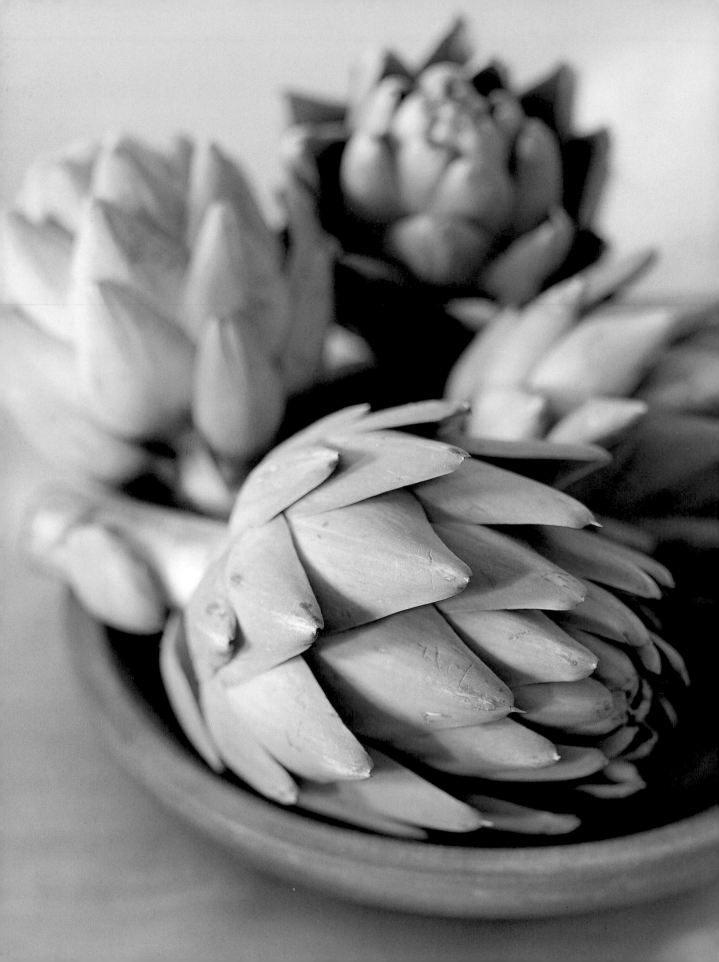

artichokes

This venerable vegetable contains several restorative nutrients. Used since ancient times as a digestive aid and for poor liver function, research reveals that artichokes may also confer cholesterol-lowering benefits.

what's in it

cynarin Cynarin is an organic acid found in artichokes that stimulates the sweetness receptors in the tastebuds of some people, causing the foods eaten afterward to taste sweeter. This phytochemical may also offer antioxidant protection against carcinogenic and environmental toxins such as pollution and smoke. Cynarin also may have a beneficial effect on the liver by helping to promote bile flow (which assists in the removal of toxic substances from the body) and by preventing fat accumulation in the liver.

folate In addition to preventing certain birth defects, this B vitamin (also known as folic acid) may help lower heart disease risk by reducing levels of homocysteine, an amino acid that has been linked to atherosclerosis. Folate may also help to prevent cancer, since low levels of folate can be harmful to DNA. (One artichoke provides 110mcg, or 28% of the Daily Value for this important vitamin.)

luteolin With the potential to prevent LDL ("bad") cholesterol oxidation, this flavonoid may reduce the risk for heart disease. Preliminary studies suggest that luteolin also may block the release of histamines, which can trigger congestion and inflammation.

maximizing the benefits

Although frozen and canned "hearts" are the most available market form of artichokes, it's best to cook and eat fresh, whole artichokes as often as possible to take advantage of the phytochemicals found in the leaves. To preserve as much of the water-soluble **folate** as possible, steam rather than boil artichokes.

add more to your diet

▶ When steaming whole artichokes, add a mixture of herbs (such as rosemary, tarragon, and thyme) to the steaming water. This will add a subtle herb flavor to the artichokes themselves.

▶ Instead of dipping artichoke leaves in melted butter, try this: Make a puree of mashed roasted garlic, black pepper, soft silken tofu, and lemon juice.

▶ For a quick artichoke appetizer, puree jarred artichokes (rinsed and drained) with garlic, light mayonnaise, and nonfat yogurt. Serve as a dip with crudités.

▶ Fresh baby Italian artichokes, available seasonally, can be steamed or stewed and eaten whole with a drizzle of lemon juice and extra-virgin olive oil.

▶ Make an artichoke relish: Steam whole artichokes, then coarsely chop the tender part of the leaves and the heart. Toss with olive oil and vinegar and use on sandwiches or with grilled fish.

health bites

Both the tender "heart" and the meaty leaves of the artichoke are edible, though it's the leaves that contain many of the vegetable's phytochemicals.

asparagus

Asparagus is delicious, low in fat, and low in sodium—a superb vegetable for those who are watching their weight. A nutrient-dense super-food, asparagus may prevent heart disease, cancer, and certain birth defects.

add more to your diet

▶ When you're trimming the tough ends from asparagus stalks, save them and cook them in water until very tender. Use this B-vitamin-enriched water to boost the nutrition of an asparagus (or other) soup or pasta sauce.

▶ Fold cooked, cut-up asparagus into macaroni and cheese.

▶ Most people don't think of roasting asparagus, but it's delicious and a good way to preserve the B vitamins. Toss trimmed asparagus with a little olive oil and a sprinkling of grated Parmesan and roast in a 450°F oven for 10 to 20 minutes.

▶ Puree cooked asparagus (thawed, frozen would be fine) with a little milk and herbs for a quick soup.

▶ Add cooked asparagus to pizzas, sandwiches, and wraps.

▶ For a twist on the classic guacamole, chop cooked asparagus very finely, add just a little avocado, and season as you would a traditional guacamole.

what's in it

fiber Insoluble fiber is important for promoting a healthy digestive tract, and soluble fiber helps to lower cholesterol. (One cup of asparagus has nearly 3g of dietary fiber.)

folate Folate is vital during pregnancy as it prevents development of neural-tube defects in the fetus. Folate is also cardioprotective, helping to reduce homocysteine, an amino acid linked to heart disease risk. Folate may also help prevent cancer (low folate levels may damage DNA and lead to cancerous changes in cells). A cup of cooked asparagus provides a remarkable 263mcg of folate, which is 66% of the Daily Value.

glutathione Functioning as an antioxidant, the enzyme glutathione may have the ability to detoxify carcinogenic substances and protect cells from free-radical damage.

rutin This antioxidant flavonoid works hand-in-hand with the antioxidant vitamin C to maintain blood-vessel health.

saponins These compounds may prevent heart disease by binding and preventing absorption of cholesterol in the digestive tract.

vitamin B$_6$ This immune-boosting vitamin required for the production of disease-fighting antibodies plays an important role in enabling the body to derive energy from food. Preliminary research suggests that vitamin B$_6$ also helps to relieve the discomfort of premenstrual tension as well as nausea in early pregnancy.

maximizing the benefits

To reap the full health benefits from this nutritional powerhouse, you should steam or microwave asparagus. Or, if you cook the stalks in water, use an asparagus cooker, which is designed to cook the asparagus with the tips facing up and not immersed in water: This is important because it's thought that most of the phytonutrients are in the tips.

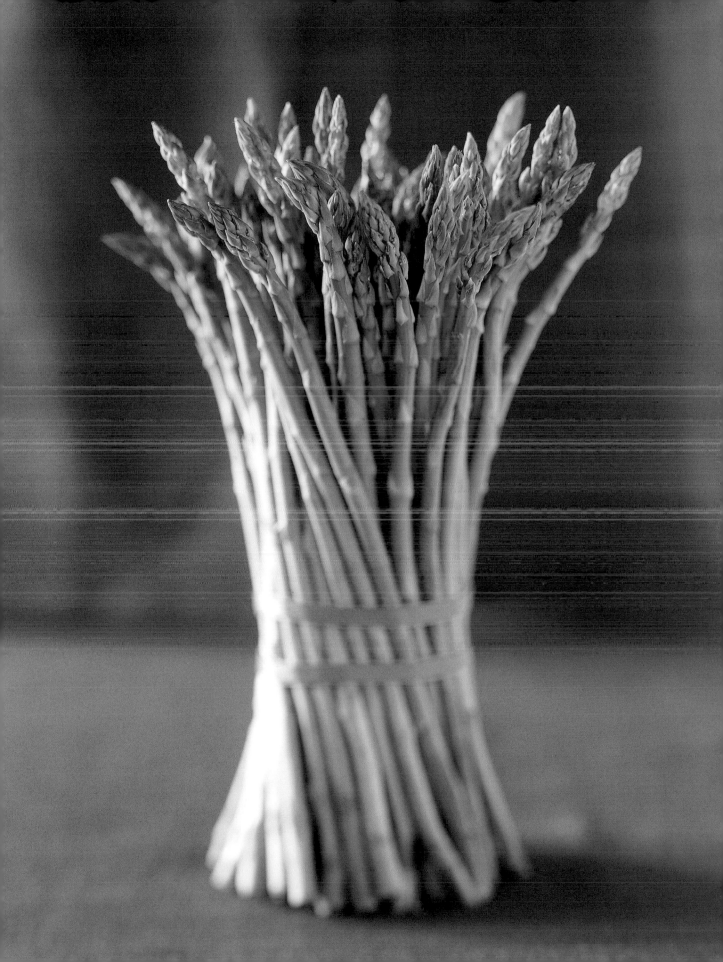

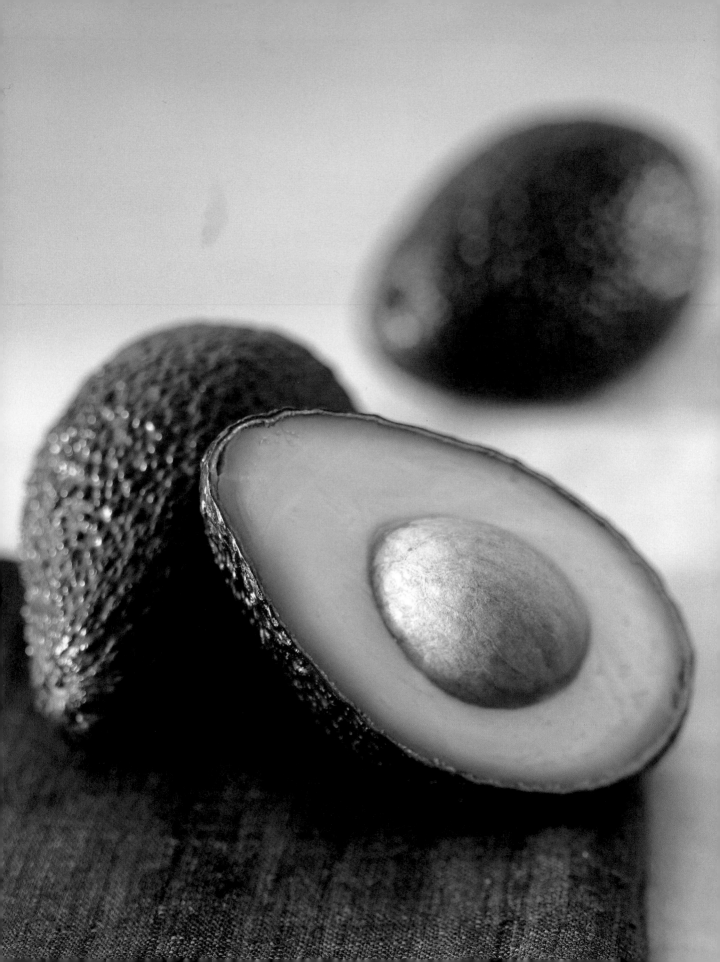

avocados

Creamy, luscious avocados are such a rich source of vitamins, minerals, healthful fats, and phytochemicals that the U.S. government has revised its nutrition guidelines to urge Americans to eat more of them.

what's in it

beta-sitosterol This compound may block cholesterol absorption as well as reduce discomfort of BPH (benign prostatic hyperplasia). It is also under review for the potential to prevent breast cancer.

fiber The fiber content of avocados is high (one avocado provides 34% of the Daily Value for dietary fiber), which is good news since soluble fiber removes excess cholesterol from your body, and insoluble fiber helps to prevent constipation by keeping your digestive system running smoothly.

folate Avocados are good sources of folate (one avocado provides 57mcg, or 28% of the Daily Value). This important B vitamin is linked to the prevention of neural-tube defects in fetuses as well as prevention of cancer and heart disease in adults.

glutathione Functioning as an antioxidant, this compound may neutralize free radicals that damage cells.

magnesium This mineral may help to reduce discomfort associated with premenstrual syndrome, migraines, anxiety, and other disorders.

oleic acid A type of monounsaturated fat in avocados, oleic acid has been linked to lower cholesterol levels when substituted for saturated fat in the diet.

maximizing the benefits

Avocado flesh turns brown rapidly, so it is a good idea to sprinkle it with lemon or lime juice to prevent discoloration.

add more to your diet

▶ Make a salad dressing: Puree avocado with plain nonfat yogurt, lime juice, or vinegar to taste, salt, and hot sauce, if you like.

▶ Make an avocado smoothie: In a blender, puree avocado, milk, a touch of sweetener, and a couple of ice cubes.

▶ Mash avocado with lime juice and use as a spread on chicken sandwiches.

▶ Try avocado for dessert: Drizzle cubes of avocado with honey and top with a sprinkling of nuts.

▶ Mash avocado with a little salt (and perhaps some mustard) and use in place of mayonnaise in a tuna or chicken salad.

health bites

Some people tend to avoid avocados because they regard them as high in fat. Avocados are indeed high in beneficial monounsaturated fat, which—when substituted for saturated fat in the diet—helps to lower LDL ("bad") cholesterol levels and the risk for heart disease.

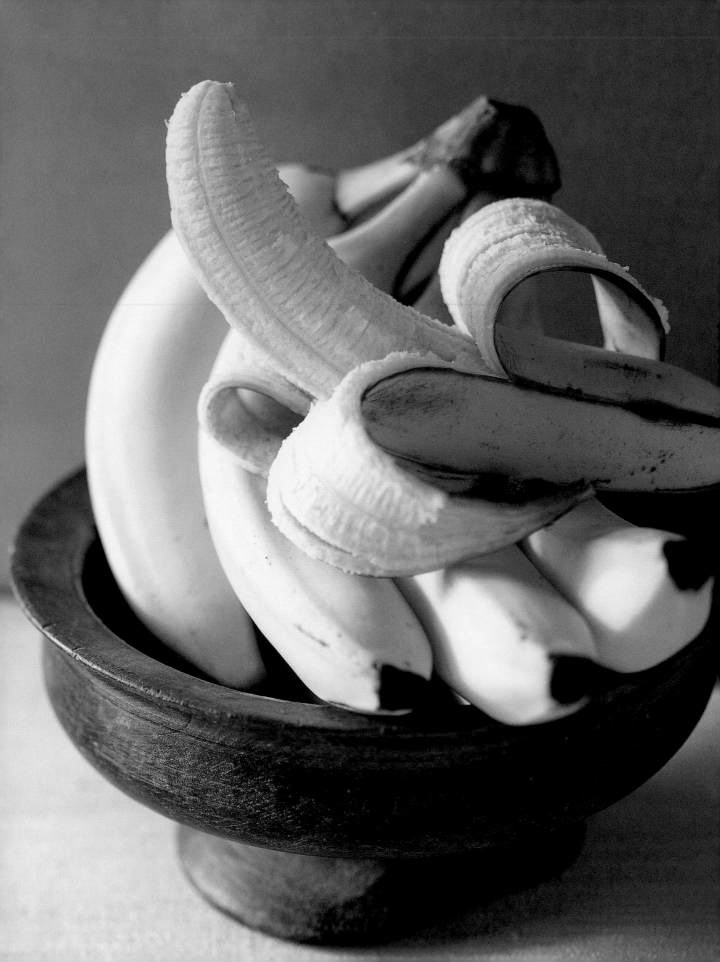

bananas

Next time you feel a bit anxious, try eating a banana. It contains vitamin B$_6$ as well as small amounts of tryptophan, both of which may promote a relaxed state of mind. This comforting fruit may also ward off heart disease, stroke, and certain gastrointestinal woes.

what's in it

pectin In addition to being heart healthy, this type of soluble fiber is helpful in controlling diarrhea.

potassium A mineral with a wide range of benefits, potassium may play a role in lowering blood pressure and preventing stroke. (One banana has 467mg of potassium, or 16% of the Daily Value.)

tryptophan An amino acid that stimulates the production of serotonin, a neurotransmitter that has a calming effect on the body, tryptophan may help to ward off depression, anxiety, and insomnia. Note that eating foods high in complex carbohydrates, such as pasta, rice, and beans, will help enhance the absorption of tryptophan.

vitamin B$_6$ This vitamin facilitates communication between muscles and nerves. It also helps to make red blood cells. It may also be useful in preventing the moodiness associated with premenstrual syndrome (PMS). Bananas are an excellent source of vitamin B$_6$ (a single banana has 0.7mg of B$_6$, which is 34% of the Daily Value).

add more to your diet

▶ Add cut-up bananas to curries for a little sweetness and to bring out the flavor of the curry spices.

▶ Bananas make a wonderful salsa: Toss diced bananas with scallions, red pepper, lime juice, and honey. Serve with a fish or poultry dish.

▶ Freeze chunks of banana and puree in a blender along with a touch of nutmeg and lime juice to make an instant sorbet.

▶ Mash bananas with minced garlic and hot sauce and serve as a condiment along with poultry or meat dishes.

▶ Banana raita, an Indian "side salad," is a sweet and cooling counterpoint to hot, spicy foods: Combine diced banana, plain yogurt, thinly sliced scallions, and a touch of curry powder. Serve chilled.

maximizing the benefits

Cooking partially destroys **vitamin B$_6$,** so if you are interested in mood enhancement, it's best to eat bananas uncooked. If you are after extra pectin, cooked bananas make this soluble fiber more available.

health bites

Initial studies suggest that sugar molecules in bananas called fructooligosaccharides (FOS) encourage beneficial bacteria growth in the intestine. This "friendly bacteria" may help to reduce toxins produced by unfriendly flora in the colon and improve nutrient absorption.

beans

A nourishing and hearty source of non-animal protein, beans may help reduce LDL ("bad") cholesterol levels, stabilize blood sugar, and help control weight. They may also prevent certain types of birth defects and cancer.

add more to your diet

▶ You don't have to rely on canned beans (which are usually very high in sodium) for convenience. Just plan ahead a bit: Cook up a big batch of beans, then freeze in small batches.

▶ Puree cooked beans with herbs and spices and use as a topping for pizza in place of tomato sauce.

▶ Make a pasta sauce by pureeing cooked beans and garlic with broth and herbs, such as oregano or cumin.

▶ Instead of mayonnaise, make a sandwich spread of pureed beans, lemon juice, and some tomato paste.

▶ Puree cooked white beans and use them in place of pumpkin puree in a pumpkin pie.

▶ Use seasoned bean puree as a filling for deviled eggs or stuffed mushrooms.

what's in it

complex carbohydrates By making you feel full more quickly, beans are a perfect food for people who are trying to control weight. Complex carbohydrates in beans also make them a great choice for people who want steady, slow-burning energy.

folate Essential for proper development of the fetus, folate also helps reduce risk for heart disease by lowering homocysteine, an amino acid linked to the development of the condition.

insoluble fiber Beans are high in this beneficial fiber (1 cup of cooked beans has nearly 8g), which helps to prevent constipation by moving food through your system more quickly.

lignans Lignans are under review for cardioprotective and anti-cancer benefits, especially for prostate and breast cancer.

protease inhibitors Protease inhibitors are being investigated for their potential to stop normal cells from becoming cancerous.

saponins These compounds may prevent cancer cells from multiplying, and they may also lower LDL cholesterol.

soluble fiber An important factor in lowering LDL cholesterol, soluble fiber may reduce heart disease risk. Fiber in beans also helps reduce blood-glucose levels, making this food a good choice for those with diabetes.

maximizing the benefits

The gas-causing culprits in beans are carbohydrates called oligosaccharides. Some theories suggest that presoaking beans, and then discarding the soaking water before cooking them, will get rid of some of the oligosaccharides.

health bites

A serving of beans will satisfy your appetite more than most foods. The rich fiber content fills your stomach and causes a slower rise in blood sugar, staving off hunger for longer and providing a steady supply of energy.

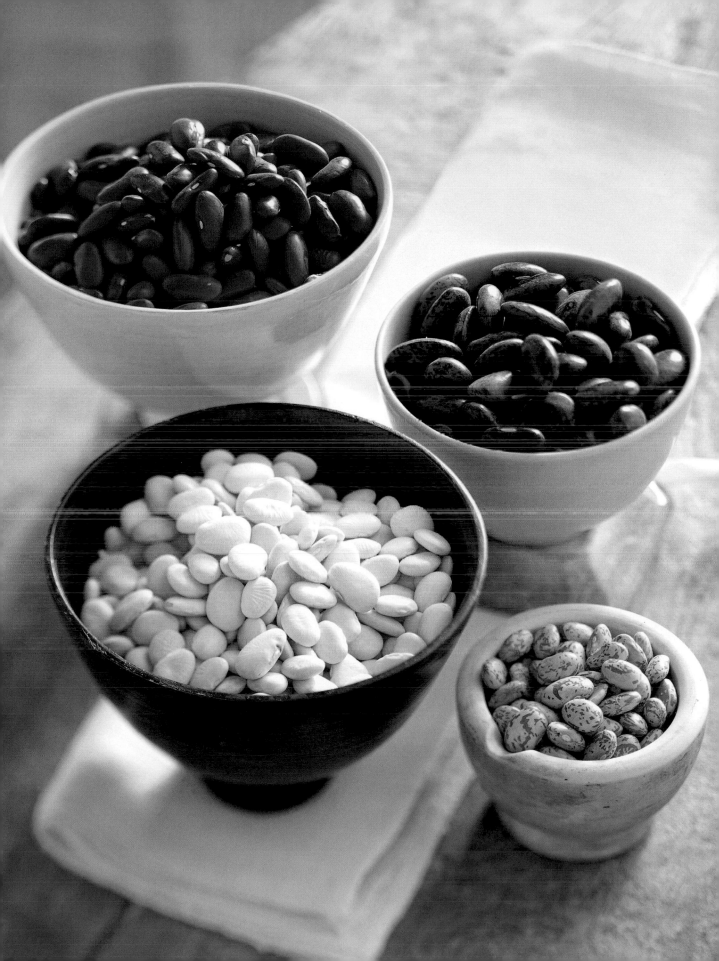

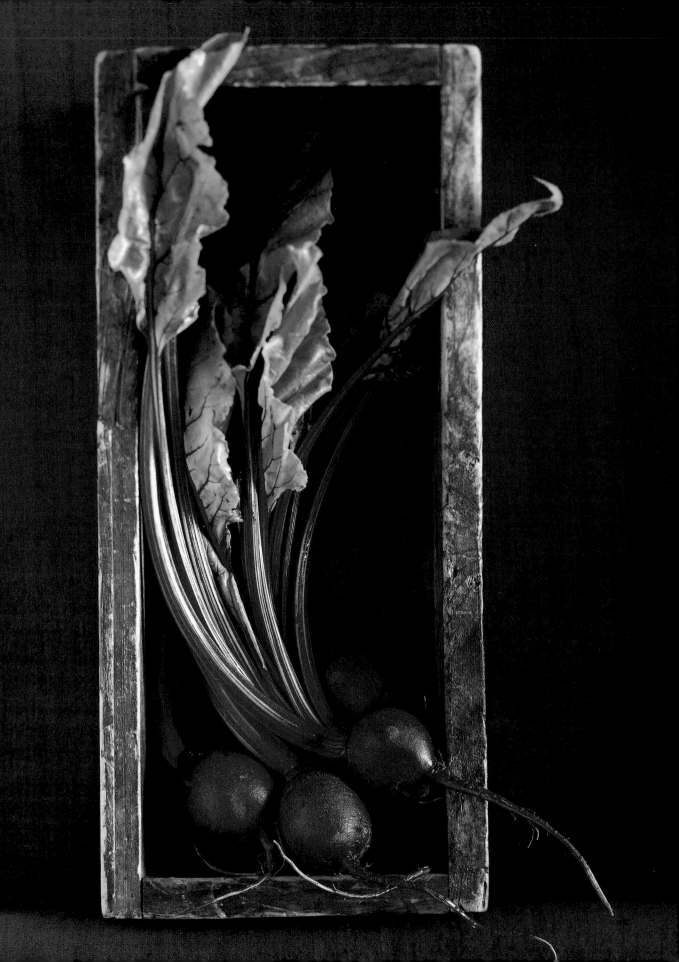

beets

Rich, sweet, and earthy in flavor, these ruby-red root vegetables are highly nutritious and provide fiber, folate, potassium, and such phytochemicals as anthocyanins and saponins.

what's in it

betacyanin A type of plant pigment, betacyanin is under review for defending cells against harmful carcinogens and is also being studied for its potential as a tumor-fighting compound.

betaine Preliminary studies suggest this substance may be helpful in lowering homocysteine, an amino acid associated with increased risk for heart disease.

fiber Soluble fiber in beets may be linked to the reduction of LDL ("bad") cholesterol levels.

folate Folate may help prevent birth defects and may also protect against heart disease and cancer. (One cup of cooked, diced beets provides 136mcg of folate, which is 34% of the Daily Value.)

oxalates If you are prone to kidney stones or gout, avoid beet greens; they are high in oxalates. Oxalates form tiny crystals that can contribute to the development of kidney stones.

saponins Available in small amounts in beets, saponins may bind cholesterol in the digestive tract, lowering the risk for heart disease.

maximizing the benefits

To preserve the **anthocyanin (betacyanin)** in beets, it's best to roast, bake, or microwave whole beets in their skins. If you cook peeled or cut-up beets, the vegetable's pigments (and thus the anthocyanins) leak out and are lost. Don't cook beets in water, as some of the water-soluble B vitamin, **folate,** will leach into the cooking water.

add more to your diet

▶ Puree beets with yogurt or reduced-fat sour cream and vinegar to taste. Chill and serve as a refreshing summer soup.

▶ Add sliced cooked (or pickled) beets to chicken or meat sandwiches in place of sliced tomatoes.

▶ Shred peeled raw beets and use in place of carrots in carrot cake, carrot bread, or muffins.

▶ Make a slaw of shredded peeled raw beets, balsamic vinegar, mustard, and dill.

▶ Combine diced, cooked beets with olive oil and lemon juice and use as a sauce for salmon.

▶ For ways to use beet greens, see *Cooking Greens* on page 63.

health bites

Some people can't properly metabolize the pigments in beets and, as a result, their urine turns a bright red. Don't be alarmed if this should happen; it is a harmless metabolic reaction.

berries

Tiny powerhouses of nutrition, berries are bursting with healthy compounds, including folate, fiber, and phytochemicals, which may help improve memory and reduce the risk for developing heart disease and cancer.

add more to your diet

▶ Do as the Italians do, and stir strawberries into savory rice dishes, such as pilaf or risotto. Stir in chopped strawberries just before serving.

▶ Make your own cranberry sauce and use it in place of jam.

▶ Add berries to tossed green salads. Or make an all-berry salad and dress it with a lemon vinaigrette.

▶ Add fresh or frozen cranberries to soups and stews.

▶ Make a quick dessert "pizza": Spread sweetened ricotta cheese over a flour tortilla, spoon berries on top, and bake in a 400°F oven for 10 minutes, just until hot.

▶ Use berries as the basis of spicy salsas, chutneys, or relishes.

what's in it

anthocyanins These natural plant pigments in berries function as powerful antioxidants, which sweep out harmful free-radical molecules, preventing them from wreaking havoc on your body.

ellagic acid Ellagic acid is believed to be effective in neutralizing carcinogenic agents. Blackberries, raspberries, and strawberries appear to be particularly good sources of this compound.

kaempferol A flavonoid found in berries, kaempferol is believed to inactivate carcinogens. Kaempferol may also help to reduce LDL ("bad") cholesterol.

quercetin This well-studied flavonoid is thought to play numerous roles, including the ability to protect against heart disease, cancer, and possibly cataracts; it may also alleviate symptoms of allergies and asthma.

tannins Tannins (also known as proanthocyanidins) in cranberries may prevent bacteria from attaching to the urinary tract. How they do this is currently under investigation. Blackberries are also rich in tannins.

vitamin C Among other functions, this important vitamin helps to strengthen the immune system and protect connective tissue. Strawberries and cranberries are good sources of vitamin C.

maximizing the benefits

Cooking does not seem to destroy **ellagic acid** in berries. However, it will destroy some of their **folate** and **vitamin C**.

health bites

Animal studies conducted at Tufts University show that blueberries help to prevent and also reverse age-related memory loss. Though the specific substance in blueberries has not yet been identified, scientists speculate that the overall antioxidant power of the fruit protects brain cells from free-radical harm.

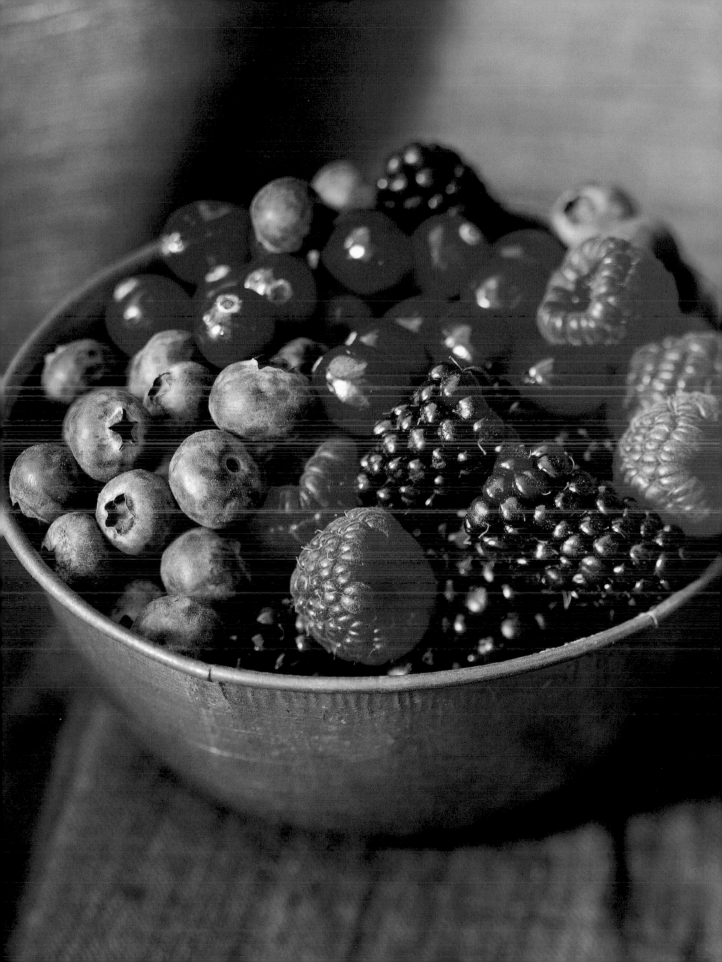

broccoli

One of the most studied of vegetables, broccoli's impressive status as a super-food is the result of its high level of phytochemicals and their potential to mobilize the body's natural disease-fighting resources.

add more to your diet

➤ Many recipes call for broccoli florets, but the stalks are delicious, too. With a paring knife, peel the stalks, then thinly slice crosswise.

➤ Puree cooked broccoli along with milk and seasonings, and serve as a soup. Top with grated Parmesan, if you like.

➤ Combine chopped, cooked broccoli and softened cream cheese and spread on flour tortillas or lavash bread. Top with sliced turkey and roll up.

➤ Puree cooked broccoli along with olive oil, garlic, and crushed red pepper flakes and use as a sauce for pasta.

➤ Make a broccoli slaw: Shred raw broccoli, toss with shredded carrots, and season as you would a coleslaw.

what's in it

beta-carotene This powerful antioxidant may help to neutralize cell-damaging free-radical molecules.

calcium Broccoli is a good nonfat, nondairy source of this bone-nourishing mineral.

dithiolethiones These anticancer agents may help to stimulate the antioxidant glutathione, a cancer-protective compound.

folate This B vitamin may help to reduce the incidence of cancer and certain birth defects. It may also help to control levels of homocysteine, an amino acid linked to heart disease. (One cup of cooked broccoli has 78mcg of folate, about 20% of the Daily Value.)

glucosinolates Once ingested, the glucosinolates in broccoli break down into various healthful compounds, including indoles, sulforaphane, and isothiocyanates, all of which may be cancer-fighters.

indoles These compounds are thought to provide protection against hormone-related cancers, such as breast and prostate cancers.

insoluble fiber This type of fiber helps food move faster and with greater bulk through the digestive tract, promoting regularity.

isothiocyanates By stimulating the body's production of its own cancer-fighting enzymes, isothiocyanates may neutralize potential cancer-causing substances. These phytochemicals also may combat carcinogens in smoke.

lutein This carotenoid may prevent colon cancer and certain eye diseases.

potassium Broccoli is a rich source of this mineral, which may help lower the risk for stroke and high blood pressure. (One cup of cooked broccoli has 456mg of potassium, or 15% of the Daily Value.)

sulforaphane This powerful phytochemical may increase the activity of cancer-fighting enzymes in the body, as well as reduce tumor formation.

maximizing the benefits

Cooking broccoli with a lot of water can diminish broccoli's **glucosinolates, folate,** and **vitamin C.** Steam, microwave, or stir-fry it instead.

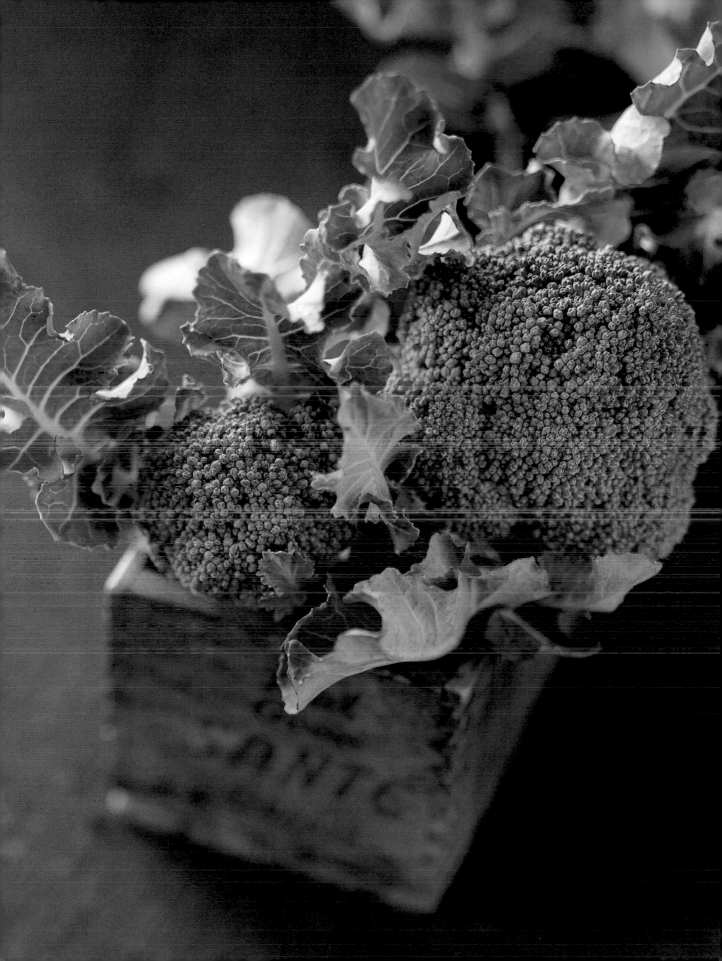

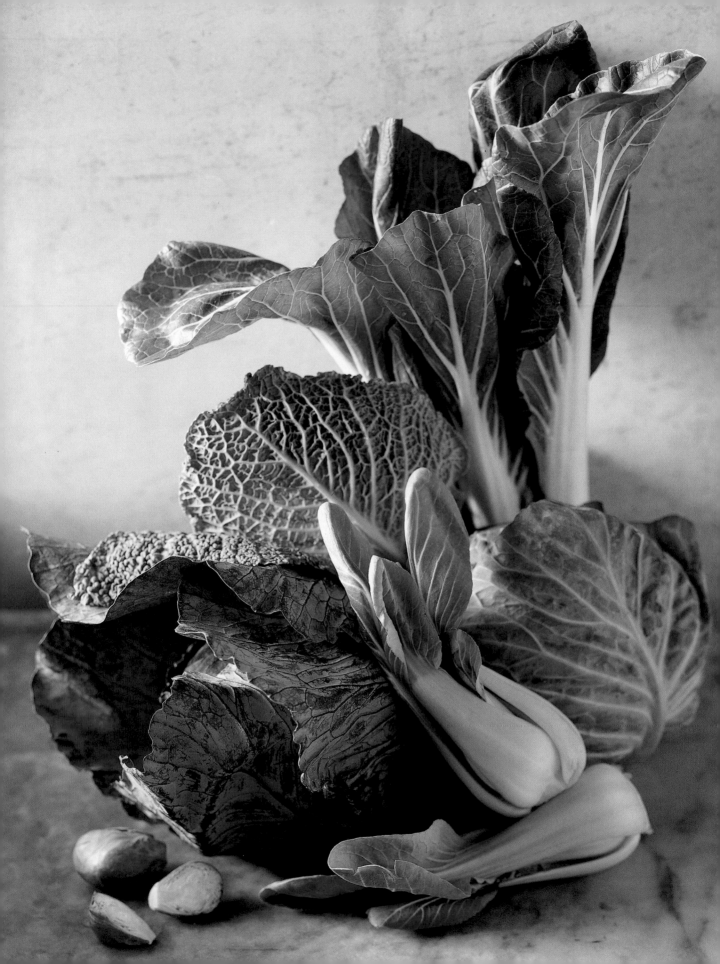

cabbage family

Cabbages are nutritional kings, as are their relatives, bok choy and brussels sprouts. Nutrient-rich and loaded with protective compounds, these members of the cabbage family may help to fight off cancer and heart disease.

what's in it

anthocyanins Found in red cabbage, these antioxidant pigments may protect cells from free-radical damage.

beta-carotene Bok choy is extremely rich in this important antioxidant and has more beta-carotene than other cabbages (1 cup of cooked bok choy has 2.6mg, while green and red cabbages have less than 0.1mg). Beta-carotene is linked to lower incidence of heart disease and certain kinds of cancer.

dithiolethiones These compounds may help protect against carcinogenic agents by increasing the body's reserve of glutathione, which has antioxidant properties.

insoluble fiber This fiber helps to alleviate constipation.

folate This important B vitamin is believed to reduce the incidence of cancer and birth defects, and lower heart disease risk.

goitrogens Raw cabbage contains these compounds, which may slow down the thyroid. Consult with your physician if you have thyroid problems and you eat a lot of raw cabbage.

indoles Thought to deactivate estrogen, which stimulates tumor growth, indoles may protect against breast and prostate cancer. Savoy cabbage is an especially good source of indoles.

isothiocyanates These compounds may stimulate the enzymes that impede hormones that promote breast and prostate cancers.

sulforaphane This isothiocyanate stimulates production of glutathione, a compound with antioxidant properties.

vitamin C Brussels sprouts supply four times the vitamin C of their cabbage cousins (97mg versus only 23mg for 1 cup). Vitamin C may help to improve immune function and fight off infections and viruses.

maximizing the benefits

For **vitamin C,** raw cabbage is best. But when cooking, it's best to steam, microwave, or stir-fry for maximum retention of other nutrients.

add more to your diet

▶ Use cabbage leaves as edible steamer wrappers: Sprinkle thick fish fillets with herbs (chervil, tarragon, or dill), wrap in cabbage leaves, and steam over seasoned broth (use more of the same herbs in the broth).

▶ Shred brussels sprouts and stir-fry with garlic, chopped nuts, and bread crumbs. Toss with cooked pasta.

▶ Steam cabbage or bok choy leaves and wrap around matchsticks of carrot and bell pepper. Serve the packets with a spicy dipping sauce.

▶ Stir-fry cabbage and onions, add to coarsely mashed potatoes, and use as a stuffing for roast chicken or turkey.

▶ Add shredded cabbage and apples to potatoes when making potato pancakes.

▶ Make a slaw with shredded brussels sprouts, carrots, red peppers, and pears. Dress the slaw with a light vinaigrette.

carrots

Gold mines of nourishment, these healthful vegetables provide impressive amounts of beta-carotene as well as a good amount of fiber. Consuming carrots may help to protect against heart disease, certain types of cancer, skin disorders, eye conditions, constipation, and high cholesterol.

add more to your diet

▶ Use carrot juice in place of water in homemade bread or pizza dough.

▶ To make a sauce to serve over grilled chicken, sauté carrots with garlic in olive oil until very tender. Puree with carrot juice and some lemon juice to taste.

▶ Stir shredded carrots into rice pudding after the pudding is cooked.

▶ Use carrots instead of shredded coconut in macaroons or other cookies.

▶ Substitute carrot juice for broths in soups, stews, and pasta sauces.

▶ Cook carrots along with potatoes when boiling potatoes for mashing.

what's in it

beta-carotene Much more than the precursor for vitamin A, beta-carotene functions as an antioxidant that helps to combat free-radical damage to cells. The more vivid the color of the carrot, the higher the levels of carotene in it. Carrots are one of the richest sources of this important carotenoid: One cup of cooked carrots provides 18mg, or 300% of the recommended intake!

calcium pectate A unique type of pectin fiber, calcium pectate is thought to lower cholesterol by attaching to bile acids, a process that helps to remove cholesterol from the body.

insoluble fiber This type of fiber helps to prevent constipation by adding bulk to digested foods. It also makes you feel full, which may be helpful for weight loss.

vitamin A When you eat carrots or other foods high in beta-carotene, your body converts what it needs of the beta-carotene into vitamin A, which is important for numerous functions, including maintaining proper eyesight, normal cell growth, and healthy mucous membranes. Vitamin A helps eyes adjust to the dark, and it also promotes healthy skin and hair.

maximizing the benefits

Cooking carrots, especially with a little bit of fat (preferably monounsaturated fat, such as olive oil), makes **beta-carotene** more available for absorption by the body.

health bites

Although research suggests that beta-carotene in pill form doesn't help prevent heart disease, other studies suggest that eating foods high in beta-carotene may indeed do the trick. A recent study indicates that high dietary beta-carotene intake may reduce risk for cardiovascular disease by about 45%.

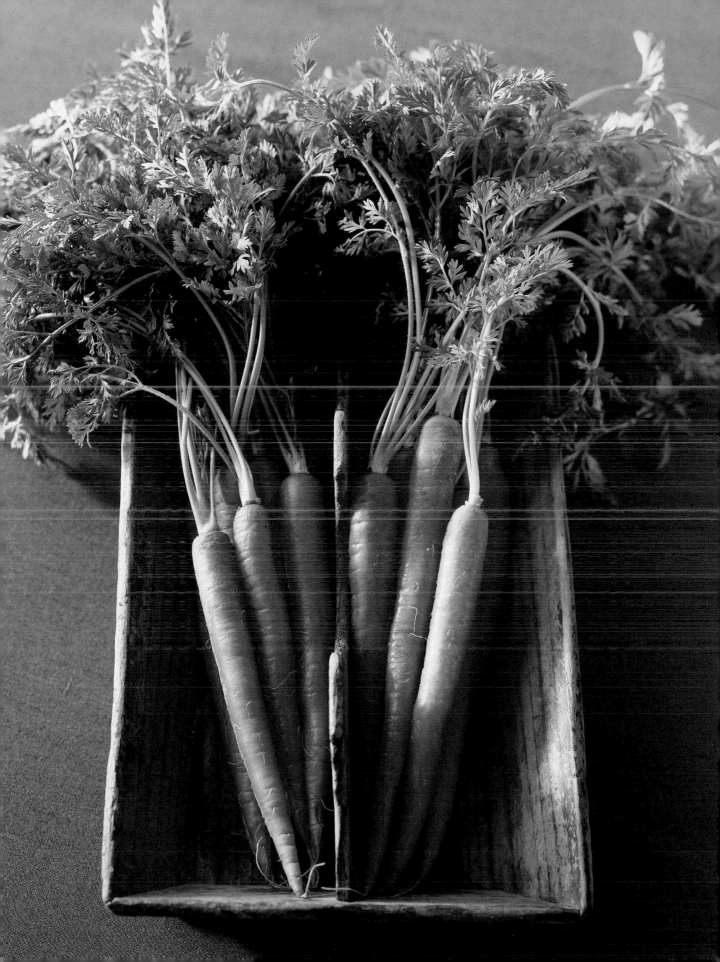

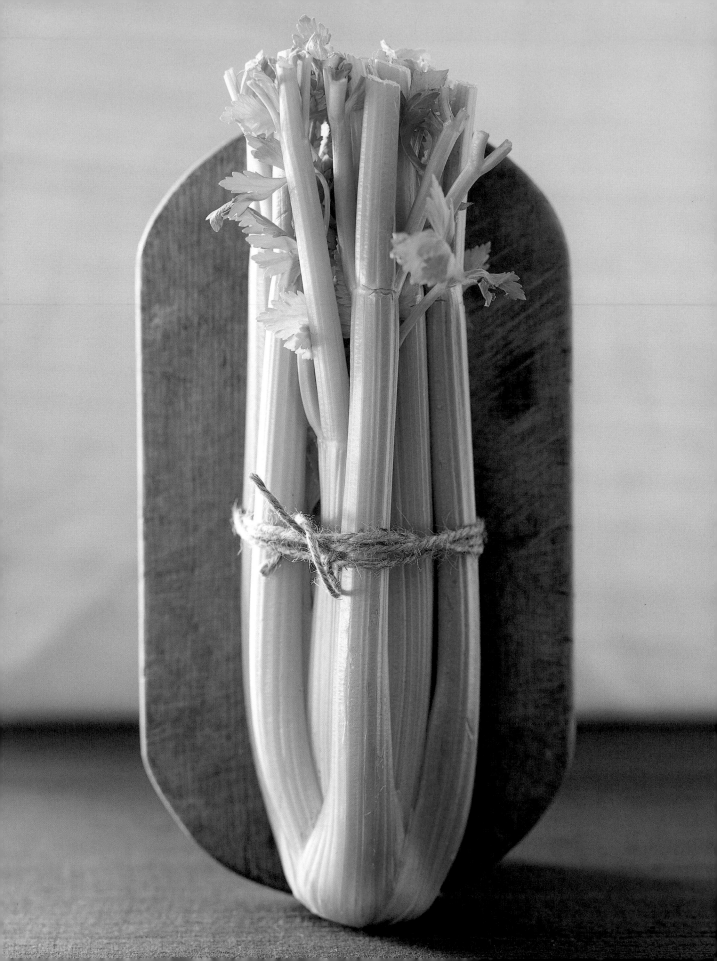

celery

Once the quintessential dieter's snack, celery has finally achieved the status of a good-for-you food. Researchers are discovering many healthful compounds in celery, including those that may help lower blood pressure or reduce the risk for certain types of cancer.

what's in it

apigenin Animal studies suggest that this flavonoid may stop tumor growth. Apigenin is also currently under investigation for potential anti-inflammatory effects.

insoluble fiber Foods that are high in insoluble fiber tend to be low in calories, and they also promote feelings of satiety (fullness). An excellent choice for those who are trying to lose weight, insoluble fiber is filling because it absorbs water and adds bulk as it moves through the digestive tract, a process that also keeps your digestive system working properly. (One cup has 1.5g of insoluble fiber.)

phthalides (3-n-butyl phthalide) Though celery is relatively high in sodium (35mg per stalk)—a possible concern for people who suffer from hypertension—it also contains a unique compound that is believed to lower blood pressure. How phthalides achieve this effect is under review, but preliminary studies indicate that these compounds may reduce the body's levels of certain hormones that constrict blood vessels and raise blood pressure.

maximizing the benefits

If possible, include the celery leaves when cooking. They contain high concentrations of nutrients, such as **potassium** and **vitamin C**.

add more to your diet

▶ For a vegetable side dish, sauté matchsticks of celery in olive oil with chopped walnuts.

▶ Make a celery relish: Finely chop celery along with onion, garlic, and parsley. Add vinegar and mustard to taste and use as a topping for burgers, grilled meat, or poultry.

▶ For a celery "tonic": In a blender, combine celery with tomato juice and horseradish, and puree.

▶ Make a triple-celery soup: Cook sliced celery, celery leaves, garlic, broth, a sprinkling of celery seeds, and herbs (such as marjoram or basil) and puree. Add milk for a creamy soup.

▶ Braise celery in seasoned broth until tender and serve as a side vegetable.

health bites

Celery seeds—whose pungency perks up the flavor of pickles or sauerkraut, or broths for cooking shellfish—contain potentially beneficial phytochemicals such as limonene, coumarins, phthalides, and apigenin. Modern science has found that celery seeds may have anti-inflammatory properties. There are also folk remedies that call for the use of celery seeds to alleviate gout and rheumatoid arthritis.

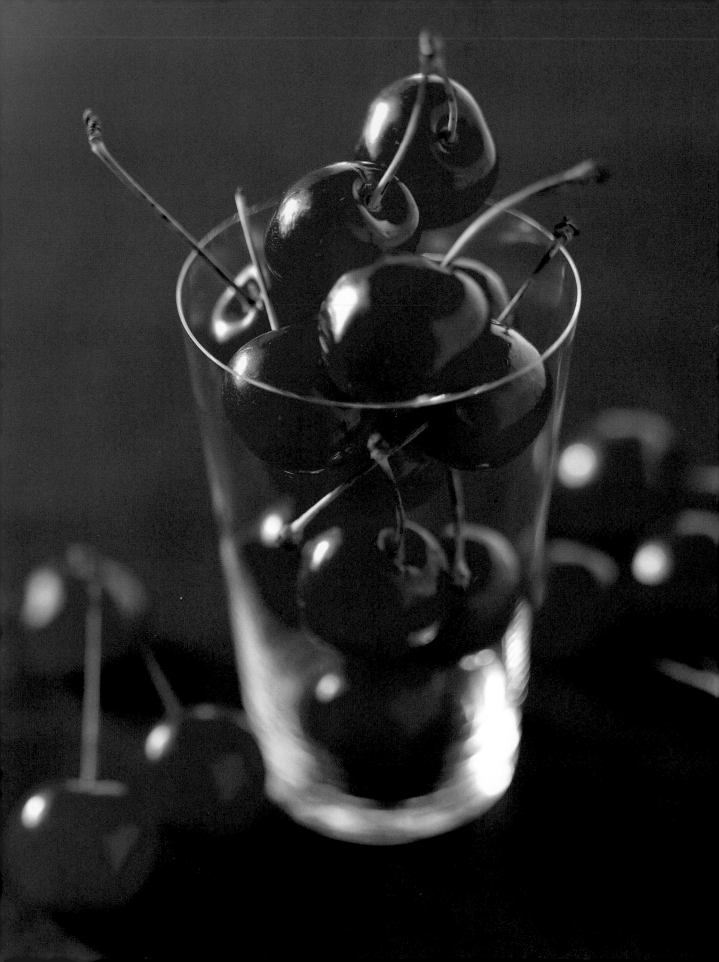

cherries

Sweet, juicy, and tantalizingly tart, cherries contain a number of healthful phytochemicals that may help prevent certain cancers and heart disease.

what's in it

anthocyanins These plant pigments may reduce LDL ("bad") cholesterol oxidation and may also help prevent heart disease.

chlorogenic acid This phenolic compound may help thwart carcinogenic environmental toxins such as nitrosamines in cigarette smoke.

cyanidin A type of anthocyanin found in cherries, this compound may inhibit inflammatory enzymes.

perillyl alcohol Research suggests that perillyl alcohol reduces pancreatic, breast, liver, and lung tumors and may cause cell death in tumor cells without harming healthy cells.

rutin Rutin may enhance the activity of vitamin C and is believed to help maintain healthy veins and capillaries.

quercetin A much-studied flavonoid, quercetin exhibits anticarcinogenic and antioxidant activities. Studies also link quercetin to a reduced risk for coronary artery disease and certain types of cancer. Cherries are believed to contain impressive amounts of quercetin.

add more to your diet

▶ Chop cherries and combine with scallions, green pepper, and celery. Toss in a spicy dressing and use as a salsa to serve with grilled meats or poultry.

▶ Add chopped cherries to your favorite brownie, cake, or cookie recipe.

▶ Add halved or chopped cherries to a savory stir-fry, stew, curry, or soup.

▶ Freeze cherry juice in ice-cube trays. Combine the frozen juice cubes with more cherry juice, cherries, and yogurt in a blender, and puree to make a smoothie.

▶ Use cherry juice in place of red wine in savory sauces.

▶ Use dried cherries in place of raisins.

maximizing the benefits

Cherries contain some **vitamin C,** which is diminished when cooked. Preliminary research shows that adding a few chopped cherries to hamburger meat reduces the level of heterocyclic aromatic amines (HAAs), the dangerous, potentially carcinogenic compounds that form when fish or meat cooks.

health bites

Although there is scant scientific evidence to support what many people believe, that cherries and cherry juice can relieve the pain of gout, some research suggests that a substance in cherries called cyanidin has anti-inflammatory properties—an attribute that might certainly help reduce the swelling and pain of gout.

citrus fruits

Far from lightweights when it comes to nutritional power, citrus fruits have an abundance of vitamin C, potassium, pectin, and phytochemicals that may benefit numerous conditions, including allergies, asthma, cancer, cataracts, heart disease, stroke, and the common cold.

add more to your diet

➤ After juicing citrus fruits, pop the empty "shells" into the freezer and you'll have zest when a recipe calls for it.

➤ Combine orange or tangerine juice with seltzer for a healthy soda.

➤ Add grated orange or lemon zest to tea bread and cookie recipes.

➤ Substitute citrus juice for vinegar in your favorite salad dressing.

➤ Stir a healthy amount of lemon juice and honey into tea for a soothing drink.

➤ Add orange, tangerine, or grapefruit segments to a green salad.

➤ Sprinkle grapefruit halves with brown sugar and broil for a quick dessert.

➤ For a tropical fruit salad: Toss sliced bananas, strawberries, kiwifruit, and mango in orange juice.

what's in it

beta-cryptoxanthin A carotenoid in oranges and tangerines, beta-cryptoxanthin may help prevent colon cancer.

hesperidin This flavonoid is found in the zest (the thin, colored portion of the citrus peel) of oranges. Hesperidin may have anti-inflammatory and cholesterol-lowering effects.

limonene Found mainly in the zest of lemons, limes, and tangerines, limonene may help prevent cancer.

naringin A flavonoid found in white grapefruit, this compound may protect the lungs against environmental toxins such as air pollution and cigarette smoke.

nobiletin This flavonoid, found in the flesh of oranges, may have anti-inflammatory actions.

folate This B vitamin is instrumental in the prevention of certain birth defects, and may also play a role in battling heart disease.

tangeretin This flavonoid, found in tangerines, has been linked in experimental studies to a reduced growth of tumor cells.

maximizing the benefits

Don't spend too much time removing the pith (the spongy white layer between the zest and the pulp), because a good amount of the fiber and phytochemicals, particularly the flavonoids, are found both in the pulp and the pith. Freshly squeezed citrus juice also has more nutrients than frozen or bottled juices.

health bites

In something known as "the grapefruit effect," compounds in grapefruit juice can increase blood levels of certain drugs, leading to dangerous side effects. If you are taking medication, it would be prudent to ask your physician if you should be avoiding grapefruit juice.

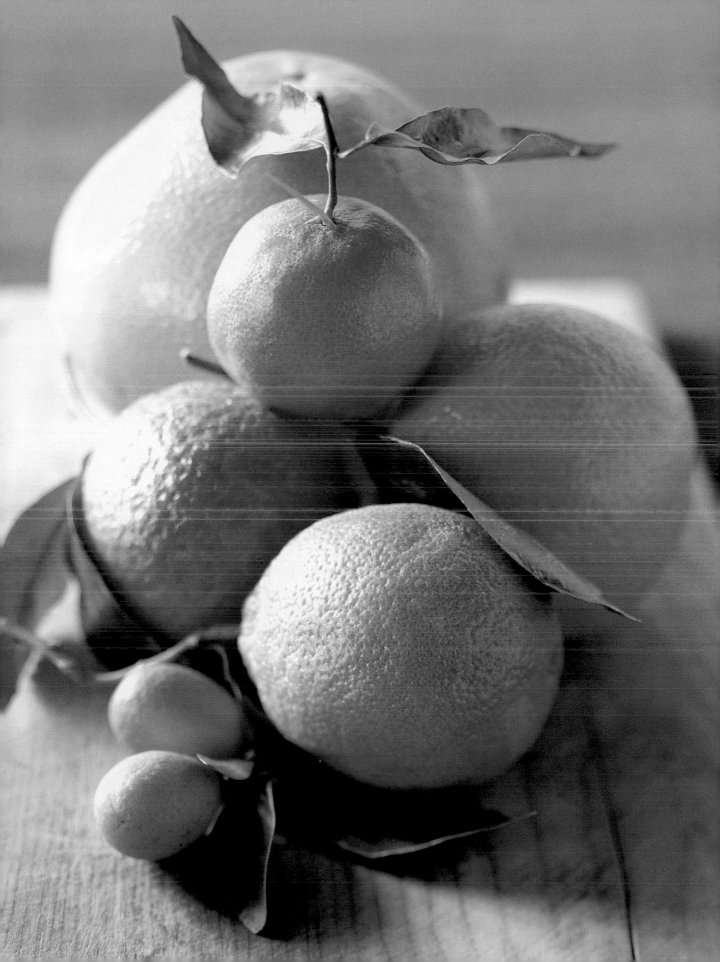

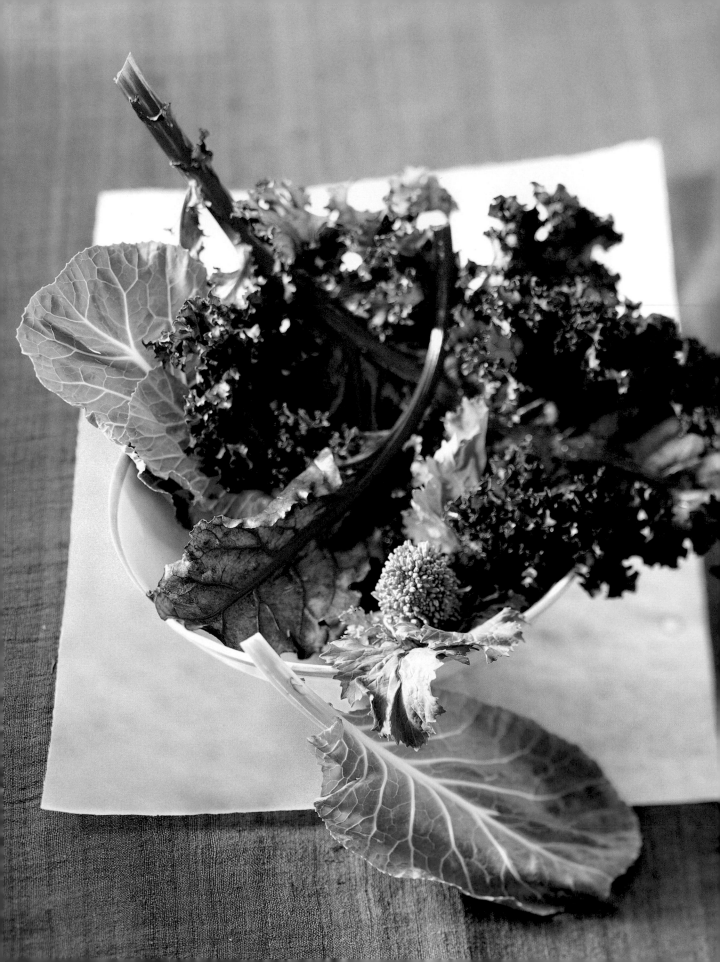

cooking greens

Cooking greens—kale, Swiss chard, and collard, beet, turnip, and mustard greens—are packed with vitamins, minerals, fiber, and an array of phytochemicals that may reduce heart disease risk, eye diseases, and certain cancers.

what's in it

beta-carotene Greens are rich sources of this antioxidant, which may help strengthen the body's defense system against harmful free-radical compounds. Kale has the most, with 5.8mg per cup of cooked (this provides 72% of the daily recommended intake).

calcium Although this mineral is found in greens, some greens, such as Swiss chard and beet greens, contain compounds called oxalates, which prevent calcium from being properly absorbed. If you are prone to kidney stones or gout, avoid foods high in oxalates.

chlorophyll This plant pigment may help to block the damaging changes that convert healthy cells to precancerous cells.

folate Cooking greens are a good source of this important B vitamin, which helps to ward off certain birth defects, cancer, and heart disease. Collards and turnip greens are the best, with over 40% of the Daily Value per cup.

indoles Indoles are thought to help protect against the risk for hormone-related cancers by blocking the action of estrogen.

isothiocyanates Partially responsible for the pungency of some leafy greens, these phytochemicals are thought to help protect against hormone-dependent cancers. These compounds are also believed to inhibit environmental carcinogens.

lutein and zeaxanthin These carotenoids are linked to the prevention of macular degeneration. Kale is an extremely rich source of these phytochemicals; collard greens are also a good source.

sulforaphane This phytochemical may help prevent harmful carcinogens from initiating cancer.

vitamin K Found in huge amounts in cooking greens, this bone-building, anticlotting vitamin may interfere with blood-thinning medications.

maximizing the benefits

To enhance the bioavailability of **beta-carotene** in cooking greens, cook them with a small amount of olive oil. If you do cook greens in water, which can diminish **folate** levels, try to use the cooking water in the recipe.

---

add more to your diet

▶ Combine chopped sautéed kale with ricotta and grated Parmesan cheese and use as a filling for lasagna or manicotti.

▶ Make a green bruschetta: Finely chop cooking greens and sauté with garlic in olive oil until melt-in-your-mouth tender. Use as a topping for thick slices of toasted Italian bread.

▶ Cook assorted greens in seasoned water with some olive oil and eat both the greens and their cooking liquid over slabs of cornbread.

▶ Chop and steam cooking greens, then fold into garlicky mashed potatoes.

▶ In a traditional Italian dessert tart—*crostata di verdure*—finely chopped, cooked greens, such as Swiss chard or kale, are combined with a sweetened custard and used as the tart's filling.

▶ Add chopped, cooked greens to your favorite meatball or meatloaf mixture.

corn

A good source of complex carbohydrates, fiber, and thiamin, corn is an excellent low-fat food that provides abundant energy and may help to fight heart disease, certain cancers, macular degeneration, and obesity.

add more to your diet

▶ Boost both the flavor and the health benefits of your next batch of cornbread by adding corn kernels to the batter.

▶ Season corn-on-the-cob with lime juice instead of butter.

▶ Combine corn kernels with chopped scallions, red bell pepper, hot pepper sauce, and lime juice, and use as a quick salsa for meat, poultry, or fish.

▶ Serve an Italian-style polenta (made from cornmeal) as a side dish in place of rice or pasta.

▶ Add cornmeal to pancake batters, tea breads, and biscuits.

▶ For an interesting take on the Spanish soup gazpacho, substitute corn kernels for the cucumbers that most recipes call for, and stir in a generous amount of chopped cilantro.

what's in it

folate This B vitamin has been found to prevent neural-tube birth defects in fetuses, and current research suggests that it also helps to reduce the risk for heart disease and cancer. (One cup of corn kernels has 51mcg of folate, or 13% of the Daily Value.)

lutein and zeaxanthin Lutein and zeaxanthin are carotenoids that may help to prevent certain eye conditions such as age-related macular degeneration, one of the leading causes of blindness in older adults. Corn is especially high in lutein (1 cup has 3mg).

protease inhibitors These compounds may help to fight cancerous tumors by stopping the division of proteins that signal uncontrolled cell growth (tumorigenesis).

soluble fiber This type of fiber may help to lower cholesterol by binding with it and blocking its absorption. And if you are trying to lose weight, it is always helpful to consume high-fiber foods because they increase bulk and make you feel full sooner and for longer.

thiamin This B vitamin is required by the body for converting food to energy; a thiamin deficiency can result in fatigue. Thiamin is also essential for proper functioning of the nervous system.

maximizing the benefits

To preserve the water-soluble B vitamins in corn (**folate** and **thiamin**), it's best to steam rather than boil it. If this isn't practical (since most people cook corn-on-the-cob by the dozen), then be sure to cook for no longer than 10 minutes in boiling water to minimize nutrient loss.

health bites

A study conducted by researchers at Harvard University showed that women with the highest intake of dietary lutein (and its companion carotenoid, zeaxanthin) had a 22% reduced risk for cataracts, while men reduced their risk by 19%.

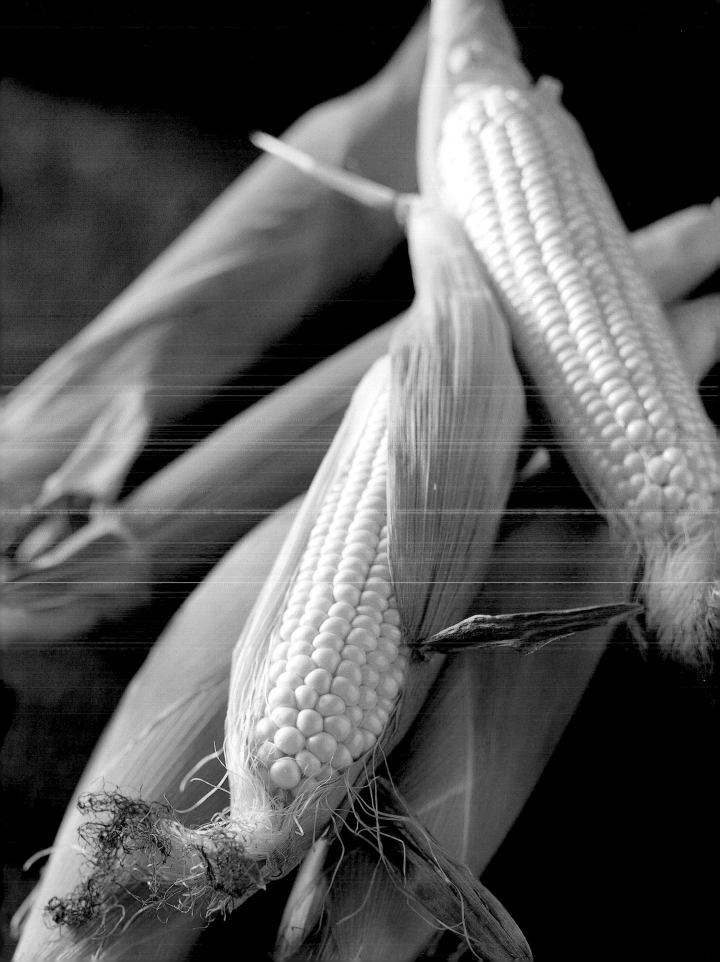

dairy

Packed with nourishing minerals, vitamins, and protein, low-fat dairy products (milk, cheese, and yogurt) and eggs may help provide protection against osteoporosis, insomnia, and headaches and may also boost the immune system.

what's in it

probiotics Probiotics are beneficial bacteria (friendly flora) found in active-culture yogurts, kefir (a fermented milk product), and acidophilus milk. Probiotics may help to improve immune function and prevent and manage yeast infections.

calcium This bone-preserving mineral is vital for all people at all stages of life. Inadequate intake of calcium can result in osteoporosis, a dangerous bone-thinning disease that can lead to fractures and spinal deformities.

lysine Preliminary studies suggest that foods high in this amino acid—including eggs, cheese, and milk—may help to reduce the severity of cold sores.

phosphorus Instrumental in forming bones and teeth, phosphorous also builds muscle and is important for metabolic activity.

potassium This mineral is linked to a reduction of blood pressure and risk for stroke.

riboflavin This B vitamin releases energy, maintains healthy red blood cells, helps create hormones, and may help prevent migraines.

tryptophan Drinking a warm glass of milk before you go to bed may help to prevent insomnia because tryptophan, an amino acid in milk and other dairy foods, is converted into serotonin, which promotes a relaxed mood. Note that eating foods rich in complex carbohydrates (pasta, beans, rice) can help to enhance proper absorption of tryptophan.

vitamin B$_{12}$ Dairy foods and eggs are good sources of this vitamin, which is essential for neurological function and red blood cell formation.

vitamin D Most milk in the United States is fortified with vitamin D, which enhances absorption of calcium, helping to prevent osteoporosis and bone fractures. Egg yolks are one of the few natural sources of vitamin D. Generally, cheeses and most yogurts are not fortified with this important vitamin.

maximizing the benefits

To reap the most benefits from the **probiotics** in yogurt, be sure to check that the yogurt contains "active" or "live" cultures.

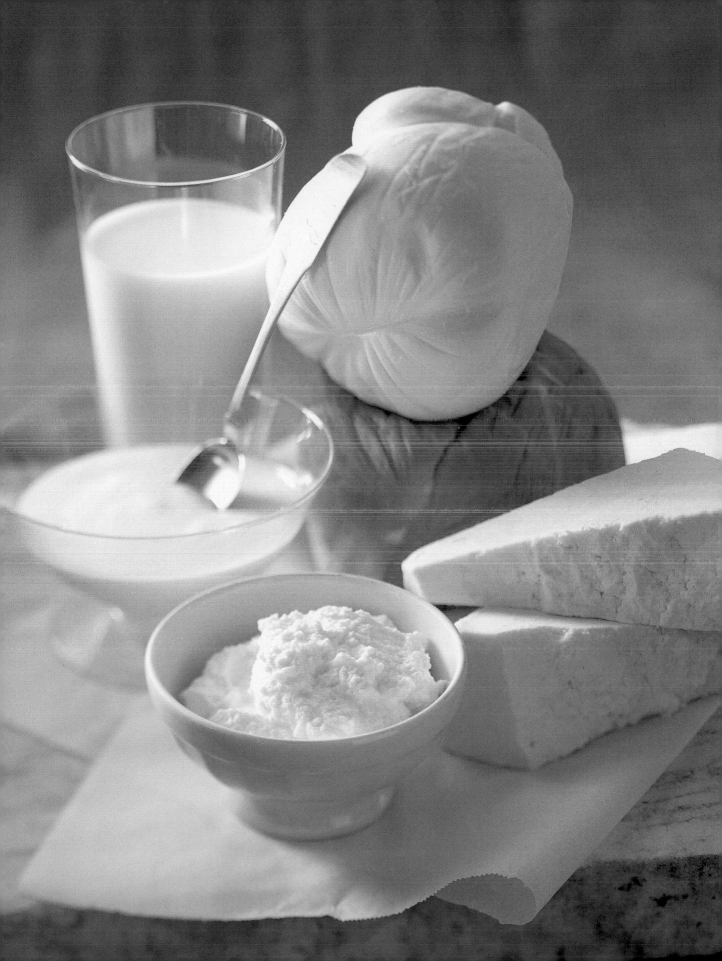

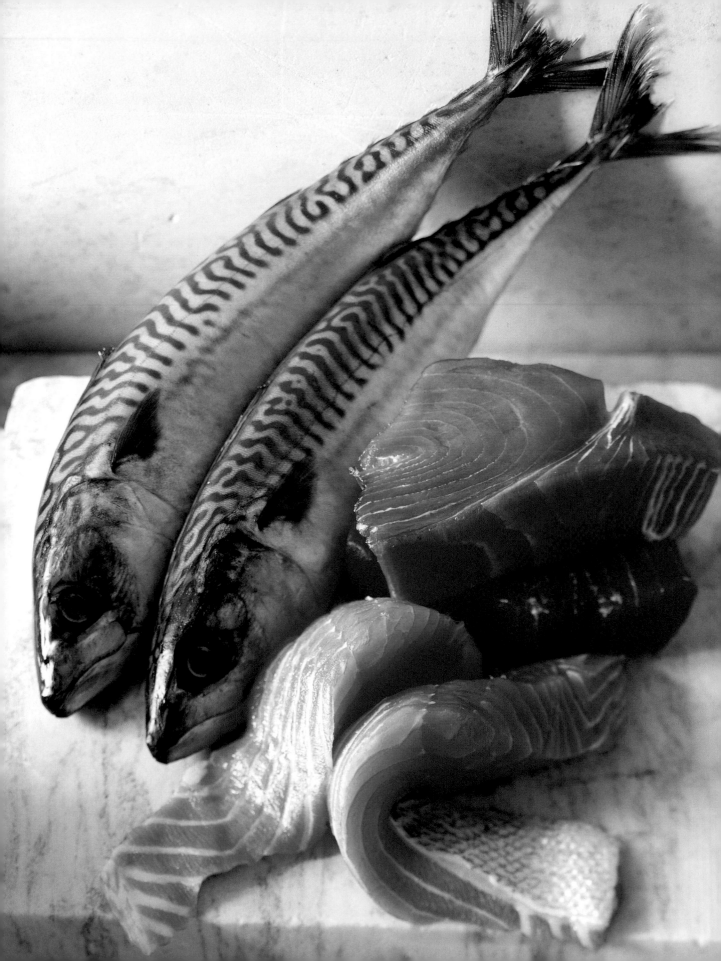

fatty fish

High in omega-3 fatty acids, fatty fish—salmon, fresh tuna, herring, mackerel, sardines, and lake trout—are important heart-healthy sources of protein, vitamins, and minerals. Fish enhance health in impressive ways.

what's in it

iron Mackerel and sardines are a good source of this vital mineral, which provides oxygen to blood and prevents anemia.

niacin Fish contain this B vitamin, which helps to release energy from carbohydrates.

omega-3 fatty acids Two main omega-3 fatty acids in fish, docosahexaenoic acid (DHA) and eicosapentaenoic acid (EPA), are linked to the prevention of asthma, depression, heart disease, high blood pressure, psoriasis, and rheumatoid arthritis.

protein Without the harmful saturated fat found in other high-protein foods, fish is an excellent source of quality protein.

tyrosine This amino acid is involved with the synthesis of neurotransmitters in the brain and may promote mental health.

vitamin B$_6$ Fish are a decent source of this vitamin, which may help to maintain a healthy immune system and improve mood.

vitamin B$_{12}$ Salmon, mackerel, and fresh tuna are good sources of this vitamin, which is required for healthy blood cells. It also helps the central nervous system to function properly.

vitamin D This bone-healthy vitamin is found in only a few foods, and salmon and mackerel are top sources.

maximizing the benefits

It is best to cook fish, since the heat will destroy parasites and potentially harmful microorganisms in raw fish. Canned **salmon** and **sardines,** with the bones, are a good source of calcium.

add more to your diet

▶ Chop pickled herring and toss with chopped walnuts, beets, diced apples, and a lemon vinaigrette.

▶ Puree canned tuna with cooked white beans and lemon juice and use as a sandwich spread.

▶ Poach fresh salmon, flake, and fold into reduced-fat sour cream along with capers and dill. Serve on crisp toasts or thick cucumber slices.

▶ Mash canned sardines into mashed potatoes. Shape into patties and broil.

▶ Puree tuna along with plain nonfat yogurt, a little mayonnaise, and fresh lemon juice and use as a sauce for cold poached chicken.

▶ Make fresh fish salads using citrus segments and/or citrus vinaigrettes.

health bites

Fish are so beneficial for cardiovascular health that the American Heart Association recommends eating two 6-ounce servings of fatty fish weekly to help lower the risk for death from heart disease.

figs

Eating figs may help to prevent such ailments as cardiovascular disease, premenstrual syndrome, and hemorrhoids. Figs are especially rich in minerals, fiber, and polyphenols, compounds that neutralize free radicals.

add more to your diet

▶ Serve fresh figs with goat cheese and thin slices of prosciutto as an appetizer.

▶ Chop dried figs and add to granola.

▶ Poach dried figs in red wine sweetened with honey, and serve as a condiment with grilled or broiled meat.

▶ Make a pasta salad with diced fresh figs, crumbled feta cheese, toasted pecans, and cooked pasta, and dress with a red wine vinaigrette.

▶ Cook dried figs in water until very tender. Puree with some of the cooking liquid and use as an all-fruit spread.

▶ Dice dried figs and add to cookie dough in place of raisins.

▶ Stuff pork loin or chicken breasts with chopped dried figs.

what's in it

fiber Figs are an excellent source of both insoluble and soluble fiber (one dried fig has over 2g of dietary fiber). Insoluble fiber may help to prevent constipation, diverticulosis, and hemorrhoids. The soluble pectin fiber in figs may help to lower blood cholesterol.

ficin An enzyme unique to figs, ficin has mild laxative properties that add to the fruit's ability to relieve constipation.

plant sterols These plant compounds may lower LDL ("bad") cholesterol and reduce the risk for heart disease.

polyphenols According to research, dried figs have up to 50 times more polyphenols than most other commonly consumed fruits and vegetables. Polyphenols neutralize damaging free radicals and help to prevent chronic disease.

potassium A diet rich in this powerful mineral may help to lower blood pressure and the risk for heart attacks and strokes. (Four fresh figs have 464mg of potassium, 15% of the Daily Value.)

vitamin B$_6$ This B vitamin may improve cardiovascular health and premenstrual syndrome (PMS). Fresh figs, in particular, are a good source: One serving (4 figs) has 0.2mg of this vitamin, which is 11% of the Daily Value.

maximizing the benefits

Fresh figs spoil quickly and should be consumed within a week of being picked. Dried figs, on the other hand, store well. And, because their water content is lower, dried figs are, ounce for ounce, more nutrient-dense than fresh.

health bites

Figs possess the highest overall mineral content of any of the most common fruits, providing significant quantities of bone-building, blood-nourishing, and cardioprotective minerals—calcium, iron, magnesium, manganese, and potassium—in amounts ranging from about 10 to 15% of the Daily Value per serving.

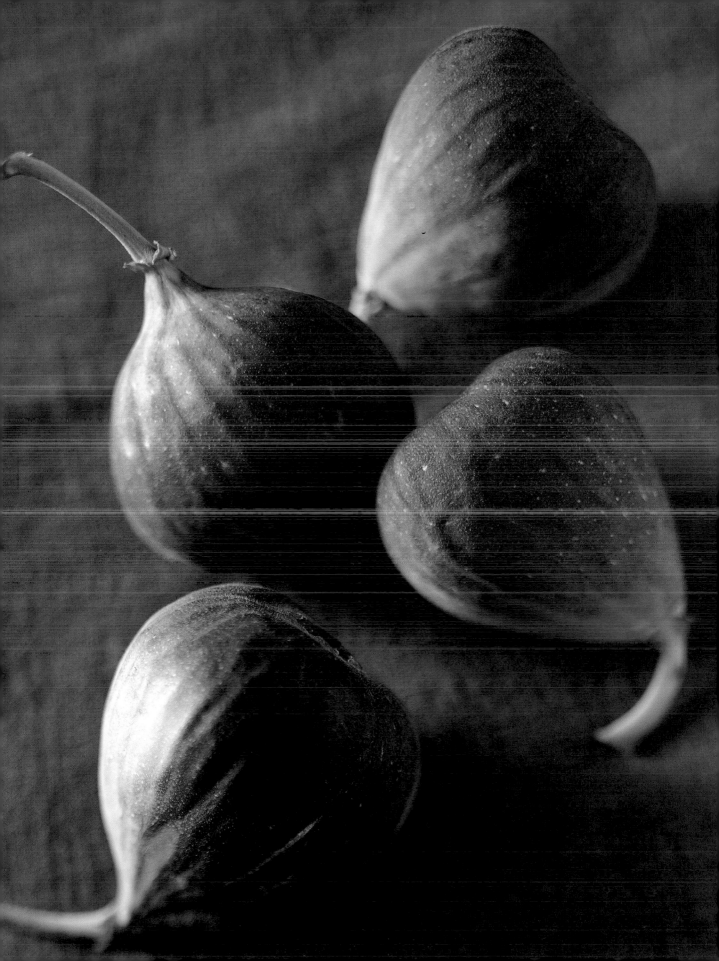

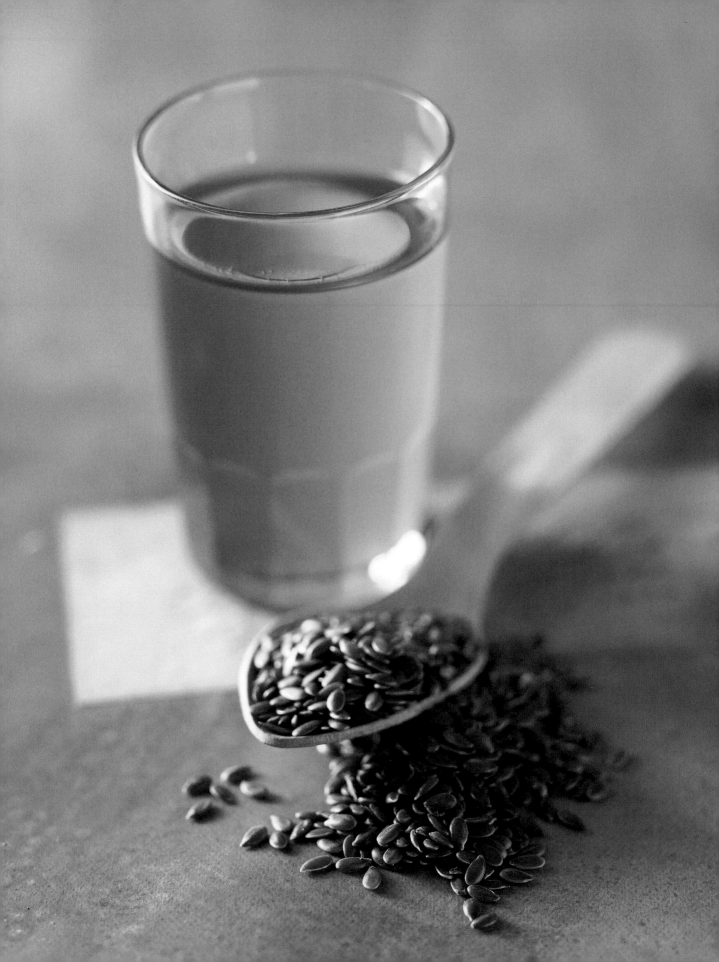

flaxseeds

The many merits of flaxseeds (and flaxseed oil) have propelled this ancient seed, which was cultivated as early as 4000 B.C., into the nutritional spotlight. Flaxseeds are being studied for the prevention or management of numerous conditions.

what's in it

alpha-linolenic acid (ALA) Because our bodies cannot manufacture this essential fatty acid, we must consume it in foods. Important for regulating blood pressure and for cell membrane health, ALA may have a wide range of beneficial health effects, including the ability to prevent heart disease by reducing the production of hormonelike substances that lead to blood clotting. ALA makes flaxseed oil healthful, though it should be noted that fiber and lignans are lost when the flaxseeds are processed into oil.

insoluble fiber This type of fiber keeps your digestive system running smoothly and helps to prevent constipation.

lignans Also referred to as phytoestrogens, lignans have mild estrogenic properties. Lignans may also play a protective role against autoimmune disorders such as systemic lupus erythematosus, rheumatoid arthritis, as well as fibrocystic breasts and some hormone-related cancers (breast, endometrial, and prostate).

soluble fiber The soluble fiber in flaxseeds forms a gel in the intestine, helping trap and usher out harmful LDL ("bad") cholesterol particles.

add more to your diet

▶ Grind flaxseeds in a mini food processor or coffee grinder and use the flaxseed meal to replace one-fourth of the flour in pancake or waffle batter.

▶ Add ground flaxseeds to cookie, bread, and pie doughs.

▶ Make a pesto with fresh basil, garlic, ground flaxseeds (in place of nuts), flaxseed oil, and grated Parmesan cheese. Toss with hot pasta.

▶ Grind flaxseeds and add to your cold cereal or stir into hot oatmeal.

▶ Add ground flaxseeds to meatballs and meatloaves.

▶ Grind flaxseeds along with toasted nuts, mix with Neufchâtel cream cheese, and use as a spread.

maximizing the benefits

To get the most out of flaxseeds, grind them (in a coffee grinder). Unless the seeds are well chewed or ground, they simply pass through the body, and you don't reap their health benefits. In addition, don't heat flaxseed oil—this will destroy its alpha-linolenic content as well as make the oil taste unpleasant.

health bites

Adding flaxseeds to your diet may help to ward off heart disease. In a recent study, men and women with high cholesterol ate muffins with either flaxseeds or a wheat bran placebo for three weeks each. Participants who ate flaxseeds showed decreases in LDL cholesterol, compared to little change in the placebo group.

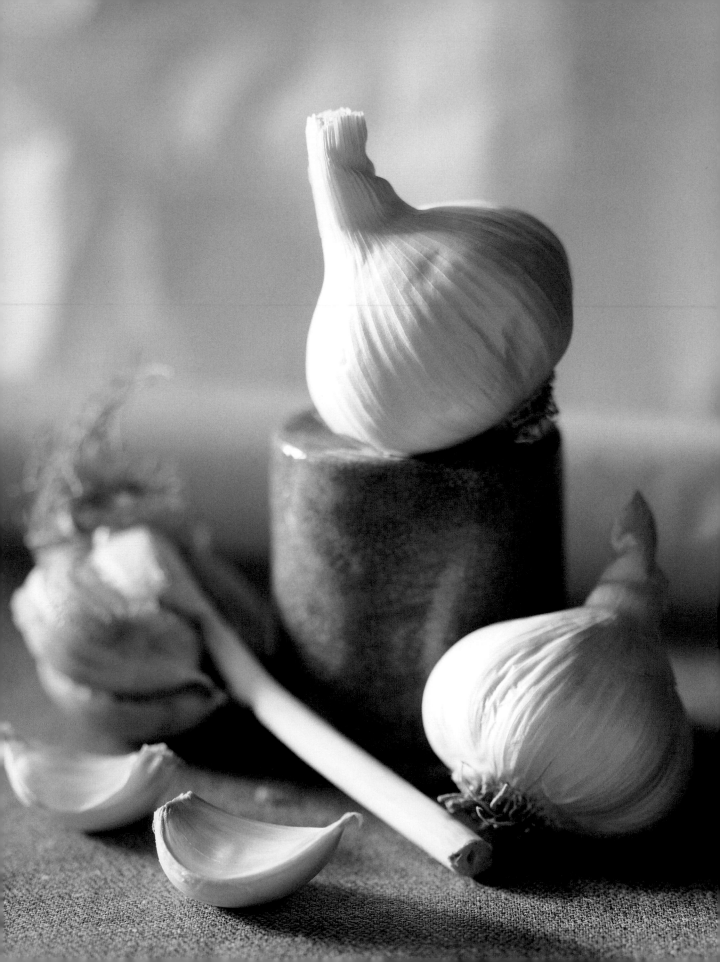

garlic

The medicinal application of garlic goes back as far as 1500 B.C., when the ancient Egyptians recommended it for a host of ailments, including heart disease, wounds, tumors, parasites, and headaches—some of the benefits modern science has also attributed to garlic.

what's in it

ajoenes Ajoenes may be responsible for garlic's antithrombotic (anticlotting) actions, and possibly may have antifungal activity.

allicin Allicin has antibacterial properties (it is also responsible for garlic's pungent smell) and is released when garlic is crushed or cut, producing numerous sulfur compounds.

allyl sulfides Believed to inhibit tumor growth, these sulfur compounds block the damaging effects of carcinogens and promote cancer cell apoptosis (cell death).

sulfur compounds These compounds, including ajoenes and allyl sulfides, may possess anticarcinogenic, anticlotting, antifungal, and antioxidant effects. Sulfur compounds also promote the activity of glutathione, a substance that may inhibit carcinogens.

maximizing the benefits

To activate garlic's full nutritional power, after chopping or crushing it, let the garlic stand for 10 minutes before cooking it. The brief standing period allows allicin and its potent derivatives to be activated.

add more to your diet

▶ Finely mince several cloves of garlic and stir into reduced-fat sour cream. Serve as a dip for crudités.

▶ Roast whole, unpeeled cloves of garlic in olive oil. The garlic will get soft and creamy and can be spread on bread.

▶ Make a garlic-walnut sauce for pasta: Combine equal amounts of peeled garlic cloves and walnuts, a little olive oil, and fresh lemon juice, and puree until smooth. Toss with hot pasta.

▶ For appetizer nuts: Mince garlic, sauté in olive oil, and toss with toasted walnuts and almonds. Sprinkle with a bit of salt.

▶ In a blender, puree garlic, yogurt, and fresh cilantro for a savory drink.

▶ Chop garlic and stir into bread, biscuit, or savory pie doughs. Or try it in corn muffins, and serve with savory soups and stews.

health bites

What's all the stink about? When garlic is digested, a portion of the sulfur compounds enters the bloodstream and is subsequently exhaled from the lungs or eliminated through the pores when we sweat. This is the price we pay to reap the benefits of the "stinking rose." And since the human nose can detect less than one part of these sulfur compounds in one billion parts of exhaled air, it's no wonder that garlic breath is so noticeable. Eating parsley might help to reduce these unpleasant odors, possibly because of its chlorophyll.

grapes

Nature's jewels, grapes contain phytochemicals that may help to reduce risk for heart disease, cancer, and strokes. Studies also indicate that in addition to grapes, red wine, grape juice, and raisins are also rich in disease-fighting compounds.

add more to your diet

▶ Stir halved seedless grapes into chicken, beef, or fish stews.

▶ Chop red grapes and combine with honey, fresh lemon juice, chopped red onion, and minced parsley, and use as a relish for meat or poultry.

▶ Cook dried fruits such as apricots and raisins in purple grape juice until tender, then puree and use as an all-fruit spread.

▶ Prepare hot mulled grape juice or wine: Add cinnamon sticks, whole cloves, allspice berries, and whole black peppercorns to grape juice and cook over low heat until warm and fragrant.

▶ Finely chop grapes and toasted walnuts, stir into Neufchâtel cream cheese, and spread over flour tortillas. Add watercress and sliced turkey or chicken and roll up for a sandwich wrap.

what's in it

anthocyanins Laboratory studies suggest that these pigments in red and purple grapes may suppress the growth of tumor cells.

ellagic acid This phenolic acid in grapes (and other berries) is thought to protect the lungs against environmental toxins.

flavonoids Grapes contain high levels of these heart-healthy antioxidant pigments, which may have the ability to prevent blood from clotting. Both red and purple grape juice are rich in flavonoids, which may help to prevent LDL ("bad") cholesterol from attaching to artery walls and creating blockages that can lead to heart attacks.

pectin This soluble fiber may help to lower LDL cholesterol.

quercetin A flavonoid linked to a reduced risk for cancer development, quercetin may also reduce clotting in blood vessels, and offer relief to people with respiratory ailments.

resveratrol This phytochemical, found in the skin of grapes, has been linked to the ability to fight cancer. It is also being studied for cholesterol-lowering effects and its ability to help prevent strokes.

maximizing the benefits

To reap the full benefits of grapes, it is best to select red or purple varieties, which seem to contain the highest concentrations of healthful compounds.

health bites

Though the French eat a high-fat diet, they have a low incidence of heart disease, a phenomenon called the "French Paradox." The conjecture is that flavonoids in red wine may protect against damage to arteries. The same heart-healthy benefits may also apply to unfermented grape juice: A recent study showed that consuming 10 to 12 ounces of purple grape juice a day could substantially reduce the risk for heart disease.

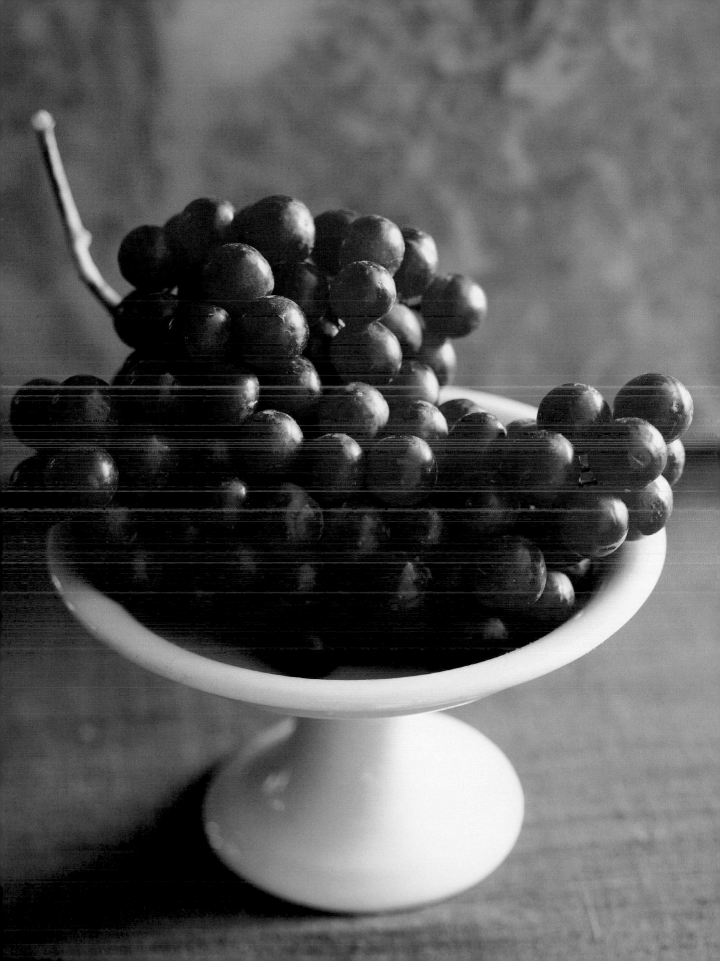

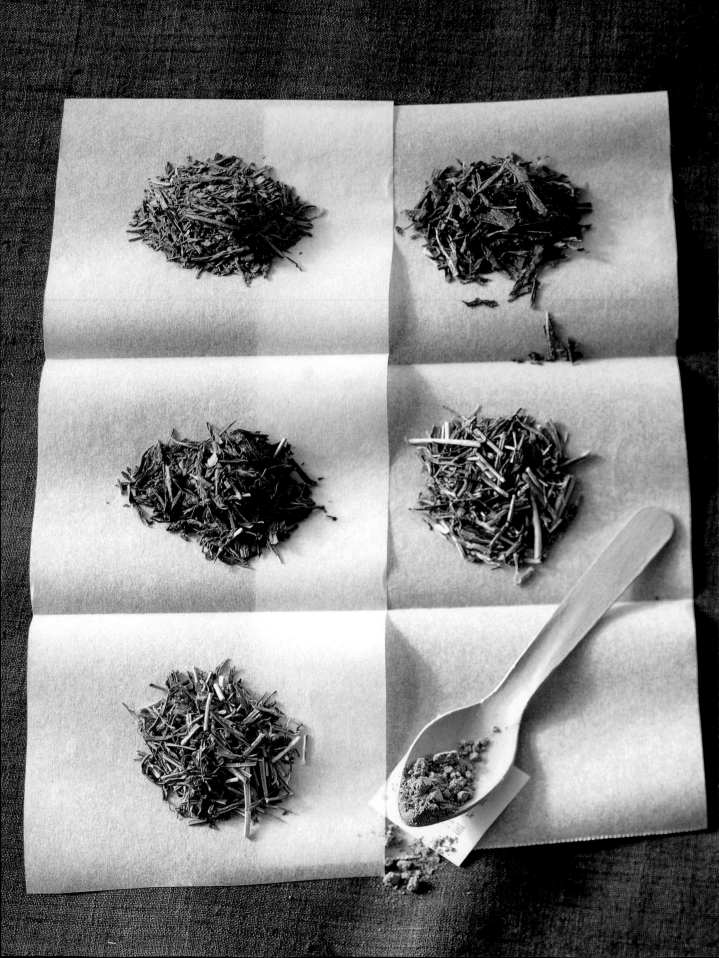

green tea

The healing powers of green tea have been valued in Asia for thousands of years. In the West, preliminary research suggests that drinking green tea may help to prevent cancer and possibly heart disease. Black tea is also under review for health benefits, though the healing agents, called catechins, may be altered in black tea during processing.

what's in it

epigallocatechin gallate (EGCG) One of a class of flavonoids called catechins, EGCG is believed to be the most potent compound in green tea. With the purported capacity to fight cancer at all stages, EGCG may have (1) antioxidant power to seek out and destroy harmful free radicals, (2) the ability to inhibit an enzyme needed for the growth of cancer cells, and (3) a capacity to induce apoptosis (cell death) in cancer cells without damaging healthy cells. Researchers are also currently examining EGCG's potential role in reducing LDL ("bad") cholesterol.

maximizing the benefits

Rest assured that adding milk to tea will not diminish the benefits associated with its healthful compounds. A study suggests that the addition of milk to black or green tea did not adversely affect antioxidant content or activity in 21 healthy study participants. Also, it might be worth buying a teapot and some loose tea, as research conducted at the USDA's Department of Food Composition Lab showed that the levels of catechins in instant teas and bottled teas were lower than in freshly brewed tea.

add more to your diet

▶ Brew green tea, sweeten with honey, chill, and serve over ice.

▶ Sweeten green tea, then follow the directions on packages of unflavored gelatin to make your own Jell-O.

▶ Steep green tea leaves in warm milk for 30 minutes, or until full-flavored. Use the milk in sweet puddings, cake recipes, soups, or pancake and waffle batter. Or use it in a vanilla ice cream recipe to make green tea ice cream.

▶ Make cubes of iced green tea and use to cool lemonade.

▶ Brew a pot of green tea and use it as the basis for a vegetable soup or broth.

health bites

Evidence suggests that drinking green tea may promote weight loss. Though the amount of green tea required to achieve weight loss has not been specified, researchers suggest that long-term consumption of green tea may decrease the incidence of obesity.

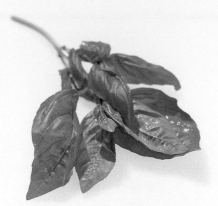

herbs

dillweed

A relative of fennel, wispy green dill weed is available both fresh and dried.

what's in it

Dill contains carvone, coumarins, flavonoids, limonene, and phthalides. Studies suggest that carvone and limonene have the potential to inhibit tumors, and flavonoids may neutralize harmful free radicals. Coumarins and phthalides show promise in stimulating cancer-fighting enzymes in the body.

add more to your diet

Use in: salads and salad dressings; creamy mustard sauces; quiche and savory turnovers. Matches well with lamb, fatty fish, and chicken.

basil

Fresh or dried basil is teeming with powerful antioxidants, responsible for basil's unique flavor.

what's in it

Flavonoid and terpene phytochemicals in basil are under review for their potential benefit in reducing total and harmful LDL cholesterol, as well as suppressing tumor growth.

add more to your diet

Use in: homemade pasta, pizza, and bread doughs; savory soups and stews; tomato sauces and pesto sauce; pilafs, risottos, and other grain dishes; stuffings and fillings for poultry or fish; and mashed potatoes. Use as whole leaves in sandwiches and wraps.

horseradish

This pungent root is a member of the mighty cruciferous family, which includes broccoli, cabbage, and watercress.

what's in it

Horseradish's bite comes from a powerful chemical called allyl isothiocyanate, which may alleviate congestion and respiratory inflammation, and possibly protect against foodborne pathogens. Kaempferol, also in horseradish, is believed to detoxify cancerous agents.

add more to your diet

Use in: salad dressings; cocktail sauces, vegetable dips, and spreads; crusts for fillets of fish, beef, and chicken; and potato salads.

cilantro

Cilantro's bold, distinctive taste is popular in Chinese, Indian, and Mexican cuisines. Fresh cilantro is far more flavorful than dried cilantro.

what's in it

Coumarin, phthalide, polyactylene, and terpene phytochemicals in cilantro are thought to stimulate anticancer enzymes in the body.

add more to your diet

Use in: salsas, relishes, condiments, and chutneys; pesto and other pasta sauces; rice, grain, bean, corn, and tomato salads; peach, pineapple, mango, plum, and papaya desserts; savory cheese pancakes and carrot muffins.

mint

Fresh or dried peppermint and spearmint add a refreshing zest to any dish.

what's in it

Mint has traditionally been used to relieve abdominal pains, bad breath, and sore throats. Powerful terpene phytochemicals present in the mint family—carvone, limonene, menthol, and perillyl alcohol—may inhibit tumor growth.

add more to your diet

Use in: teas and drinks; yogurt or mild-cheese sauces and spreads; sautéed vegetables; vinaigrettes; pasta sauces; and poached fruit. Matches well with lamb, beef, and chicken.

oregano/marjoram

Quintessential Italian herbs, oregano and marjoram are similar in aroma and taste, as well as disease-fighting antioxidant power.

what's in it

Research suggests that quercetin and galangin, two antioxidant flavonoids in oregano, may inhibit the initial development of cancer in cells. Terpene compounds in both marjoram and oregano show promise in elevating levels of cancer-protective enzymes in the body.

add more to your diet

Use in: herb rubs and marinades; chili, pasta sauces, and soups. Matches well with mushrooms, potatoes, and summer squash.

parsley

A relative of the carrot, parsley is one of the most versatile and widely available fresh herbs. Choose flat-leaf (not curly) parsley for the best flavor, and avoid dried parsley altogether.

what's in it

Flavonoid, coumarin, and terpene phytochemicals in parsley are powerful antioxidants that are thought to stimulate the immune system and block cancer-causing substances. Parsley's high chlorophyll content may explain its use as a breath freshener.

add more to your diet

Use in: stuffings, grain, and rice dishes; soups and stews; salads; and pasta dishes.

rosemary

The distinctive taste of rosemary is faintly piney. It's available fresh and dried.

what's in it

Rosemary is rich in such anticancer compounds as carnosol, rosmanol, and a variety of flavonoids. Carnosol may be particularly protective against breast cancer. Additional anticancer substances in rosemary—cineole, geraniole, and pinene—show promise in blocking tumor growth.

add more to your diet

Use in: pizza and bread doughs; rubs and marinades for meat or poultry.

sage

The bold, faintly earthy flavor of sage is a customary poultry seasoning. Sage is available as fresh whole leaves, or dried or "rubbed" leaves.

what's in it

Powerful anticancer terpene substances in sage may lower heart disease and cancer risk. Studies suggest that cineole and perillyl alcohol (terpene compounds) possibly suppress tumor growth. A flavonoid, luteolin, shows promise in preventing cancerous changes in cells.

add more to your diet

Use in: pork and poultry dishes; homemade pizza, pasta, and bread doughs; grilled vegetables, sauces, and marinades.

tarragon

The bold, satisfying flavor of this fine French herb traditionally accompanies fish and is used to flavor vinegar and béarnaise sauce.

what's in it

Tarragon contains cancer-protective terpene phytochemicals that may interfere with tumor growth and help to stimulate cancer-protective enzymes in the body.

add more to your diet

Use in: beans and grain dishes; homemade vinegars, mustards, and relishes; poached and stewed fruit; sandwich and cheese spreads. It matches well with fish, poultry, carrots, artichoke, eggplant, and peas.

thyme

Fresh or dried thyme leaves are popular in French, Cajun, and Creole cuisines.

what's in it

Terpene compounds—cineole, limonene, and pinene—may suppress tumor growth and increase the body's production of protective anticancer enzymes. The flavonoid luteolin, common to peppermint, sage, and thyme, has shown promise in blocking cancerous changes in cells.

add more to your diet

Use in: soups, stews, and chowders. Matches well with shellfish, chicken, and turkey.

kiwifruit

This fuzzy, egg-shaped fruit, in addition to providing spectacular amounts of vitamin C, is richly endowed with phytochemicals that help to boost your immune system and may stave off certain eye conditions, cancer, and heart disease.

what's in it

actinidin This enzyme is believed to aid digestion by helping to activate natural digestive reactions.

chlorogenic acid This compound is an antioxidant with the potential to prevent development of cancerous tumors.

chlorophyll Though not much is known about chlorophyll's health benefits, it is currently under review for its potential to prevent certain chemicals from causing DNA damage to cells.

fiber Pectin is a type of soluble fiber that protects against heart disease and diabetes, while insoluble fiber keeps the digestive tract running smoothly and prevents constipation. (One kiwifruit has 2.6g of dietary fiber—10% of the recommended daily intake—and nearly half of that is soluble fiber.)

lutein This important carotenoid may possibly reduce the risk for colon cancer, cataracts, and macular degeneration.

potassium Kiwifruit is an excellent source of potassium, a mineral that helps the heart work more efficiently, and plays a key role in controlling blood pressure. (One kiwi has 252mg of potassium, which is 8% of the Daily Value.)

vitamin C Kiwifruit is an exceptional source of this important vitamin, which functions as a powerful antioxidant. Vitamin C is believed to protect against nasal congestion and heart disease. It also helps to build and repair the immune system and may protect against certain types of cancer. The antioxidant power of vitamin C is also thought to help prevent cataracts. (One kiwifruit has about 75mg of vitamin C.)

maximizing the benefits

To preserve the **vitamin C** content in kiwifruit, it is best to eat the fruit uncooked. If you combine kiwifruit with meat, poultry, or fish, as in a salad, you should not let the mixture sit too long before serving; kiwi's enzyme, actinidin, will begin to "tenderize" the animal protein and turn it mushy.

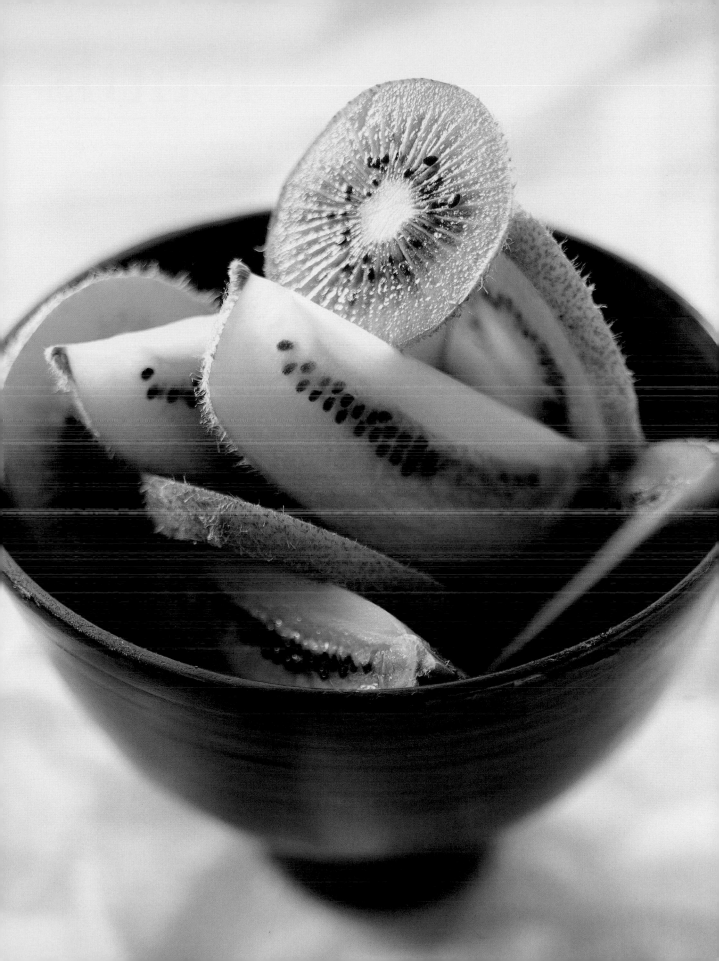

lentils

These low-fat, protein-rich legumes offer substantial phyto-chemical power, folate, and an impressive amount of fiber, more than a quarter of which is the heart-healthy soluble type. They also have decent amounts of iron and calcium.

what's in it

fiber Lentils are rich in insoluble fiber, which may stave off hunger and alleviate constipation. The soluble pectin and gum fiber in lentils helps to lower cholesterol and stabilize blood sugar. (A half cup of cooked lentils has a total of 7.8g dietary fiber, with 1.3g of it soluble.)

folate A half cup of cooked lentils provides almost half of the daily requirement for this B vitamin, which may be instrumental in pre-venting birth defects, cancer, and heart disease.

iron Most lentils are good sources of this mineral, which is vital for immunity, healthy pregnancy, and anemia prevention.

isoflavones These phytoestrogens may lower the risk for heart disease and manage some of the symptoms of perimenopause and menopause.

plant sterols Similar in structure to cholesterol, these com-pounds help reduce blood cholesterol levels by competing with dietary and body-synthesized cholesterol for absorption.

protease inhibitors Found in lentils (and other legumes), these plant chemicals may inhibit tumor growth by short-circuiting processes necessary for cancer cell survival.

saponins Plentiful in lentils, saponins may prevent cardiovascular disease by binding cholesterol in the digestive tract. Laboratory studies suggest that these phytonutrients may also inhibit cancer by increasing the number of nat-ural killer immune cells, and by blocking cancerous changes in cells.

tyrosine kinase inhibitors These compounds may work with fiber to stabilize blood-sugar levels. Preliminary studies suggest that tyrosine kinase inhibitors may lower levels of a chemical in the blood that contributes to pre-mature cardiovascular disease in diabetics.

maximizing the benefits

Eat foods high in **vitamin C** along with lentils to enhance **iron** absorption. To protect the **B vitamin** content, do not cook lentils in too much water, and if there is any cooking liquid that needs to be drained off, try to use it in the recipe or save for soups or other dishes. **Soluble fiber** in lentils is made available as the lentils cook and the fiber dissolves (this also softens the lentils).

add more to your diet

▶ Cook lentils, puree along with garlic, yogurt, and fresh lemon juice, and use as a dip or spread.

▶ Stir cooked lentils into pancake batter along with a touch of curry powder for a vegetarian, Indian-style main course.

▶ Mash cooked seasoned lentils; add an egg white and enough bread crumbs so the mixture can be formed into patties. Sauté as you would a burger.

▶ Toss cooked lentils in a lemony dressing along with cherry tomatoes and diced red pepper.

▶ Make a lentil soup using carrot juice instead of water for the base.

▶ Add cooked lentils to pasta sauce.

▶ Stir cooked lentils into hamburger or meatloaf mixtures.

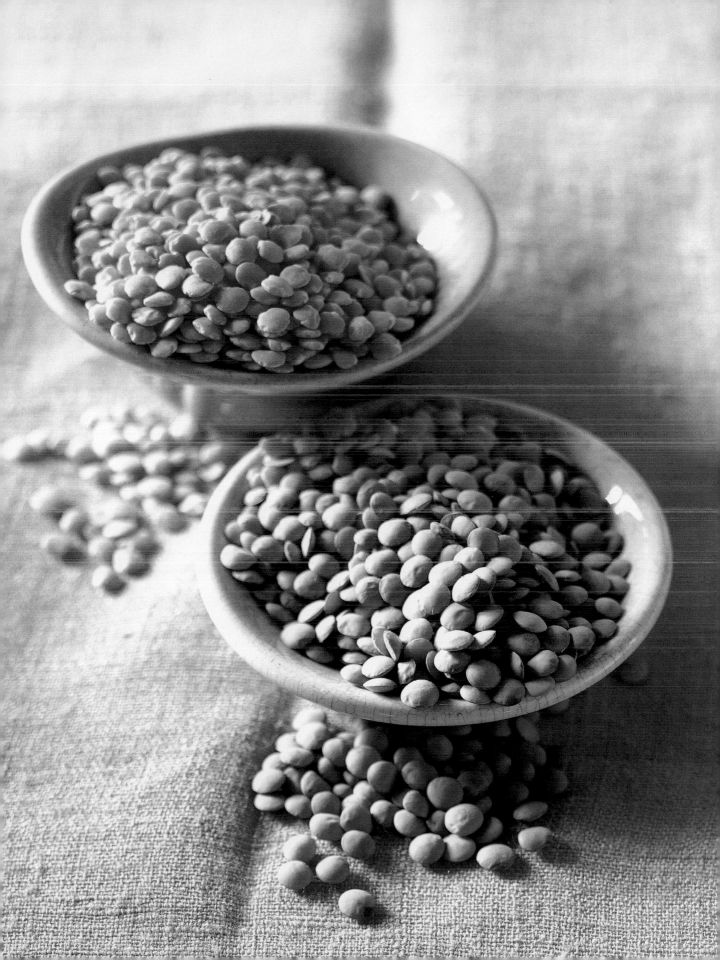

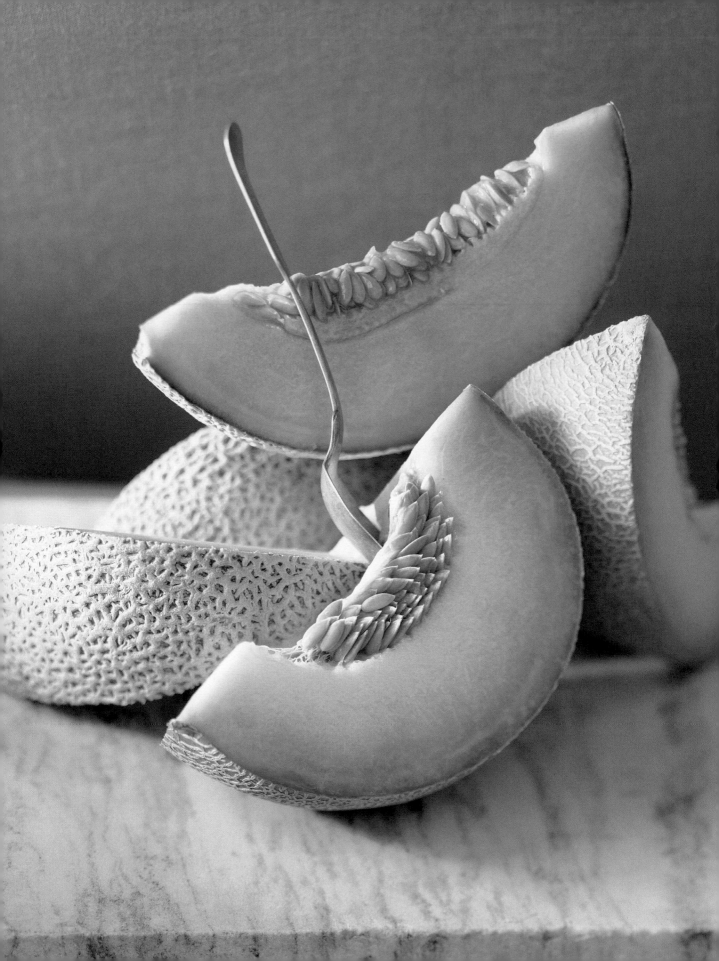

melons

The subtle scent of these fragrant fruits belies the muscularity of their nutritional powers. Melons—from cantaloupe to watermelon—may help prevent acne, cardiovascular disease, certain cancers, respiratory illness, and vision loss.

what's in it

beta-carotene Because of its orange hue, cantaloupe is the best melon source of this healthful orange-yellow pigment, which may protect against acne, certain forms of cancer, and vision loss. (One cup has 3mg of beta-carotene, 38% of the day's supply.)

lycopene Studies link a lycopene-rich diet with a low risk for heart disease and cancer, particularly prostate cancer. One cup of watermelon is a particularly good source of this antioxidant pigment, which lends reddish color to watermelon flesh.

pectin The soluble pectin fiber in melons (about 0.4g per cup) helps to lower cholesterol.

potassium Cantaloupe and honeydew are especially good melon sources of this vital mineral, which is linked to lower blood pressure and a reduced incidence of heart disease and stroke. (One cup of these melons has about 360mg, or 12% of the Daily Value.)

vitamin C Melon is a good source of this antioxidant vitamin, which may enhance the immune system and may be beneficial for respiratory infections. Cantaloupe and honeydew are particularly high, with an average of 50mg per cup.

zeaxanthin A vital component in the retina of the eye, this carotenoid helps to shield against damaging ultraviolet radiation, protecting against vision loss. Honeydew is the best melon source of zeaxanthin.

maximizing the benefits

To best preserve nutrient content, buy melons whole (some markets offer halves, quarters, or cubes). Certain nutrients, especially **vitamin C,** are diminished by exposure to the air.

add more to your diet

▶ Serve watermelon wedges with slices of feta cheese.

▶ Puree honeydew with fresh lime juice, honey, and mint, and chill. Serve as a dessert soup.

▶ Make a salad with cut-up plum tomatoes, cantaloupe, and cubes of mozzarella cheese, and toss with a balsamic vinaigrette.

▶ Freeze chunks of assorted melon, then puree to make a sorbet.

▶ Make a fresh melon salsa with cantaloupe or honeydew, chopped fresh basil, lemon or lime juice, and pickled jalapeños. Serve with fish or chicken.

▶ Add small chunks of cantaloupe to tomato sauces.

▶ Garnish hot tomato soup with a chilled, diced cantaloupe or honeydew.

health bites

An excellent choice for weight loss, these nutrient-dense (and water-dense) fruits average 50 calories and 0.5 grams of fat per cup of cubes and provide ample fiber and just enough sweetness to satisfy the appetite.

mushrooms

The mushroom's ancient tradition as a healing food continues as modern science uncovers its disease-fighting compounds, which may help manage cancer, heart disease, high blood pressure, high cholesterol, and viral infections.

add more to your diet

▶ Mushrooms and potatoes taste especially good together, so add cooked mushrooms to potato salads or roast them along with roast potatoes.

▶ Use mushrooms, especially shiitakes, to add a meaty texture to vegetarian stews and chilis.

▶ Make a relish: Sauté a mixture of finely chopped mushrooms, scallions, and garlic in olive oil; add vinegar and use as a topping for burgers, steaks, and sandwiches.

▶ Add finely chopped mushrooms to a meatloaf or burgers (especially turkey loaf or burgers, where the mushrooms will help keep the mixture juicy).

▶ Grind dried mushrooms to a powder and use along with bread crumbs to coat chicken or fish before sautéing.

▶ Top portobello mushroom caps with shredded cheese and chopped tomato and serve as appetizer "pizzas."

what's in it

B vitamins Though they lack vitamin B_{12}, mushrooms are high in riboflavin, niacin, and vitamin B_6, which may help to manage depression, heart disease, and migraines. (One cup of fresh shiitakes has over 10% of the Daily Value for each of these B vitamins.)

ergosterol This vitamin D precursor may promote bone health.

eritadenine Found in shiitakes, this compound may lower cholesterol by promoting cholesterol excretion.

lentinan Present in small amounts in shiitakes, this polysaccharide compound is under review for immune-enhancing properties.

lentinula edodes mycelium (LEM) These compounds in shiitake mushrooms may prevent cancer, heart disease, high cholesterol, high blood pressure, infection, and liver disease.

selenium This antioxidant mineral is thought to protect against cancer and macular degeneration.

thioproline Preliminary research suggests that this anticancer compound in shiitake mushrooms may block the formation of cancer-causing nitrogen compounds in the body.

maximizing the benefits

Since the **B vitamins** in mushrooms leach into water when heated, if you soak dried mushrooms to reconstitute them, it's best to use the soaking water in the recipe. Since some people may react to the allergens in raw mushrooms, it's best to eat them only in small amounts.

health bites

In a small study, Japanese men who ate about 4 ounces of fresh shiitakes (or 2 ounces of dried) experienced a substantial reduction in cholesterol within 1 week. A similar study among healthy women demonstrated a significant drop in cholesterol after a week of eating about 3 ounces of fresh shiitakes daily.

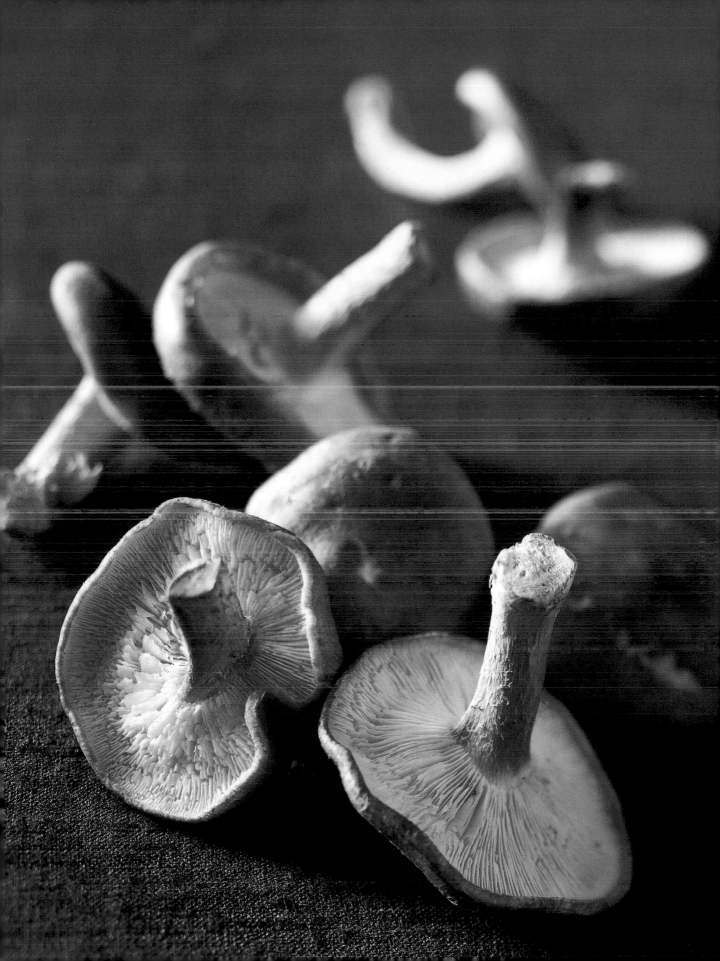

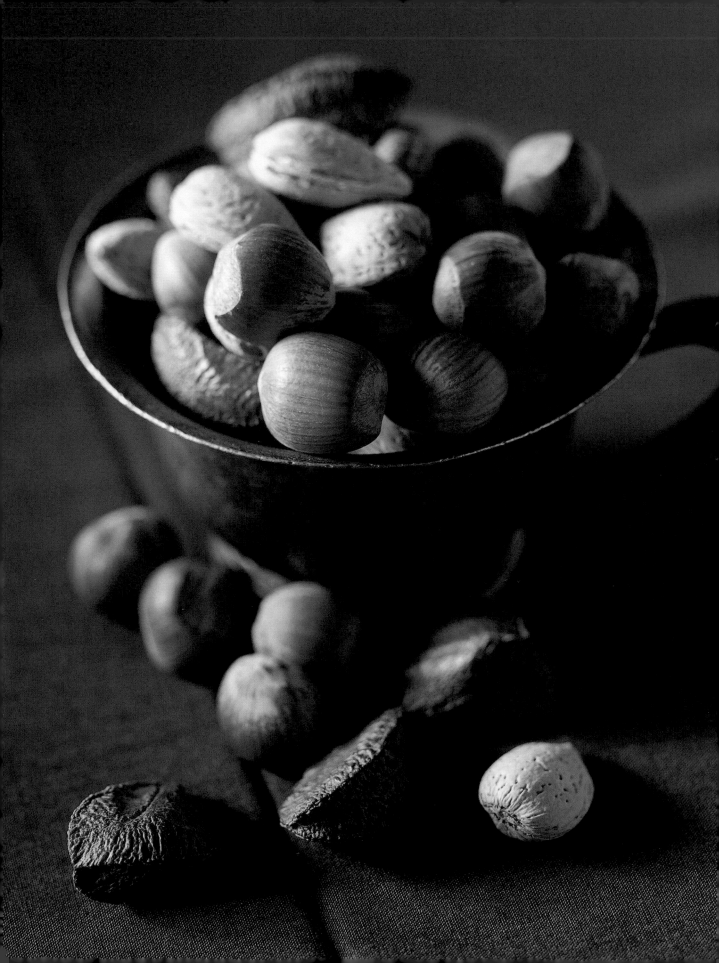

nuts

Energy-packed and protein-rich, nuts may also lower the risk for cancer and cardiovascular disease. In addition to the nutrients listed below, nuts are an excellent source of the cardio-protective amino acid, arginine, and also offer B vitamins.

what's in it

alpha-linolenic acid (ALA) Found in walnuts, this omega-3 fat may alleviate arthritis and lower risk for heart attack and stroke.

ellagic acid Walnuts are an especially good source of this anti-oxidant compound, which may inhibit the growth of cancer cells.

plant sterols Especially rich in pistachios, plant sterols help defend against certain forms of cancer and cardiovascular disease.

potassium High in pistachios (1 ounce provides 10% of the Daily Value), potassium may lower blood pressure and stroke risk.

resveratrol Found in peanuts, this phytochemical may prevent cancer, high cholesterol, and stroke.

saponins These cancer-fighting phytochemicals may boost immunity and promote healthy levels of blood sugar and cholesterol.

selenium Brazil nuts are extraordinarily rich sources of this powerful antioxidant, which helps to prevent cancer, certain eye disorders, and heart disease. (A half ounce of Brazil nuts has 420mcg, or about 600% of the Daily Value.)

vitamin E Nuts are one of the best food sources of this antioxidant vitamin, which may help prevent cardiovascular disease and cataracts. (Almonds and hazelnuts contain the most, with 34% of the Daily Value per ounce.)

maximizing the benefits

Refrigerate or freeze nuts to prevent their oils from going rancid. To enhance the flavor of nuts, toast them in the oven for 5 to 10 minutes, or until fragrant.

add more to your diet

➤ Sauté finely chopped nuts in olive oil along with bread crumbs and toss with freshly cooked pasta.

➤ Make your own nut butters: Place nuts in a food processor and process until pureed; add salt if you like.

➤ Toast and finely chop nuts, sweeten with maple syrup, and use as a topping for ice cream or frozen yogurt.

➤ Stir peanut butter into stews or curries to help enrich and add flavor.

➤ Use finely chopped nuts as a coating for pan-fried fish fillets or poultry cutlets.

health bites

Often maligned for their fat and calorie content, nuts have been redeemed by research, which touts their phytochemicals and heart-healthy monounsaturated fat. Studies show that when nuts are eaten in place of unhealthy saturated and trans fats, cholesterol levels improve and the risk for clogged arteries is slashed.

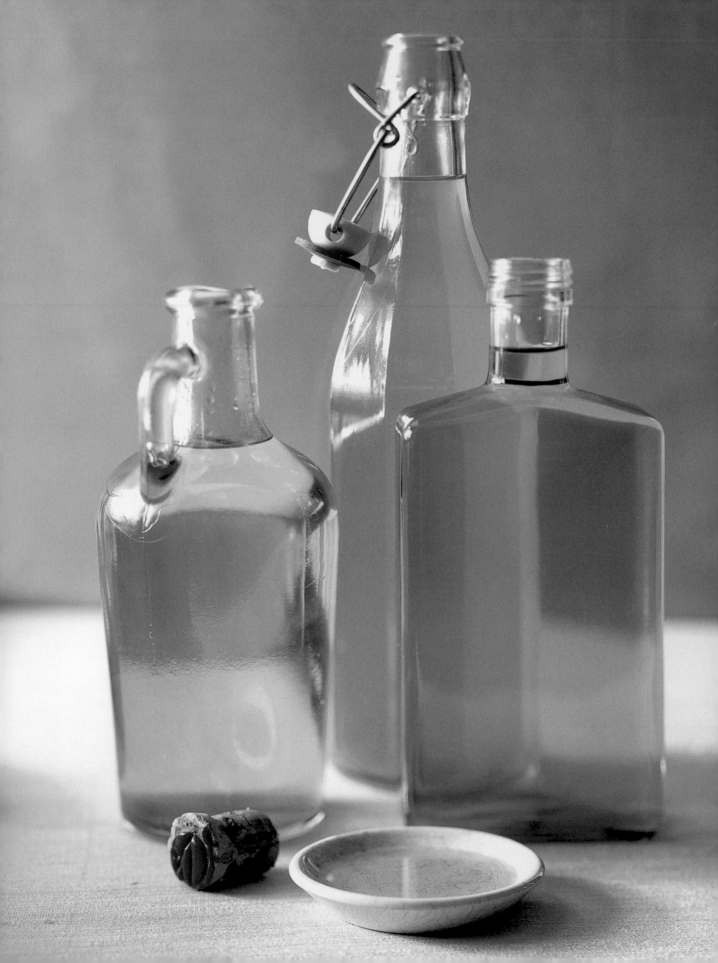

olive oil

Olive oil is rich in unique disease-fighting phytochemicals, vitamin E, and monounsaturated fat, which all help to clear cholesterol from arteries. Research also suggests that olive oil may manage diabetes, rheumatoid arthritis, stroke, and breast and colon cancer.

what's in it

hydroxytyrosol and oleuropein These antioxidant phytochemicals may work together, according to laboratory studies, to help protect against breast cancer, high blood pressure, infection-causing bacteria, and heart disease.

lignans Present in extra-virgin olive oil, these potent antioxidants may protect against breast, colon, and prostate cancer by suppressing early cancer changes in cells.

monounsaturated fat When substituted for saturated fat, this cardioprotective fat helps to lower total and LDL ("bad") cholesterol and may increase HDL ("good") cholesterol levels. Research suggests that a diet deriving most of its fat calories from monounsaturates may reduce the risk for chronic disease, including arthritis, certain cancers, and cardiovascular disease. At 73% monounsaturated fat, olive oil has the highest percentage among common cooking oils: By contrast, coconut oil has 6% and corn or soy oil 24%.

vitamin E Olive oil is one of the best dietary sources of this food-scarce vitamin, which shields against damaging free radicals. (One tablespoon of olive oil provides 8% of the Daily Value for vitamin E.)

maximizing the benefits

To preserve flavor as well as disease-fighting compounds, store olive oil in an airtight container in the refrigerator or other cool, dark place, and use as soon as possible. Refrigerated olive oil will solidify, so you will have to let it reach room temperature before it's pourable.

add more to your diet

▶ Steep chili peppers, or herbs, or orange, lemon, or lime zest (or any combination of these seasonings) in olive oil for two weeks, then strain. Use the flavored oil in pastas, salads, or drizzled on pizza.

▶ Substitute a light, mild-flavored olive oil for other oils or melted butter in baked goods and baked desserts.

▶ Serve a fruity olive oil instead of butter at the table for drizzling on bread.

▶ Don't forget whole olives, which also add healing oils and delicate flavors to food. Chop and add to pasta sauces, salad dressings, stews; or fold into bread or pizza dough.

▶ Use olive oil for sautéing pancakes or cooking waffles.

health bites

Since the heat and chemicals used in processing olive oil can diminish nutrient content, it's best to choose those oils that are minimally processed, such as extra-virgin or cold-pressed.

onion family

All members of the onion family—onions, chives, leeks, scallions, and shallots—are noted for their powerful phytochemicals and healthful fiber, which may protect against cancer, cardiovascular disease, and constipation.

add more to your diet

➤ Cook sliced red onions in olive oil over low heat with a sprinkling of sugar until the onions are very tender, sweet, and golden brown. Use as an accompaniment to meat, fish, or poultry, or as a sandwich relish.

➤ Stuff large, cored red onions with a seasoned rice mixture and bake as you would stuffed peppers.

➤ Make an onion pizza: Omit the tomato sauce and top a pizza shell with grated cheese and cooked onions and scallions.

➤ Add cooked onions, scallions, or cooked diced leeks, along with chopped dill, to homemade bread doughs.

➤ Stir sautéed leeks and scallions into mashed potatoes.

➤ Make a salad dressing: Cook chopped onions until meltingly tender, then steep in vinegar. Whisk olive oil into the onion mixture to make a vinaigrette.

➤ Core apples, stuff with cooked red onions, and bake until tender. Serve as a side dish with meat or poultry.

what's in it

diallyl sulfide Most abundant in onions but also found in other members of the onion family, this cancer-protective phytochemical appears to increase levels of cancer-fighting enzymes, particularly in the stomach. In Vidalia, Georgia, where large amounts of onions are consumed, the death rate from stomach cancer is significantly reduced, and diallyl sulfide intake is thought to be a factor.

fiber The onion family is a source of both insoluble and soluble fiber, which may confer protection against constipation, hemorrhoids, high cholesterol, and possibly weight gain.

fructooligosaccharides (FOS) Shallots are a significant source of FOS, the indigestible carbohydrates that encourage growth of beneficial bacteria in the colon.

kaempferol This anticancer substance, found in leeks, may help to block the development of cancer-causing compounds.

lutein and zeaxanthin Present in the green tops of leeks and scallions, these pigments work together to help prevent cell damage that may lead to vision loss and cancer.

quercetin Found in red onions, this antioxidant has shown promise (in laboratory studies) in inhibiting growth of breast, blood, and skin-cancer cells and in helping prevent cardiovascular disease.

maximizing the benefits

High-heat cooking significantly reduces the benefits of **diallyl sulfide.** Fresh, raw onion has the most health benefits, and mincing (even chewing) the onion helps to release the phytochemical power.

health bites

Population-based studies have found a significantly reduced risk for lung cancer among people who eat quercetin-rich foods, such as red onions. Studies also show that quercetin is better and more efficiently absorbed from onions than from other foods.

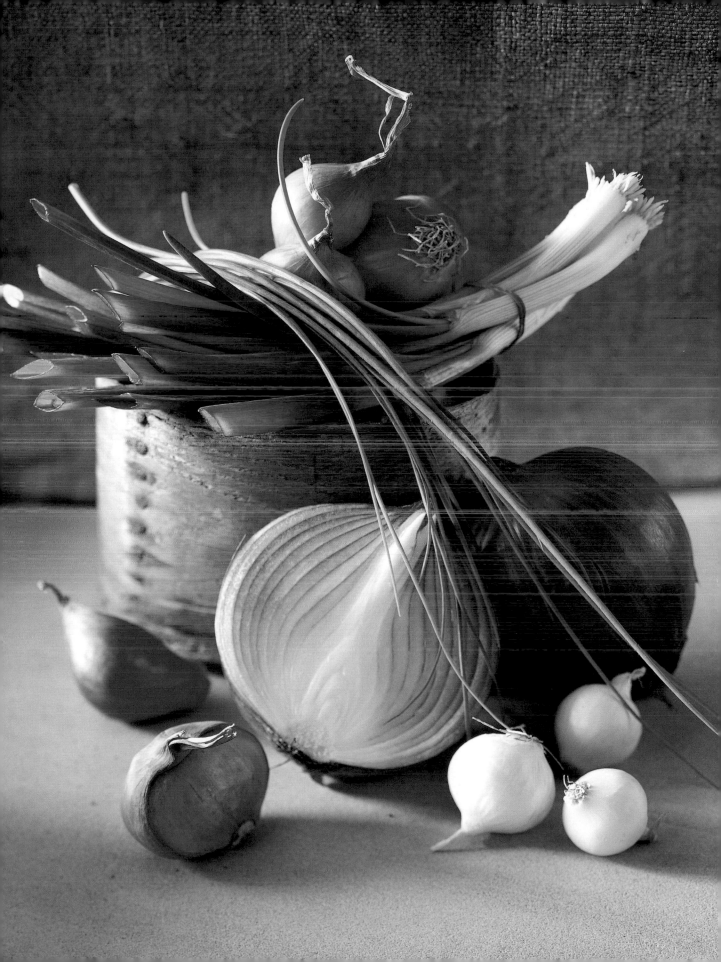

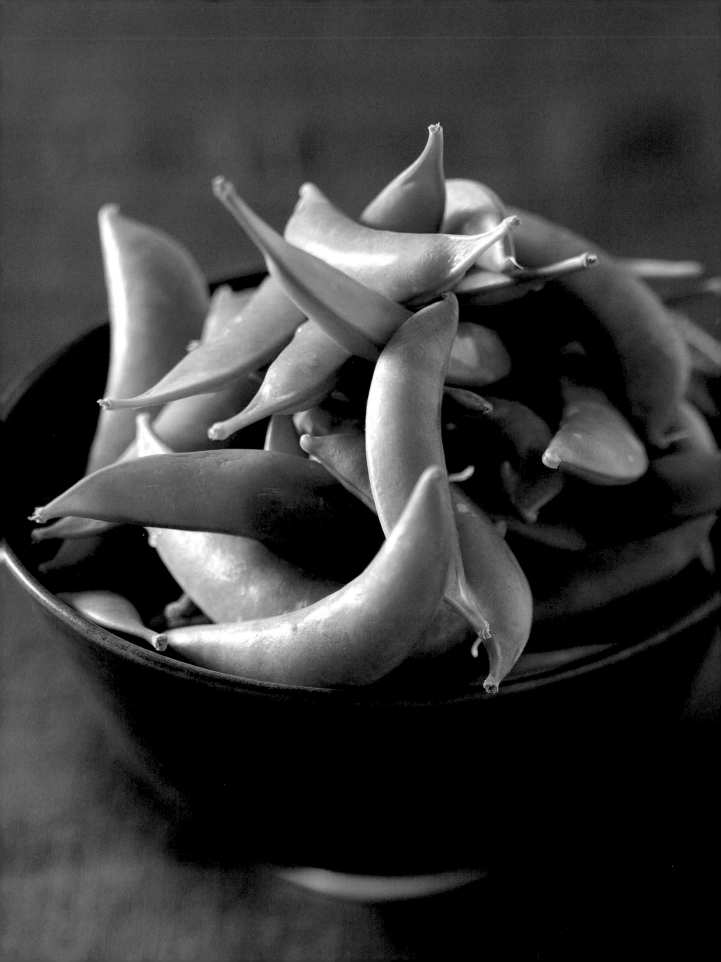

peas

Fresh, sweet garden peas are a good source of plant-based protein and nonheme (plant-derived) iron, making them an excellent food for vegetarians. Peas may help reduce the risk for developing certain cancers, depression, high cholesterol, and macular degeneration.

what's in it

chlorophyll Though the health benefits of chlorophyll are not fully understood, some studies suggest that it may deter certain chemicals from causing DNA damage to cells.

folate Important for all stages of life, this B vitamin is linked to reduced incidence of certain birth defects, cancer, heart disease, and possibly depression.

lutein This carotenoid may prevent colon cancer and eye diseases such as macular degeneration and possibly cataracts.

lysine A building block for the manufacture of protein, this essential amino acid is vital for collagen synthesis and tissue repair. It may also help to manage cold sores.

protease inhibitors These compounds may help to diminish the rate of division in cancer cells.

saponins Believed to lower LDL ("bad") cholesterol levels, saponins can bind cholesterol in your digestive tract and usher them out of your body.

tryptophan Found in small amounts in peas, this amino acid helps to maintain proper levels of serotonin, which regulates mood.

vitamin B$_6$ Preliminary studies show that this B vitamin may boost serotonin levels, which may prevent depression.

vitamin C As an antioxidant, vitamin C may protect against cataracts by fighting the harmful effects of free radicals.

maximizing the benefits

Heat-sensitive **vitamin C** and water-soluble B vitamins (**folate** and **B$_6$**) are best preserved if you either quickly steam or microwave peas.

add more to your diet

► Steam peas, stir into cottage cheese, and use as a filling for stuffed twice-baked potatoes.

► For a twist on the classic guacamole, add mashed cooked peas to avocado along with the usual seasonings.

► Cook peas in a small amount of water with thyme and scallions. Puree the peas with their cooking liquid, add milk, and serve as a soup.

► Buy edible-pod peas (such as sugar snaps) and eat as a snack.

► Stir cooked peas, chopped cilantro, and diced jalapeño jack cheese into pancake batter for a Mexican-style vegetarian main-dish pancake

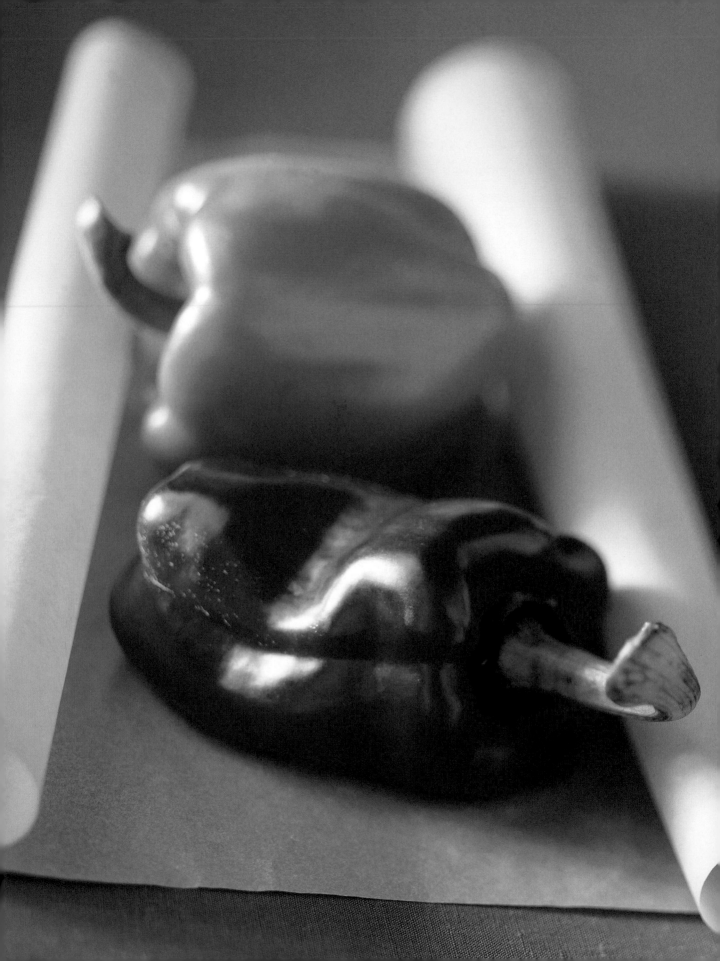

peppers

Sweet bell peppers and spicy chili peppers add color and zest to your favorite dish, while offering protection against heart disease, vision loss, and nasal congestion.

what's in it

beta-carotene This antioxidant pigment may help prevent eye diseases, certain cancers, and heart disease. Red peppers are particularly rich in beta-carotene, providing nearly 5mg per cup.

capsaicin This pungent phytochemical, which supplies the "heat" in chili peppers, may ease congestion by increasing secretions in the nose and airways. Studies suggest that capsaicin may also detoxify cancer-causing compounds and encourage cancer-cell death. The hotter the chili pepper, the greater the capsaicin content.

chlorophyll Preliminary research suggests that this plant compound may stop healthy cells from mutating into cancerous cells and may protect against environmental carcinogens.

lutein and zeaxanthin A diet rich in lutein and its antioxidant partner, zeaxanthin, may protect against certain forms of cancer, heart disease, macular degeneration, and possibly cataracts. One cup of diced fresh red peppers offers tremendous quantities of lutein, while orange peppers are a top source of zeaxanthin.

vitamin C Peppers are a major source of this essential vitamin, which may enhance our defense against respiratory ailments. The combined antioxidant power of beta-carotene and vitamin C in peppers may help to prevent cataracts and macular degeneration. One cup of fresh bell peppers supplies even more vitamin C (133mg) than 1 cup of fresh orange juice (82mg).

maximizing the benefits

For **vitamin C,** eat uncooked peppers, since this vitamin is easily destroyed by heat. To maximize the bioavailability of **beta-carotene,** cook peppers until they are crisp-tender, and eat with a little monounsaturated fat, such as olive oil.

add more to your diet

▶ Fill bell pepper wedges with bean puree and serve as an appetizer.

▶ Add roasted, peeled red bell peppers and spicy chipotle peppers to mashed potatoes for a side dish. Or thin the potato-pepper mixture with milk to make a soup.

▶ Add diced chili peppers to muffins or cornbreads.

▶ Puree homemade or bottled roasted red peppers with a little tomato paste, garlic, salt, and pepper, and serve as a vegetable dip. Or thin the mixture with a little olive oil and use as a pasta sauce.

▶ Make a hot and sweet pepper salsa: Mince red, green, and orange bell peppers along with chili peppers (jalapeño, chipotle); add minced red onion, vinegar, and cilantro. Serve the salsa with meat or poultry, or toss it with freshly cooked pasta.

health bites

A population-based study in California found that women who consumed large quantities of vegetables, including bell peppers, had the lowest incidence of a type of brain tumor called a glioma.

pineapple

Long used as a folk remedy to settle intestinal upsets and relieve constipation, this tropical fruit is also noted for its anti-inflammatory enzyme and healing nutrients, which help bolster immunity and bone and cardiovascular health.

add more to your diet

▶ Make a pineapple salsa: Chop pineapple, bell peppers, and red onion. Toss with ginger, honey, and lime juice. Serve with meat, poultry, or fish.

▶ Use pineapple juice instead of vinegar in a salad dressing.

▶ Cook crushed pineapple in unsweetened pineapple juice until thick and use as a no-sugar-added all-fruit spread.

▶ Add thin slices of pineapple and spicy mustard to roast chicken or turkey sandwiches.

▶ Make a barbecue sauce substituting chopped pineapple and pineapple juice for half of the tomato in the recipe.

▶ Make a pineapple drink: Puree pineapple with buttermilk or yogurt and a touch of honey.

what's in it

bromelain This anti-inflammatory enzyme is plentiful in pineapple and may help to control tissue swelling and inflammation associated with bronchitis, cough, osteoarthritis, rheumatoid arthritis, varicose veins, strains, and sprains. Preliminary research suggests that bromelain's anti-inflammatory property may reduce blood clots, which may lower the risk for stroke and heart attack.

ferulic acid Pineapple is a good source of this phytochemical, which helps prevent the formation of cancer-causing substances.

manganese One cup of pineapple provides 2.6mg of manganese, which is 128% of the daily requirement for this bone-building mineral.

plant sterols These plant compounds may help to lower cholesterol and reduce the risk for heart disease.

soluble fiber Pineapple is high in pectin fiber and gum fiber, which have cholesterol-lowering properties and also promote healthy bowel function. (One cup of fresh pineapple has 0.2g of soluble fiber.)

vitamin C Fresh pineapple is a good source (24mg per cup) of vitamin C, which may enhance immunity and wound healing, while also preventing heart disease and serious eye disorders.

maximizing the benefits

To preserve the **vitamin C** content, eat pineapple uncooked. The **soluble pectin fiber** in pineapple becomes available when the pineapple is cooked.

health bites

Preliminary research suggests that bromelain may reduce traveler's diarrhea by inhibiting *E. coli*, one of the bacteria responsible for the illness. Scientists believe bromelain may displace *E. coli* from receptors in the intestinal wall.

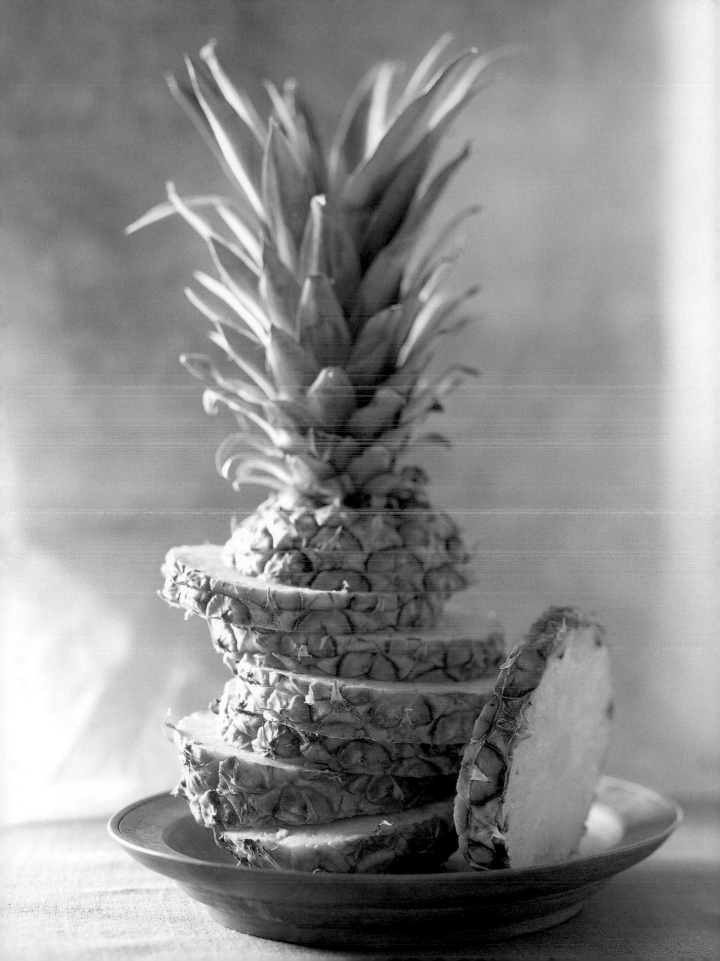

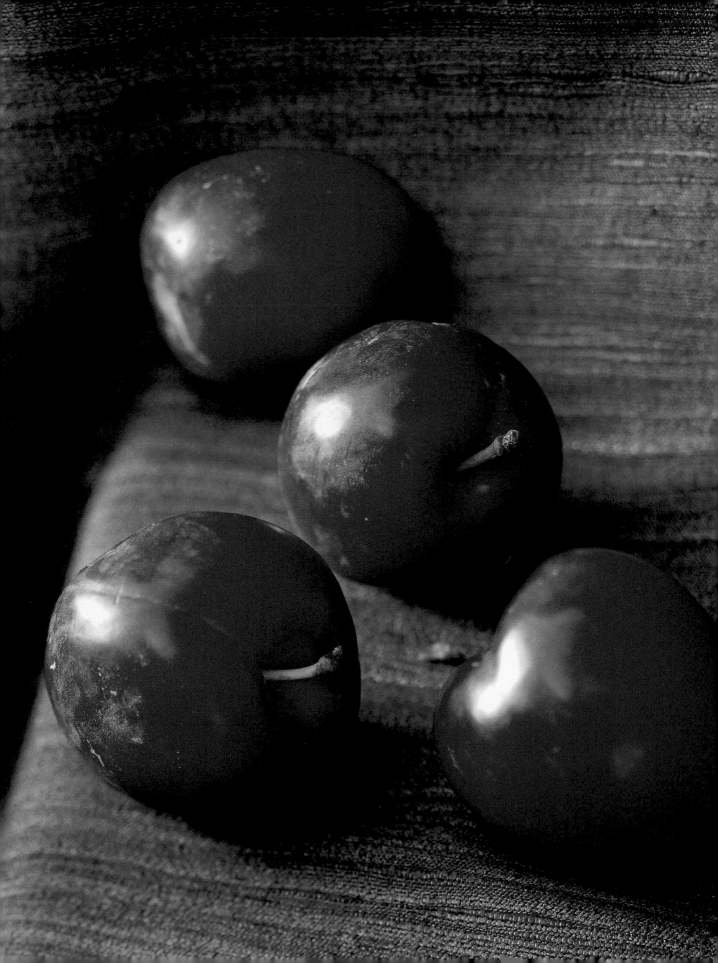

plums & prunes

Juicy, vividly colored plums and prunes (dried plums) are packed with disease-fighting antioxidants and natural sugars. Prunes and prune juice are a delicious, natural choice for relieving constipation (and boosting heart health).

what's in it

anthocyanins Reddish blue pigments that lend intense color to plums, anthocyanins may protect against cancer and heart disease by mopping up harmful free radicals.

chlorogenic acid A phenolic phytochemical, this potent antioxidant quenches damaging free radicals and is thought to help detoxify carcinogenic environmental agents, such as nitrosamines in cigarette smoke.

insoluble fiber The insoluble fiber in plums and prunes helps to bulk up the stool and ease elimination.

potassium A potassium-rich diet is associated with lower blood pressure and a reduced risk for kidney stones and stroke. (A quarter cup of prunes has 317mg of potassium, or 9% of the Daily Value.)

quercetin A potent free-radical fighter, quercetin may help to prevent estrogen dependent cancer, including breast cancer, and may help to block oxidation of harmful LDL ("bad") cholesterol, a process that could lead to heart disease.

soluble fiber Plums and prunes are rich in soluble fiber, which helps to relieve constipation and lower cholesterol levels.

sorbitol A naturally occurring sugar, sorbitol may help to relieve constipation by absorbing water and bulking up the stool. Note that sorbitol can irritate the colon, especially in those with irritable bowel syndrome.

maximizing the benefits

If you stew prunes, be sure to eat the liquid or include it in the recipe to retain the **sorbitol,** which leaches into cooking water.

add more to your diet

▶ Make a fruit soup: In a blender, mix prune juice, reduced-fat sour cream, and a little fresh lemon juice. Chill and serve with diced fresh plums and minced fresh mint.

▶ Buy prune butter and use it as a fruit spread, a filling for layer cakes, or for stirring into plain yogurt.

▶ Cook diced pitted prunes in vinegar and sugar along with onions and garlic and serve as a condiment alongside meat or poultry.

▶ Make a barbecue sauce: Cook diced pitted prunes in prune juice along with honey, vinegar, minced fresh ginger, and hot sauce.

▶ Add sliced fresh plums to savory soups and stews.

▶ Instead of cream cheese and jelly: Spread bread with Neufchâtel (reduced-fat) cream cheese and top with thin slices of ripe plums.

health bites

Prune juice is an antioxidant-rich constipation remedy. Drinking prune juice at bedtime may promote a morning bowel movement (or one in the evening if you drink prune juice at breakfast).

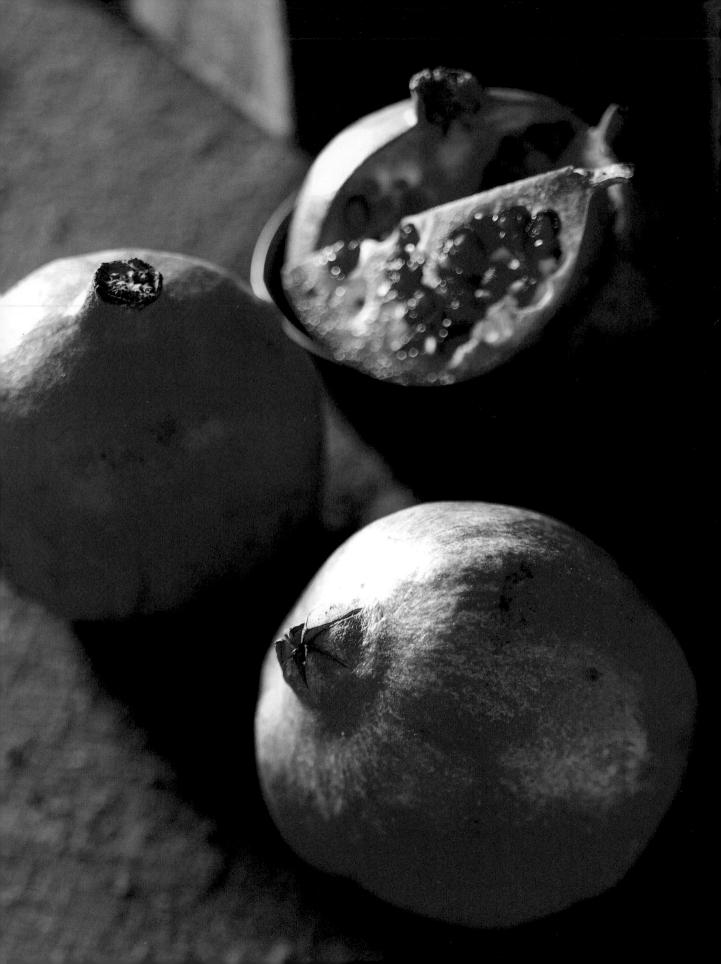

pomegranates

The word pomegranate is old French for "seeded apple," an apt name for this apple-sized fruit packed with jewel-like clusters of crimson seeds. The pomegranate is touted as an anti-aging fruit that may prevent hardening of the arteries.

what's in it

anthocyanins By protecting against free-radical cell damage, these pigments may help to prevent cancer and heart disease. Some evidence suggests that anthocyanins strengthen capillaries, which is beneficial for hemorrhoids and varicose veins. Research has shown that pomegranate juice has two to three times the antioxidant capacity of equal amounts of red wine or green tea, and anthocyanins make an important contribution to the pomegranate's antioxidant power.

catechins These phytochemicals may defend against cancer, heart disease, and infectious agents by protecting cells from dangerous free radicals.

ellagic acid Abundant in pomegranates, ellagic acid may work with other antioxidants to protect the body from environmental toxins.

fiber Both soluble and insoluble fiber present in pomegranates help to relieve constipation, satisfy hunger, and lower cholesterol.

manganese Pomegranates have lots of this mineral, which is essential for strong teeth and bones. (One pomegranate provides 0.9mg, or 44% of the Daily Value.)

potassium Linked to lower blood pressure, potassium-rich foods may also reduce the risk for heart disease, kidney stones, and stroke. (One pomegranate has 399mg of potassium, which is 11% of the Daily Value.)

maximizing the benefits

You can eat the pomegranate's seeds (its skin is inedible) as is, or crush them in a strainer to separate the juice from the kernels.

add more to your diet

▶ Keep a bottle of pomegranate molasses (found in gourmet stores and Middle Eastern groceries) on hand for a variety of uses. This condensed, syrupy form of pure pomegranate juice has a high concentration of antioxidants.

▶ Use pomegranate molasses in place of vinegar in a salad dressing.

▶ Brush red onion slices with pomegranate molasses and a touch of brown sugar and broil.

▶ Add pomegranate juice to orange juice for a refreshing drink.

▶ Stir pomegranate juice or pomegranate molasses into a barbecue sauce.

▶ Toss diced pomegranate seeds and citrus fruit in a dressing of pomegranate molasses and olive oil, and use as a salsa for grilled poultry or fish.

health bites

A recent study suggests that drinking as little as one-quarter cup of pomegranate juice daily may improve cardiovascular health by significantly reducing oxidation of LDL ("bad") cholesterol.

potatoes

This versatile American favorite, served in its high-fiber skin, is a nourishing, satisfying source of healing compounds. Spare yourself the added calories by enjoying potatoes in their low-fat, naturally filling, unprocessed form.

add more to your diet

▶ Add potatoes to soups and stews and, once cooked, mash some of the potatoes to help thicken the dish.

▶ Make a quick, cold potato soup: Cook sliced, unpeeled potatoes until tender. Mash with buttermilk (enough to make the potatoes the consistency of a thick but spoonable soup) and salt. Stir in chopped fresh dill and scallions.

▶ When making mashed potatoes, cook potatoes in their skin and use some of the potato cooking water when mashing. Save the remaining water to use in soups and stews.

▶ Make a salad dressing using mashed potatoes as a substitute for some of the oil, then stir in chopped garlic and lemon juice or vinegar.

▶ For a colorful potato salad, use purple, red, blue, yellow, and white potatoes, and leave the skins on.

▶ Add small cubes of cooked potato to meatloaf and hamburger mixtures.

what's in it

anthocyanins Found in purple, blue, and red potato skin, these antioxidant pigments may be cancer- and cardioprotective.

caffeic and ferulic acids Present in the potato skin, these phytochemicals may team up to help destroy harmful carcinogens.

chlorogenic acid This phytochemical may help prevent cancer by blocking the formation of cancer-causing nitrogen compounds.

complex carbohydrates These energy-producing nutrients may help manage depression, heartburn, and memory function.

potassium Potassium-rich foods such as potatoes are linked to enhanced cardiovascular health and a lower risk for kidney stones.

protease inhibitors These compounds show promise in suppressing cancer at both the primary and secondary stages.

saponins These may reduce heart disease and cancer risk.

vitamin B$_6$ This cardioprotective B vitamin may lessen symptoms of depression, insomnia, and premenstrual syndrome (PMS).

vitamin C Because such vast quantities of potatoes are eaten, they are a leading source of vitamin C in the American diet. This important antioxidant vitamin may protect against free radicals and enhance immune function.

maximizing the benefits

For the most nutrients, eat potatoes with their skin, and bake, microwave, or steam. If peeling, remove the thinnest layer possible. If boiling, leave the skin on and try to reuse the cooking water, where many of the **B vitamins** wind up.

health bites

A study of healthy elderly people with poor memory found that eating 1 cup of mashed potatoes significantly improved their short- and long-term memory. Scientists hypothesize that potatoes may enhance the production of memory-enhancing brain chemicals.

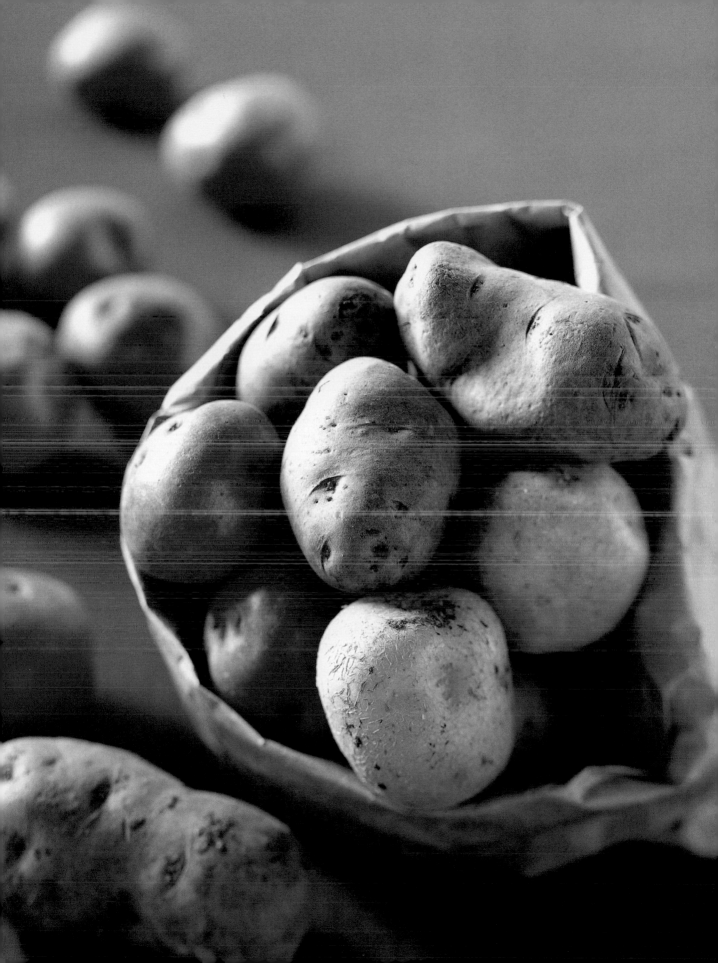

poultry

A lean source of high-quality protein, chicken, duck, and turkey are loaded with essential amino acids, B vitamins, and minerals, which help to ensure healthy skin, immunity, and proper brain and digestive function.

▶ Boneless duck breast is exceptionally lean when it's served without the skin. It has a rich, meaty flavor not unlike beef, but is far lower in fat and calories. Remove the skin, season, and cook the duck breast as you would a beef steak.

▶ Buy skinless, boneless turkey breast and grind it in a food processor—you'll get leaner meat than store-bought ground turkey, which often has turkey skin added to it.

▶ For moist turkey burgers, add cubes of whole-wheat bread or very finely chopped mushrooms to the mixture before shaping into patties.

▶ Turkey legs are great for homemade stock and soups: Remove the skin from the legs and cook with water, herbs, and spices. Once the turkey has cooked, remove the meat from the bones. Use the meat in the soup or in a salad.

what's in it

iron Duck and dark-meat turkey are excellent sources of this blood-nourishing mineral, present in its most absorbable ("heme") form.

lysine An essential amino acid, lysine may help to prevent and manage cold sores.

niacin Three ounces of cooked, skinless chicken breast supply nearly 12mg of niacin—over half the day's requirement. Duck and turkey are also excellent sources of this vitamin, which ensures healthy digestive and nervous systems.

selenium Plentiful in poultry, selenium may help to protect against cancer, cataracts, heart disease, and macular degeneration. Dark-meat turkey is particularly high in this mineral (3 ounces of cooked turkey have 35mcg of selenium, or 50% of the Daily Value).

tryptophan A precursor to niacin, this essential amino acid may help ease anxiety, depression, and insomnia.

vitamin B_6 Though all poultry has ample B_6, light-meat chicken and turkey are the best sources (3 ounces cooked provides 0.5mg, which is 25% of the Daily Value). This vitamin may ease allergies, asthma, and depression and help prevent heart disease.

vitamin B_{12} Available only in animal foods, this vitamin may be beneficial for anemia, cardiovascular health, depression, and healthy pregnancy.

zinc Essential for immune cell development, this mineral may also improve fertility and skin health, and help to alleviate premenstrual syndrome. Turkey, duck, and dark-meat chicken provide generous amounts of zinc (3 ounces of any of these provide over 2mg of zinc, which is about 15% of the Daily Value).

maximizing the benefits

Dark-meat poultry is the best choice for flavor, as well as certain nutrients such as **iron** and **selenium.** But the dark meat is also higher in fat: three to five times higher, depending on the bird. In addition to fat found in poultry meat, there is also a substantial amount in the skin (about half the total fat is in the skin). It's all right to roast, broil, or grill poultry with the skin on to preserve moisture, but the skin should be removed before eating. If the poultry is cooked in a soup, stew, stir-fry, or casserole, the skin should be removed before cooking.

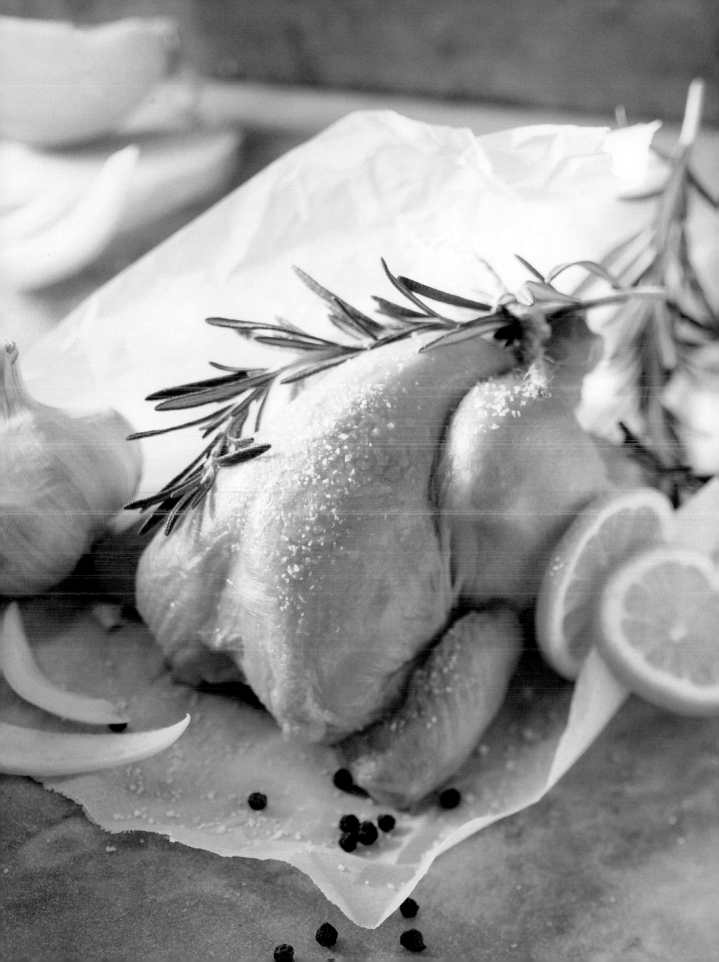

rice

A staple ingredient in cuisines worldwide, rice is an important source of complex carbohydrates, fiber, and essential nutrients. Free of gluten, rice is a natural choice for people with celiac disease or wheat gluten allergies.

add more to your diet

▶ Have rice for breakfast: Combine rice and chicken broth and cook very slowly until the rice breaks down and the mixture becomes a porridge.

▶ Add cooked rice to pancake batter, along with herbs, to make a savory rice pancake to serve alongside main dishes.

▶ Add cooked rice to a cornbread batter to add an interesting texture.

▶ Make a rice pie crust: Combine cooked rice, an egg white, and some grated cheese, and bake as you would a savory pie crust.

▶ Make puddings with rice milk (sold in health-food stores) instead of dairy milk.

what's in it

complex carbohydrates Energy-providing complex carbohydrates help to absorb fluids, contributing to white rice's reputation as a remedy for diarrhea and heartburn.

folate Enriched white rice is an excellent source of this B vitamin, which helps to lower the risk for birth defects and heart disease. (One cup of cooked rice has 92mcg, or 23% of the Daily Value.)

magnesium Brown rice provides high levels of this mineral, which may improve PMS and kidney stones. (One cup of cooked brown rice provides 84mg, or 21% of the Daily Value.)

oryzanol Research is exploring this compound's potential to relieve menopausal hot flashes, lower cholesterol levels, and prevent the harmful conversion of nitrogen compounds into cancer-causing nitrosamines. Oryzanol—a mixture of different forms of ferulic acid and terpene phytochemicals—is found in the bran layer of brown rice.

selenium This antioxidant mineral is associated with prevention of allergies, asthma, cataracts, infertility, and prostate problems. (One cup of cooked brown rice has 19mcg, or 27% of the Daily Value.)

vitamin B$_6$ This vitamin may help to thwart allergies, anxiety, asthma, depression, and heart disease. Brown rice provides substantial quantities: 0.3mg (14% of the Daily Value) per cup of cooked brown rice.

maximizing the benefits

When cooking rice, do not rinse it before (or after), because that washes away essential nutrients. Also avoid cooking with excess water to retain **B vitamins**. Serve rice with beans, peas, and other legumes for a complete protein.

health bites

Choose brown rice because it has more vitamins and minerals than plain milled white rice—stripped of many of its nutrients—and is also high in oryzanol and insoluble fiber. However, in the United States, white rice is "enriched" by adding back many of the nutrients.

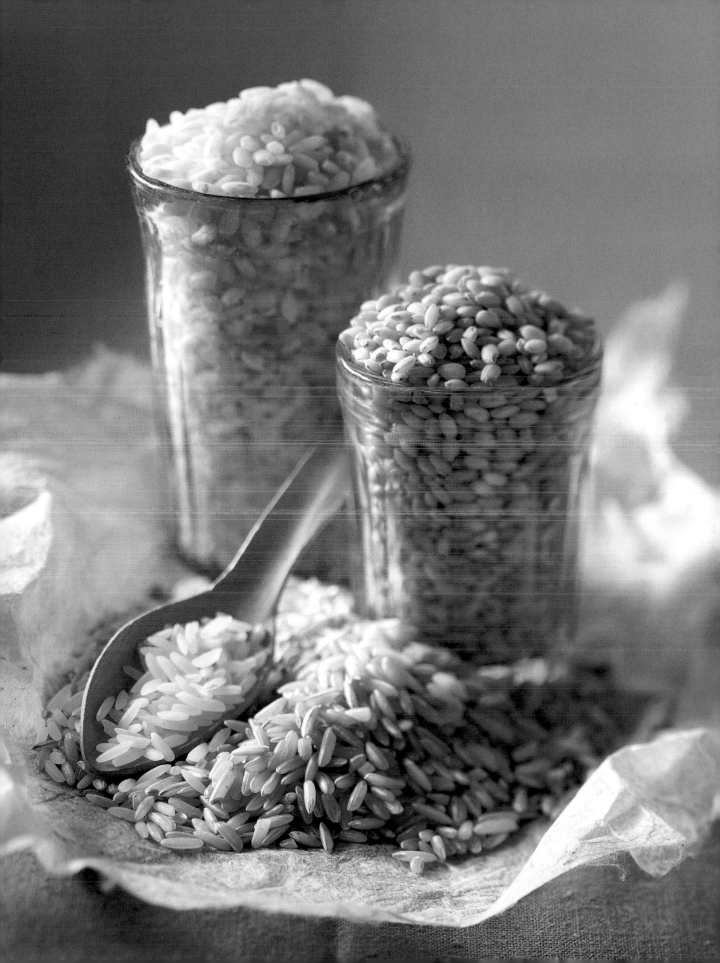

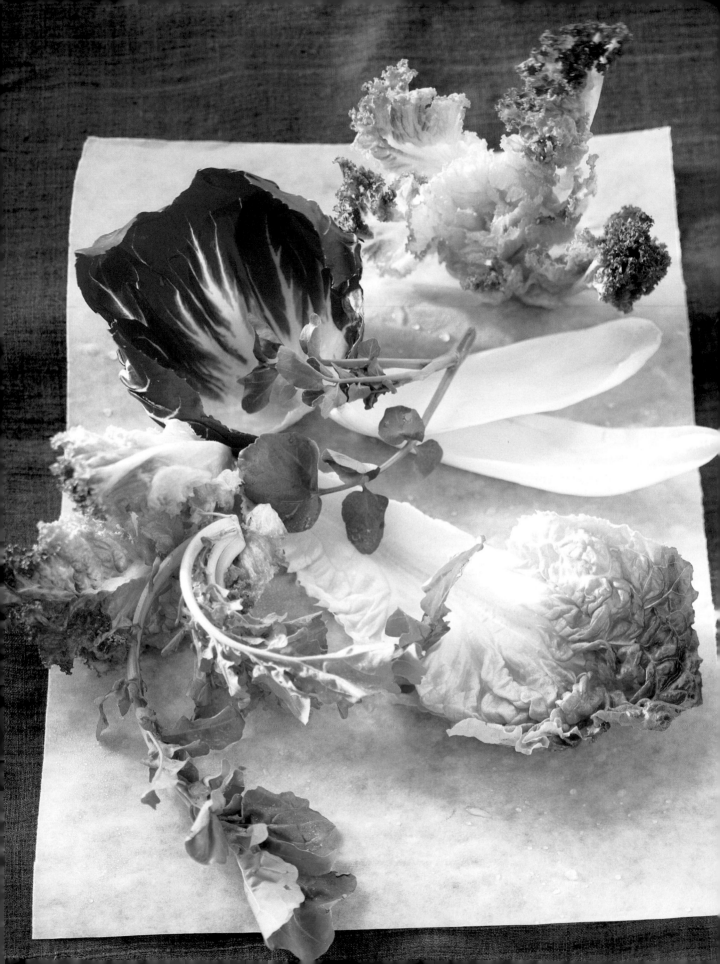

salad greens

Toss your salad with a variety of greens to elevate your fiber intake and antioxidant levels. Arugula, chicory, dandelion greens, escarole, radicchio, and watercress offer myriad nutrients and health benefits.

what's in it

beta-carotene Watercress, escarole, and especially chicory and dandelion greens, are excellent sources of this healing pigment, which may help to prevent acne, cancer, and vision loss.

insoluble fiber This type of fiber may satisfy your appetite and relieve constipation by improving intestinal function.

folate One cup of raw chicory provides almost half the daily requirement for folate, which helps to protect against cardiovascular disease and birth defects. Arugula also supplies ample folate.

fructooligosaccharides (FOS) and inulin These indigestible carbohydrates may promote the growth of beneficial bacteria in the digestive tract. FOS and inulin from chicory are currently under review for their potential to protect against cancer, constipation, diabetes, diarrhea, heart disease, obesity, and osteoporosis.

potassium Salad greens, particularly chicory, provide appreciable amounts of this cardioprotective mineral. (One cup of chopped chicory provides 756mg of potassium, or 22% of the Daily Value.)

vitamin C Chicory, dandelion greens, and watercress are very good sources of this antioxidant, which may benefit immunity and cardiovascular health.

vitamin E Chicory and dandelion greens contain appreciable amounts of vitamin E compounds, which may protect against cancer and vision loss.

maximizing the benefits

Oil enhances the absorption of **beta-carotene,** so salad dressings are beneficial partners to beta-carotene-rich greens.

add more to your diet

▶ Sauté watercress or arugula in olive oil with garlic and red pepper flakes and serve as a hot vegetable side dish.

▶ Toss chicory with crisp turkey bacon and whole-wheat croutons in a warm red wine vinaigrette.

▶ Make a sauce for pasta: Sauté dandelion greens in olive oil with golden raisins and pine nuts, and toss with pasta and grated Parmesan cheese.

▶ For a cool summer soup, combine tomato juice, watercress, vinegar, and a couple of ice cubes in a blender and puree until smooth.

▶ Serve hot foods, such as chicken, meat, or fish on a bed of cool, dressed salad greens.

▶ Add bitter salad greens such as arugula, watercress, or radicchio to sweet fruit salads.

health bites

A preliminary study suggests that smokers who eat 6 ounces (about 3 cups) of watercress each day may gain lung cancer protection from the phytochemical phenyl ethyl isothiocyanate (PEITC).

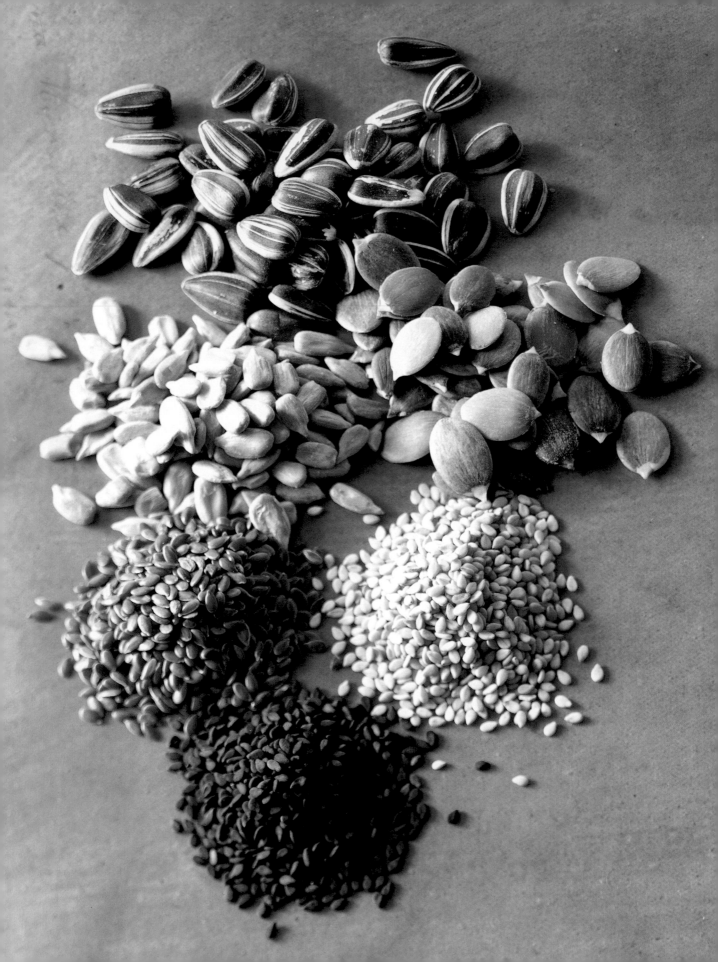

seeds

Rich in heart-healthy fat, pumpkin, sesame, and sunflower seeds possess an enormous amount of phytonutrients that may protect against cancer, cardiovascular disease, cataracts, chronic fatigue syndrome, and macular degeneration.

what's in it

essential fatty acids Seeds are rich in these nourishing fat compounds, which may improve fibrocystic breasts, cardiovascular health, immunity, and skin health.

magnesium One ounce of sunflower or pumpkin seeds supplies more than one-fourth of the Daily Value for this mineral, which may prevent chronic fatigue syndrome, heart disease, and kidney stones.

plant sterols Pumpkin seeds are particularly high in these compounds, which may lower both total and LDL ("bad") cholesterol, and may prevent the development of BPH (benign prostatic hyperplasia).

selenium This antioxidant mineral works with vitamin E to fight the free-radical cell damage that can lead to cancer, heart disease, and vision problems. (One ounce of sunflower seeds provides 17mcg of selenium, which is 24% of the Daily Value.)

sesaminol compounds Sesame seeds contain sesaminol, sesamolinol, and pinoresinols—all precursors to lignans (phytoestrogens under review for anticancer and cardioprotective potential).

syringic acid Present in sesame seeds, this phytochemical is under review for its potential to work with other plant antioxidants in the seeds to help combat UV sun damage in skin cells.

thiamin Sunflower seeds are a good source of this essential B vitamin (0.7mg per ounce, or 43% of the Daily Value); thiamin promotes brain function, including memory.

vitamin E Seeds are one of the best dietary sources of this antioxidant vitamin, which may help to protect against cancer, cataracts, heart disease, high cholesterol, and macular degeneration. (One ounce of sunflower seeds supplies a lot: 14mg per ounce, or 71% of the Daily Value.)

zinc Pumpkin and sesame seeds provide generous amounts of this vital mineral, which may enhance immune function and reproductive health.

maximizing the benefits

To preserve their **essential fats** and nutrients (and to prevent them from going rancid), refrigerate or freeze seeds in airtight containers.

---

add more to your diet

▶ Puree toasted pumpkin seeds with lime juice, garlic, cilantro, and some pumpkin seed oil. Use as a sauce for pasta, fish, or chicken.

▶ Substitute sunflower or pumpkin seeds for walnuts in a chocolate chip cookie dough.

▶ Substitute pumpkin seed oil for half of the olive oil in a salad dressing.

▶ Coat thin fish fillets or chicken cutlets in a mixture of crushed sunflower and pumpkin seeds, and pan-fry.

▶ For a super-quick pasta sauce: Stir dark sesame oil into plain yogurt and toss with hot pasta. Garnish with sliced scallions and toasted sesame seeds.

▶ Add sesame seeds or chopped pumpkin or sunflower seeds to pie crusts.

▶ Whisk together soy sauce and dark sesame oil or pumpkin seed oil and drizzle over grilled fish.

shellfish

More than a culinary delicacy, these gifts of Neptune are satisfying, rich sources of protein filled with nutrients that may help to protect against anemia, arthritis, cancer, cardiovascular disease, cataracts, depression, and infertility.

add more to your diet

▶ Stir cooked scallops and shrimp into store-bought salsa and use as a filling for tortillas.

▶ For a white seafood pizza, top prepared Italian bread shells with shredded part-skim mozzarella cheese and minced cooked clams or shrimp.

▶ Extremely high in vitamin B_{12}, use bottled clam broth for cooking rice pilafs, or for adding to fish or shellfish soups, chowders, and stews.

▶ Add cooked shrimp, clams, or mussels to your favorite pasta sauce.

▶ Make a seafood quesadilla with shredded cheese, crabmeat, diced peppers, and scallions.

▶ Make a shrimp salad with grapefruit sections and tomatoes, and toss in a lemony dressing.

what's in it

iron Shellfish possess the more bioavailable (so-called "heme") form of this blood-nourishing mineral, which helps to prevent anemia.

omega-3 fatty acids These heart-healthy fats nourish the skin and may reduce risk for cardiovascular disease, including high blood pressure and stroke.

selenium This mineral with anticancer potential may also prevent cataracts, infertility, and prostate problems. Shellfish provide tremendous amounts of this powerful antioxidant. (A half dozen oysters has 46mcg, which is 65% of the Daily Value.)

vitamin B_{12} Found only in animal foods, vitamin B_{12} may help to ward off anemia, depression, and heart disease. Clams are especially rich sources of this hard-to-find but necessary vitamin, supplying 43mcg, which is 716% of the Daily Value.

zinc Shellfish are excellent sources of zinc, a mineral that helps to maintain immunity and reproductive health. Oysters are far and away the best: 6 medium oysters provide 178% of the Daily Value.

maximizing the benefits

Omega-3 fatty acids deteriorate rapidly, so buy live shellfish and cook the same day. Avoid eating raw shellfish because they may harbor dangerous bacteria, viruses, and parasites.

health bites

Despite a reputation for being high in cholesterol, shellfish, particularly shrimp, are actually good for your heart. Shellfish are rich sources of heart-healthy omega-3 fats and contain very little saturated fat—the true culprit in raising cholesterol for most people. Research indicates that eating omega-3-rich food is cardioprotective, particularly reducing the risk for heart attack.

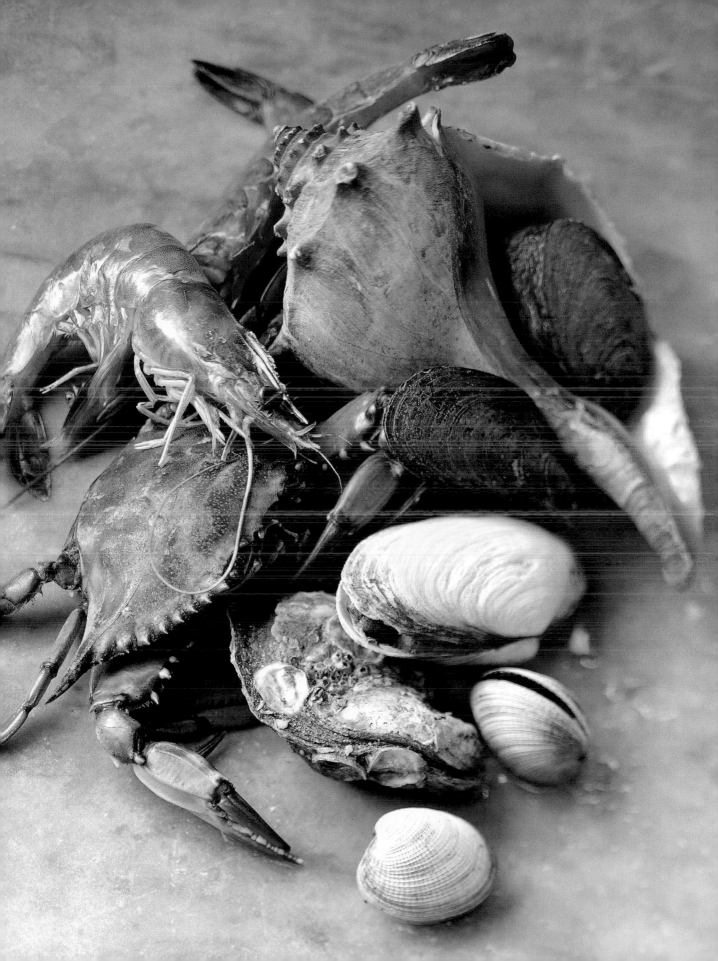

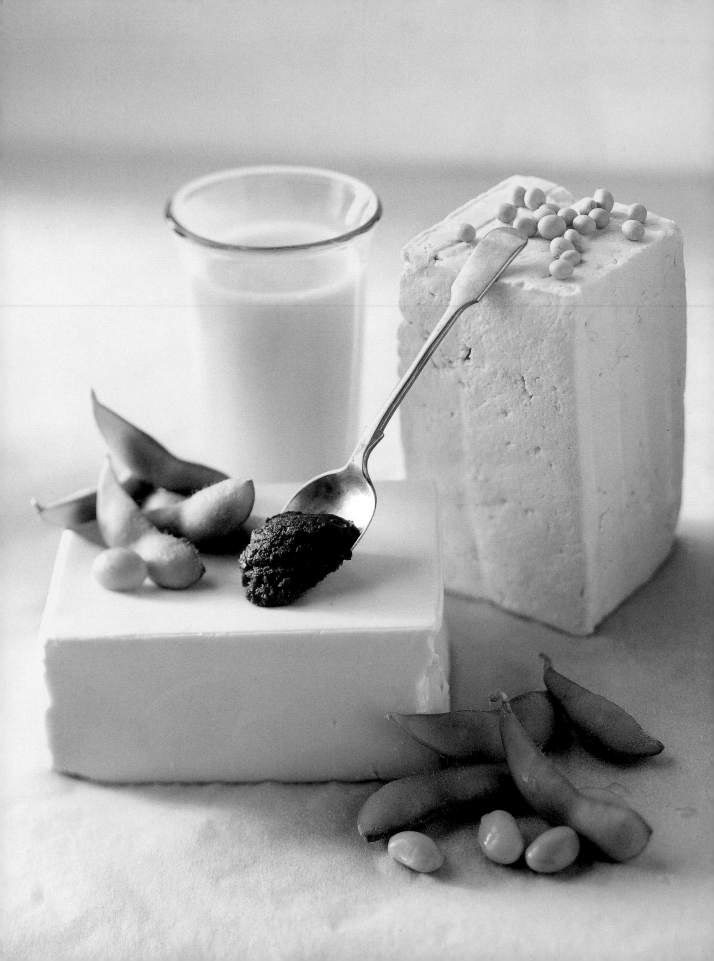

soy foods

The richest dietary sources of phytoestrogens, soy foods —tofu, edamame, dried soybeans, soy milk, miso, tempeh— possess high-quality plant protein, lots of soluble fiber, and a wealth of phytonutrients.

what's in it

beta-sistosterol A type of plant sterol, beta-sistosterol is under review for its potential to lower cholesterol and to relieve symptoms associated with prostate enlargement.

genistein and daidzein These two powerful isoflavone phytoestrogens may protect against osteoporosis by inhibiting calcium loss from bones and increasing bone mineral density and content. Genistein and daidzein may also help to prevent heart disease, prostate cancer, and some forms of breast cancer. Soy foods are the richest sources of the isoflavones genistein and daidzein.

lignans Experimental research suggests that these phytoestrogens with antioxidant properties may prevent harmful changes in cells, particularly those leading to breast, colon, and prostate cancer.

phytic acid This phytochemical may neutralize cancer-causing free radicals in the intestines.

protease inhibitors Preliminary research indicates that a protease inhibitor unique to soy foods, Bowman-Birk Inhibitor (BBI), may slow enzyme production in cancer cells and reduce intestinal tumors.

saponins These plant compounds have anticancer and cardioprotective properties and may help to raise levels of cancer-fighting immune cells, prevent bile acids from becoming cancerous agents in the colon, and lower cholesterol levels.

add more to your diet

▶ Use diced tofu to replace some of the cheese in lasagna or macaroni and cheese.

▶ Substitute soy milk for cow's milk in puddings, custards, or smoothies.

▶ Steam edamame (fresh soybeans) in their pods, then shell them. Add the beans to grain or vegetable salads.

▶ Make a miso-carrot salad dressing: Whisk a couple of tablespoons of shiro miso into carrot juice along with a couple of teaspoons of sesame oil, some ground ginger, and some wasabi paste.

▶ Use soybeans in classic bean recipes such as chili or baked beans, but precook them before starting the recipe, because they can take several hours to soften.

▶ Puree soft silken tofu with basil, garlic, almonds, and a little Parmesan, and use as a pasta sauce.

▶ Cut up firm silken tofu, drizzle honey over it, and serve in a fruit salad with melon and grapes.

maximizing the benefits

To preserve **phytoestrogen** content, minimize cooking time for tofu and miso by adding them late in the cooking process.

health bites

Soy products containing at least 6.25 grams of soy protein per serving carry an FDA-approved label stating that daily consumption of soy protein (at least 25 grams), in conjunction with a low-fat diet, can lower cholesterol levels in people with high cholesterol.

spices

caraway

Caraway is part of the carrot family and is available as a whole seed. It is the seed used to flavor rye bread and other Middle European dishes, such as sauerkraut and goulash.

what's in it

Limonene in caraway may prevent cancer. Caraway also has small amounts of perillyl alcohol, which may have the potential to prevent breast cancer.

add more to your diet

Use in: savory soups and stews; salad dressings and relishes; savory muffins and bread doughs. It matches well with cabbage, carrots, beets, ham, and pork.

cayenne

This is a fiery spice derived from the dried pods of a particular variety of chili pepper.

what's in it

Cayenne may help to reduce discomfort from allergies, colds, and flu. Capsaicin is the compound that gives cayenne pepper its bite, and it is thought to reduce congestion by opening up the nasal passages.

add more to your diet

Use in: tomato sauces and salsas; chilis, stews, and soups; chocolate sauces, cookies, and cakes; salad dressings and fruit salad; spice rubs, marinades, and barbecue sauces.

cinnamon

Derived from the inner bark of a tree, cinnamon is a sweet, warm, aromatic spice, most commonly used in baking.

what's in it

Cinnamon may have antibacterial and antimicrobial properties, and it may also reduce discomfort from heartburn. Cinnamaldehyde in cinnamon may ward off bacteria such as *H. pylori*, which has been linked to ulcers.

add more to your diet

Use in: savory soups, stews, and chilis; tomato sauces; meat marinades; pancake and waffle batters; and hot cocoa mixes.

cloves

A strong and highly fragrant spice, cloves are the dried flower bud of a clove tree. They are available whole or ground.

what's in it

Cloves may fight off bacteria, such as *E. coli*, that can cause food poisoning. Eugenol in cloves may prevent heart disease by preventing blood from forming too many clots. Cloves are also used as a natural breath freshener.

add more to your diet

Use in: spice rubs and barbecue sauces, tomato sauces and salsas, sweet fruit-poaching liquids. It matches well with ham and other smoked meats.

coriander seed

Coriander seed comes from the cilantro plant and has a mild, citruslike flavor. Coriander is used in curry powder and as a pickling spice.

what's in it

Coriander seed is thought to be helpful in relieving stomach cramps and may have the ability to kill bacteria and fungus. It contains limonene, which is a flavonoid thought to help fight cancer.

add more to your diet

Use in: yogurt and sour cream sauces; savory soups and stews; spice rubs and marinades. It matches well with fish and poultry.

cumin

Cumin is used in Indian and Mexican cooking and is available as the whole seed or ground.

what's in it

Examined for its potential to ward off bacteria and foodborne microbes, such as *E. coli*, cumin is also currently being investigated for potential antioxidant and anticancer effects.

add more to your diet

Use in: savory soups, stews, and chilis; spice rubs and marinades; salsas, chutneys, and relishes; bread doughs and savory pancake batters; pasta and rice salads. It matches well with corn, cabbage, carrots, onions, lentils, beans, and potatoes.

ginger

Ginger is sold as the fresh root, powdered, pickled, and sugar-preserved. All forms of ginger have an aromatic spiciness.

what's in it

Substances in ginger—gingerol, shogaol, and zingiberene—have antioxidant capabilities, which may help to prevent heart disease and cancer. Ginger is thought to reduce motion sickness, nausea, and vomiting; and it has also been shown to possess anti-inflammatory properties.

add more to your diet

Use in: hot apple and pineapple ciders; cakes, cookies, and muffins; fruit desserts; savory soups, curries, and stews.

mustard seed

Mustard seed and mustard powder have a pungent, slightly smoky flavor. Note that some brands of prepared mustard contain turmeric, which make it bright yellow.

what's in it

Mustard seeds contain allyl isothiocyanates, which studies suggest inhibit the growth of cancer cells. The volatile oils in mustard may clear congestion due to colds and flu.

add more to your diet

Use in: relishes and salsas; pickling and preserving; cabbage and carrot slaws; salads and salad dressings; curries and stews.

nutmeg

Nutmeg is the seed of a tropical fruit. Its sweet, aromatic, warm flavor tends to be strong, so it is advisable to use small amounts.

what's in it

Eugenol, a monoterpene in nutmeg, is thought to prevent heart disease by preventing blood cells from forming too many clots. Nutmeg may also have antibacterial properties that may destroy the foodborne bacteria *E. coli*.

add more to your diet

Use in: cookies, cakes, and pies; puddings and custards; cheese sauces and white sauces. It matches well with spinach, green beans, broccoli, carrots, and sweet potatoes.

saffron

One of the most expensive spices in the world, saffron has a flavor that is unique, delicate, and difficult to compare with any other spice. Use in minute amounts as it is fragrant and intense.

what's in it

Laboratory studies suggest that saffron may be an important disease-fighting spice, due possibly to the substance crocetin, as well as carotenoids, compounds that are believed to fight heart disease and cancer.

add more to your diet

Use in: soups, chowders, and stews; fresh pasta, pizza, and bread doughs; in white sauces. It matches well with fish, shellfish, and chicken.

turmeric

The spice that gives curry powder its deep yellow color, turmeric has a delicate flavor.

what's in it

The curcumin in turmeric is thought to have a wide range of beneficial effects, and its antioxidant properties may fend off heart disease and cancer. Studies also show that curcumin holds promise in reducing cataract development.

add more to your diet

Use in: curries, savory soups, and stews; spice rubs and marinades; pickled vegetables and condiments; and yogurt sauces.

spinach

Popeye's favorite food is not a great source of iron, but it *does* have a tremendous wealth of disease-fighting carotenoids and phytochemicals that team up with vitamins to help protect against cancer, high cholesterol, and vision loss.

add more to your diet

➤ For a quick soup, puree steamed spinach with garlic and yogurt and top with scallions.

➤ Steam spinach, then puree with parsley and lemon juice, and use as a sauce for chicken or pasta.

➤ Steam spinach with mint and thinly sliced scallions, and stir into mashed potatoes.

➤ Make a spinach pesto: Puree raw spinach with almonds, garlic, olive oil, and Parmesan cheese. Toss with pasta and chickpeas.

➤ Make a spinach salad dressing: Steam spinach and puree along with parsley, basil, and garlic. Whisk in olive oil and lemon juice.

what's in it

beta-carotene A half cup of cooked spinach provides 4.4mg, which is close to a full day's supply of this antioxidant. Beta-carotene may help to protect against cancer and macular degeneration.

folate Two cups of raw spinach provide 116mcg of folate, almost a third of your daily requirement for this B vitamin, which helps protect against anemia, birth defects, and possibly heart attacks.

lutein and zeaxanthin Spinach is a rich source of these two carotenoids, which may work together to help prevent macular degeneration and possibly cataracts and colon cancer.

oxalates Oxalates inhibit absorption of calcium and iron from spinach. Spinach and other foods high in oxalates are not recommended for people with gout and certain types of kidney stones.

plant sterols Researchers believe these plant substances may help to prevent cancer and high cholesterol.

vitamin C This antioxidant vitamin may help to prevent macular degeneration, osteoarthritis, and stroke.

maximizing the benefits

Serve spinach either raw or cooked, but avoid overcooking. To preserve loss of water-soluble **B vitamins,** steam or stir-fry spinach. Cooking helps to convert **protein, lutein,** and **beta-carotene** in spinach into more bioavailable forms. To enhance **carotenoid** absorption, eat spinach with some heart-healthy fat.

health bites

Phylloquinone is the most common form of vitamin K found in green vegetables and is particularly high in dark greens, such as spinach. Vitamin K is necessary for proper blood clotting and possibly may play a role in preserving bone health. However, if you are on blood-thinning medications, consult with your physician before consuming vegetables high in vitamin K. High amounts may interfere with the anticlotting action of the medication.

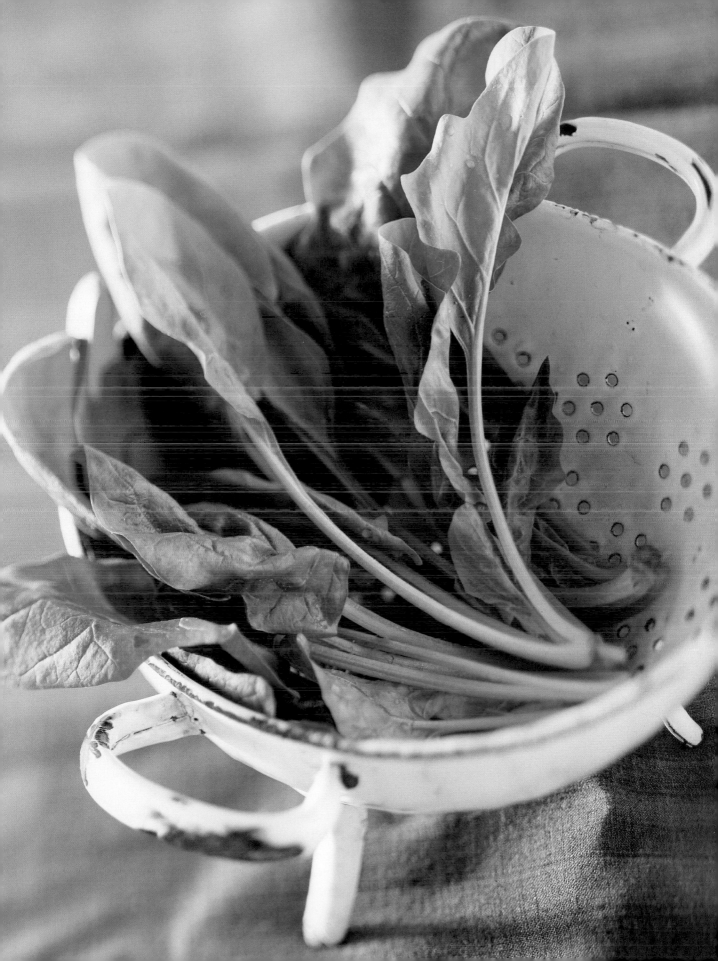

super grains

Ancient high-protein foods with healing properties, so-called super grains—amaranth, buckwheat, teff, and quinoa—are filling and rich in fiber, B vitamins, and phytonutrients.

add more to your diet

▶ Add teff flour to pancakes and biscuits, using 2 parts wheat flour to 1 part teff flour.

▶ Cook buckwheat, quinoa, or amaranth and make a salad with feta cheese, green peppers, tomatoes, and cucumber. Toss with a lemon dressing.

▶ Grind amaranth in a mini food processor and use the amaranth flour to replace up to one-fourth of the wheat flour in a muffin recipe.

▶ Make a pilaf with quinoa, onions, dried cherries, and toasted pecans. Serve as a side dish instead of rice.

▶ Stir cooked buckwheat groats or quinoa into savory tea-bread batters.

what's in it

complex carbohydrates Amylopectin and amylose, carbohydrates in buckwheat, may help to control blood-sugar levels.

lignans These phytoestrogens may help to lower LDL ("bad") cholesterol and risk for breast, colon, ovarian, and prostate cancer.

lysine Quinoa is a good source (0.7g per half cup) of this essential amino acid, which may help to prevent and manage cold sores.

magnesium Amaranth and quinoa are good sources of heart-healthy magnesium, which may also help to prevent allergies, asthma, kidney stones, and premenstrual syndrome (PMS). (A serving of quinoa or amaranth provides about 40% of the Daily Value.)

phytic acids These phytochemicals may help to protect against free-radical cell damage in the intestines.

plant sterols These may help significantly reduce cholesterol.

protease inhibitors These cancer-fighting compounds may inhibit the formation of cancer cells.

rutin Present in buckwheat, rutin may help minimize cancer risk by detoxifying cancer-causing substances and preventing cancer agents from taking hold in the body. Rutin is also under review for its ability to help lower blood pressure, strengthen blood vessels, and reduce levels of harmful cholesterol.

saponins Quinoa is an especially good source of these substances, which may help to prevent cancer and heart disease.

vitamin E Working with other antioxidant phytochemicals in super grains, vitamin E may help to prevent cancer, cataracts, heart disease, and macular degeneration. Quinoa is a particularly good super grain source of vitamin E.

maximizing the benefits

To preserve nutrients, cook grains without excess water and until just tender; overcooking diminishes phytochemicals.

health bites
Animal studies suggest that buckwheat protein has a cholesterol-lowering property comparable to, and possibly more effective than, soy protein.

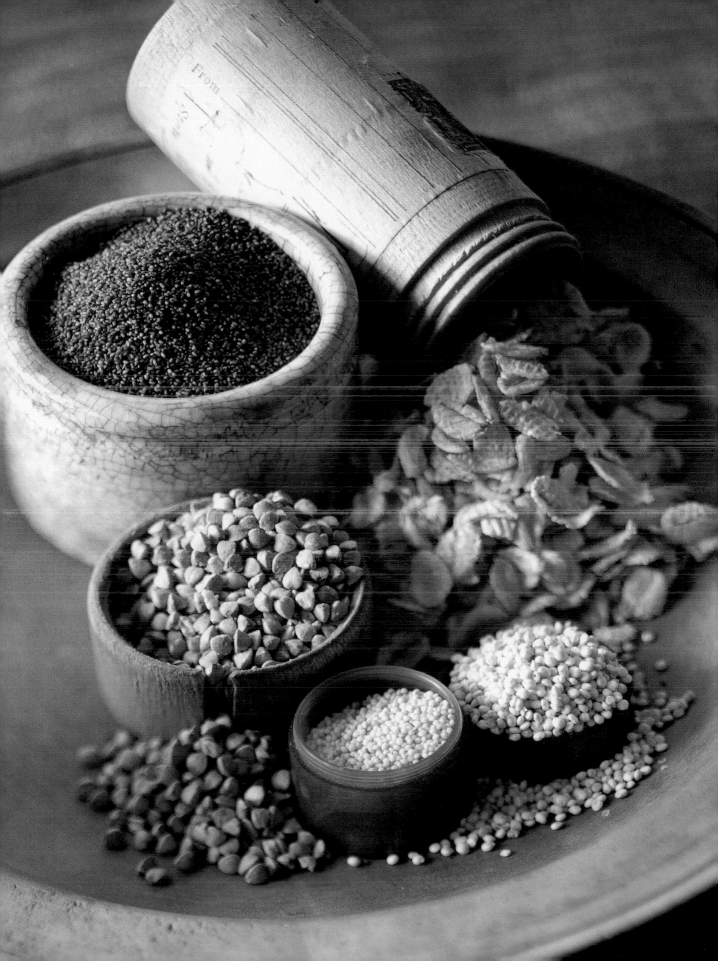

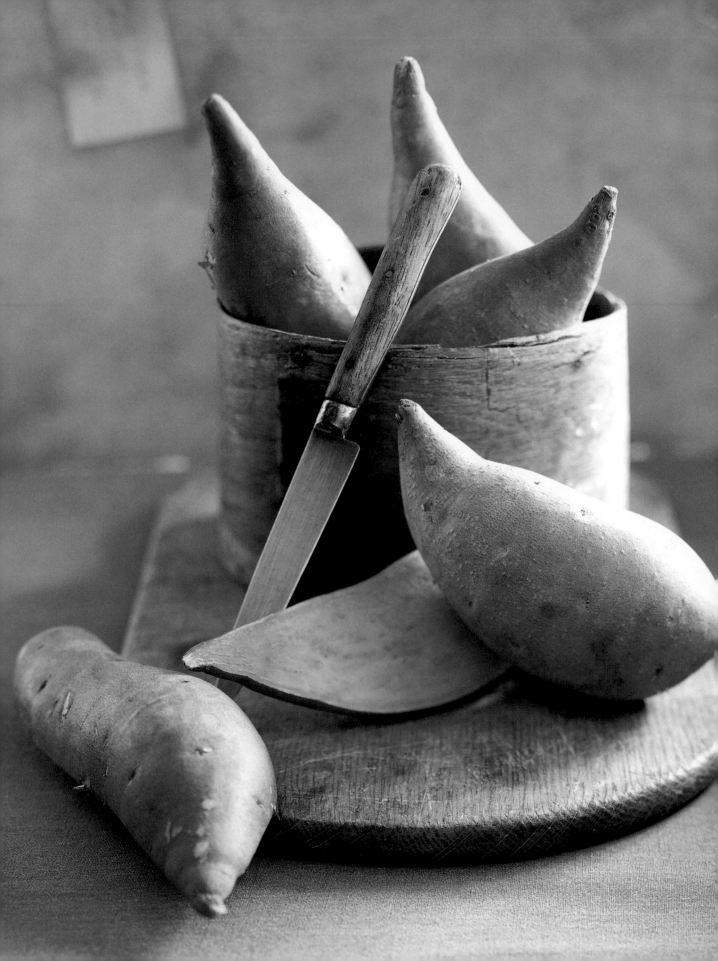

sweet potatoes

Vibrantly colored with carotenoids and filled with fiber, sweet potatoes are one of the most nutrient-dense vegetables. These roots may help prevent cancer, degenerative eye disease, depression, and heart disease.

what's in it

beta-carotene Sweet potatoes are an exceptionally rich source of this plant pigment (one sweet potato has 187% of the recommended intake for beta-carotene). Beta-carotene may help to prevent certain cancers (stomach, pancreas, mouth, and gums) and macular degeneration.

caffeic acid This phenolic compound shows promise in fighting cancer and the AIDS virus.

chlorogenic acid Preliminary studies suggest this anticancer phytochemical may help detoxify harmful carcinogens and viruses.

insoluble fiber When eaten with its skin, a sweet potato is an excellent source of insoluble fiber, which may help to prevent constipation, diverticulosis, hemorrhoids, and weight gain. (A medium sweet potato provides over 2g of insoluble fiber.)

lutein and zeaxanthin These two carotenoid pigments lend bright orange color to sweet potatoes and may help to protect against atherosclerosis, certain types of cancer, and eye diseases.

pectin About half of the fiber in sweet potatoes is soluble pectin fiber, which may control cholesterol.

plant sterols These cholesterol-lowering compounds may reduce cancer risk by binding carcinogenic agents in the digestive tract.

potassium This heart-healthy mineral, found in abundance in sweet potatoes (397mg per potato), is associated with lower blood pressure and a lowered risk for heart disease, kidney stones, and stroke.

vitamin B6 Sweet potatoes provide good amounts of B6, which may help to prevent heart disease, stroke, depression, and insomnia.

vitamin C Plentiful in sweet potatoes, vitamin C may help to bolster immunity and wound healing, as well as prevent degenerative eye conditions.

maximizing the benefits

Eat sweet potatoes with their skin to get more **beta-carotene** and **fiber.** Baking or broiling enhances beta-carotene and sweetens the potato as its starches turn to sugar.

add more to your diet

▶ Mash sweet potatoes with maple syrup for an unusual dessert.

▶ Make sweet potato chips: Thinly slice sweet potatoes, drizzle with olive oil, and bake in a 400°F oven until tender.

▶ For a twist on mashed potatoes, use half sweet potatoes and half regular all-purpose potatoes.

▶ Add slices of cooked sweet potatoes to savory sandwiches.

▶ Mash cooked sweet potatoes with grated Parmesan cheese and use in place of half the cheese in lasagna.

▶ Substitute mashed sweet potatoes for pumpkin in pies.

▶ Shred raw sweet potatoes and use in place of shredded carrots in cakes, muffins, and tea breads.

▶ Make a sweet potato salad: Cook sweet potatoes and while the potatoes are still warm, peel and cut into chunks. Toss in a dressing of lime juice, olive oil, minced scallions, curry powder, and salt.

tomatoes

Heartily indulge in phytochemical-rich tomatoes (as well as tomato products), because the nutrients in this vegetable seem to work in concert to protect against cancer (particularly prostate cancer), clogged arteries, and skin ailments.

add more to your diet

▶ Cook fresh tomatoes with sugar, cinnamon, and orange zest for a sweet and savory jam.

▶ Combine tomato juice and carrot juice and chill. Serve as a refreshing summer soup garnished with chopped tomatoes and a dollop of yogurt.

▶ To give a nutritional boost to savory soups, replace half of the water with tomato or tomato-vegetable juice.

▶ Make a quick sauce for pasta salad: Combine tomato paste, tomato juice, olive oil, balsamic vinegar, and chopped fresh basil, mint, or parsley.

▶ Brush bread with olive oil and garlic, top with tomato paste and broil. Top with chopped fresh tomatoes.

what's in it

beta-carotene This bioactive pigment may help to prevent acne, certain forms of cancer (stomach, pancreas), and vision loss.

caffeic and ferulic acid These anticancer chemicals may help enhance the production of the body's cancer-fighting enzymes.

chlorogenic acid Found in greatest amounts in freshly picked tomatoes, this compound may be cancer-protective by inhibiting environmental toxins such as nitrosamines in cigarette smoke.

lutein and zeaxanthin These carotenoids present in tomatoes may team up to help prevent vision loss and possibly cancer.

lycopene Abundant in red tomatoes, this pigment may be a stronger antioxidant than beta-carotene and may prevent cell damage that leads to heart attacks and cancer. One study found that men who consumed lycopene-rich diets cut their heart attack risk in half, and several studies indicate lycopene may protect against prostate cancer. Tomato juice is a particularly concentrated source of lycopene.

vitamin C Present mainly in the jellylike substance around tomato seeds, vitamin C may protect against heart disease, respiratory infections, skin cancer, and vision loss.

maximizing the benefits

Lycopene is best absorbed from concentrated forms of tomatoes, such as tomato paste, juice, ketchup, sauce, and soup. The more concentrated the tomato source, the more concentrated the lycopene. Heat and oil enhance absorption of lycopene and **beta-carotene,** though some **vitamin C** is lost.

health bites

Lycopene-rich food may protect against prostate cancer. In a six-year study of 48,000 men who consumed 10 or more servings (1 cup of tomato juice is a serving) per week of tomato products, participants experienced a 45% reduction in prostate cancer.

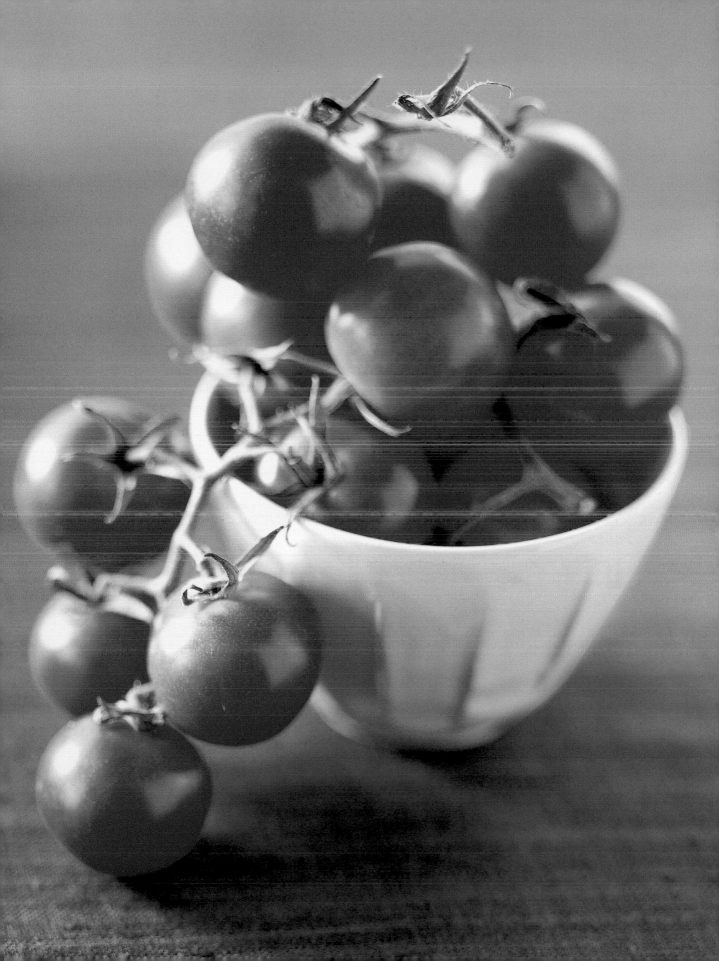

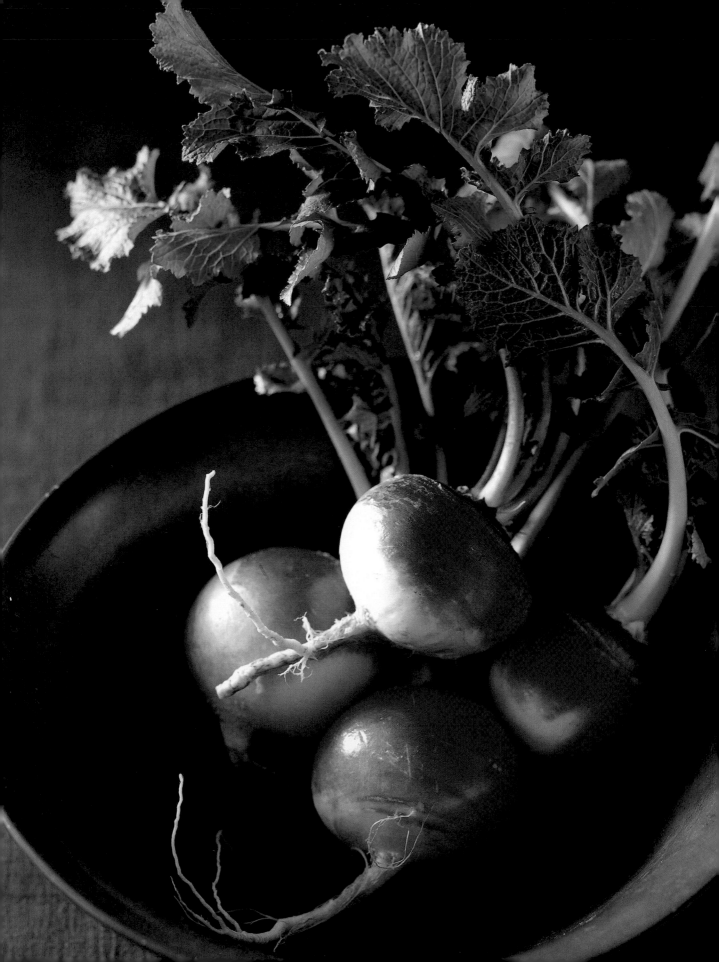

turnips

Earthy roots, with a sweet, smoky flavor, turnips (including the yellow rutabaga) are surprisingly full of vitamin C and some essential amino acids. Complex carbohydrates and fiber add to the healing power of this cabbage relative.

what's in it

complex carbohydrates An excellent fuel source for the body, complex carbohydrates tend to release a slow, steady supply of energy. They may also enhance memory, absorb stomach acid associated with heartburn, and improve tryptophan absorption.

goitrogens Found in raw turnips and other cruciferous vegetables, these compounds may suppress thyroid function.

insoluble fiber Insoluble fiber helps to alleviate constipation, and possibly varicose veins and hemorrhoids.

lysine Part of the turnip's protein content, this essential amino acid may help to prevent and manage cold sores.

soluble fiber This type of fiber helps to soak up cholesterol, lowering blood levels of artery-damaging LDL ("bad") cholesterol.

tryptophan A precursor to the B vitamin niacin, this essential amino acid may help to ease anxiety, depression, and insomnia.

vitamin C Acting as a powerful antioxidant, vitamin C helps to control damaging free radicals and may enhance immunity.

add more to your diet

► Combine sliced rutabaga, carrots, and potatoes and cook as for mashed potatoes.

► Shred rutabaga or white turnips, add to shredded potatoes along with chopped fresh dill, and make turnip-potato pancakes.

► Sauté cubed white turnips in olive oil with garlic and shredded turnip greens.

► Shred turnips and toss with shredded red and green apples, and a mixture of apple cider, apple cider vinegar, and Dijon mustard. Serve as a slaw.

► Roasted rutabagas have an earthy, nutty flavor: Peel rutabagas and cut into chunks. Toss with olive oil, wrap in foil, and bake at 400°F for 20 to 30 minutes, or until tender.

maximizing the benefits

Cooking appears to deactivate **goitrogens** and some **vitamin C** may be lost; on the other hand, cooking increases the availability of **soluble fiber.**

health bites

Goitrogens are present in raw cruciferous vegetables, including turnips, and may interfere with the synthesis of thyroid hormone. These compounds do not pose a risk for healthy people who eat moderate amounts of cruciferous vegetables, but individuals with hypothyroidism may want to cook cruciferous vegetables to deactivate goitrogens. Conversely, those with hyperthyroidism may want to increase intake of raw cruciferous vegetables.

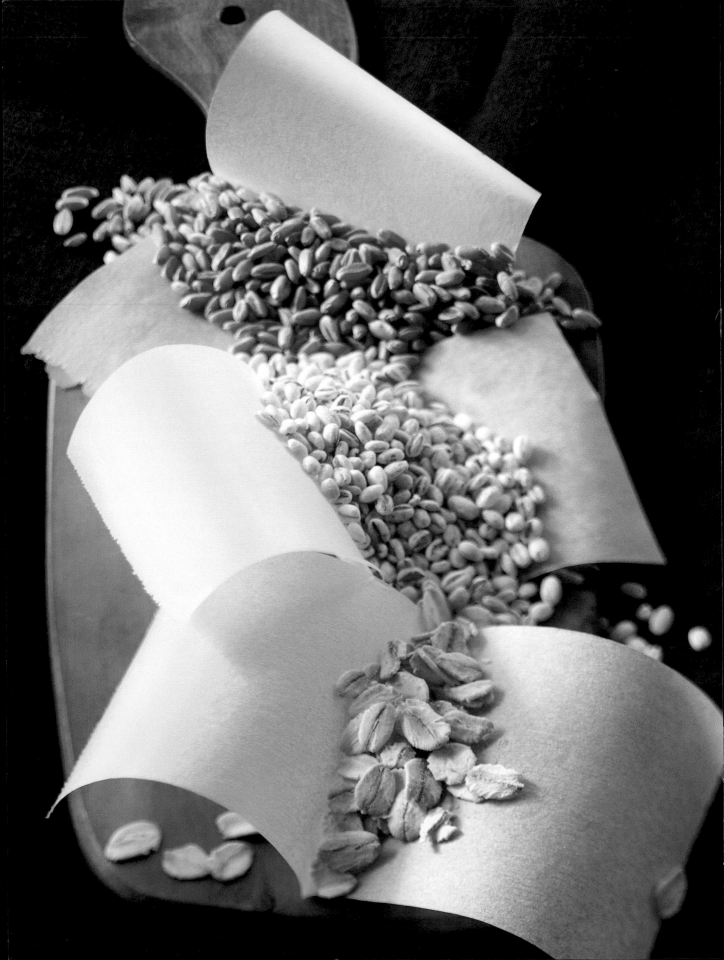

whole grains

The nutritious germ and bran layers of a whole grain are packed with phytochemicals and insoluble fiber. Whole grains—barley, oats, rye, and wheat—are linked to a lower risk for cancer, cardiovascular disease, and diabetes.

what's in it

beta-glucan Experts believe that about 1 to 1½ cups of cooked oatmeal or about 1 cup of cooked oat bran, both rich in soluble beta-glucan fiber, may help to reduce total cholesterol by as much as 5%. Barley also has beta-glucan fiber.

complex carbohydrates These substances may be why one study found that 1 cup of barley improved memory function in healthy elderly adults. Indigestible oligosaccharide carbohydrates may help prevent cancer, cardiovascular disease, and diabetes.

flavonoids These antioxidant compounds in the bran and germ may help to prevent cancer, diabetes, heart disease, and vision loss.

gluten A protein found in barley, oats, rye, and wheat, gluten is not recommended for people with celiac disease.

lignans Estrogenlike substances found in the bran and germ layers, lignans may lower cholesterol and help inhibit the damaging effects of estrogen, protecting against breast cancer.

phytic acids These compounds may protect against free-radical cell damage and may slow starch digestion, thus helping to stabilize blood-sugar levels.

plant sterols These substances may help reduce total and LDL ("bad") cholesterol by binding it in the digestive tract.

saponins Oats are an especially good source of these substances, which may bind cholesterol and interfere with cancer growth.

selenium Barley is an outstanding source of this antioxidant mineral, which partners with vitamin E to fight damaging free radicals. (A half cup of barley provides 38mcg of selenium, which is 54% of the Daily Value.)

vitamin E This antioxidant may help to prevent cancer, heart disease, skin disorders, and vision loss. Wheat germ is an exceptionally concentrated source. (Just a quarter cup provides about 25% of the Daily Value.)

maximizing the benefits

Cook these grains in a minimum of water and only until tender; overcooking will diminish the nutrient content.

---

add more to your diet

► Cook cracked wheat or soften bulgur (precooked cracked wheat) in boiling water. Use in salads, pilafs, stuffings, soup, salads; or add to a meatloaf as a meat extender.

► Cook whole wheatberries or rye berries until soft, and fold into home-made whole-wheat bread dough.

► Substitute barley for rice in a rice pudding recipe (the cooking times will be longer for barley).

► Toast oat groats (this brings out flavor), then grind them to make a flour. Use the toasted oat flour to make cookies and cakes.

► Coat fish fillets or chicken cutlets in egg whites, dip into wheat germ, and sauté until crisp and cooked through.

► Cook old-fashioned rolled oats until soft, then puree. Use to replace some of the oil in salad dressings.

► Add wheat germ to homemade pizza doughs and savory pie doughs.

winter squash

The Halloween jack-o'-lantern and its orange-fleshed relatives—acorn and butternut squash—are colorful and delicious vegetables that may help to prevent acne, heart disease, macular degeneration, and weight gain.

add more to your diet

▶ Add peeled and diced butternut squash to chili, soups, or stews.

▶ Buy frozen pureed winter squash, thin it with milk, and serve as a soup.

▶ Add peeled, shredded squash to pancake batter.

▶ Use pumpkin or squash puree in a cheesecake.

▶ Combine cooked, pureed butternut squash with grated Parmesan cheese and herbs, and use as a sauce for pasta.

▶ Stir cooked squash into sweet or savory rice or grain dishes.

▶ Make a squash chutney: Cook chunks of squash with sugar, raisins, red pepper, and spices until tender. Serve alongside meat, fish, or poultry dishes.

what's in it

beta-carotene Pumpkin and butternut squash supply extraordinary amounts of this nourishing orange-yellow pigment, which may help to prevent acne, cancer, and macular degeneration. (One cup of cooked butternut has 8.5mg of beta-carotene, or 107% of the recommended intake. Pumpkin has 7.8mg, or 98% of the Daily Value.)

fiber Squash contains appreciable amounts of soluble fiber, which helps to lower harmful LDL cholesterol. Insoluble fiber in squash helps to make you feel full and to relieve constipation.

lutein Pumpkin is a particularly significant source of this carotenoid, which may stave off macular degeneration and possibly help prevent cataracts and colon cancer.

magnesium Acorn and butternut squash are good sources of this vital mineral, which may be beneficial for allergies, asthma, cardiovascular health, high blood pressure, kidney stones, and premenstrual syndrome (PMS).

potassium A diet high in this mineral may help to lower the risk for high blood pressure, kidney stones, and stroke. Acorn and butternut squash supply generous amounts of potassium. (One cup of cooked acorn squash provides 25% of the Daily Value for potassium.)

thiamin A serving of acorn squash (1 cup cooked) contributes very good amounts of this necessary brain-boosting B vitamin, which may help to improve memory and mood.

vitamin B$_6$ Acorn squash supplies an impressive quantity of this essential B vitamin, which is linked to a reduced risk for heart disease and possibly depression. (One cup cooked has 0.4mg, or 20% of the Daily Value.)

vitamin C This powerful antioxidant may prevent cataracts and chronic disease. Butternut is the best winter squash source of vitamin C, with just 1 cup providing 31mg.

maximizing the benefits

For **beta-carotene,** boiling, steaming, baking, or broiling are all fine; but **B vitamins** will be lost if the squash is cooked in water.

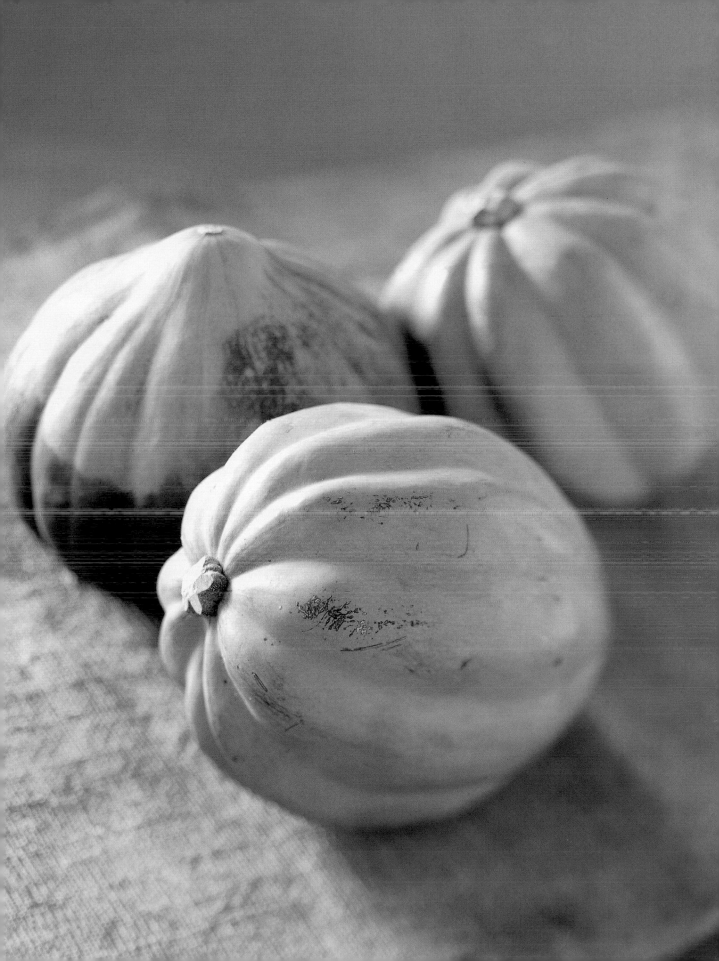

what ails you?

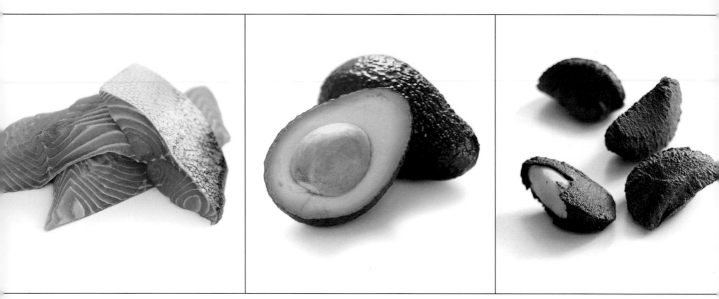

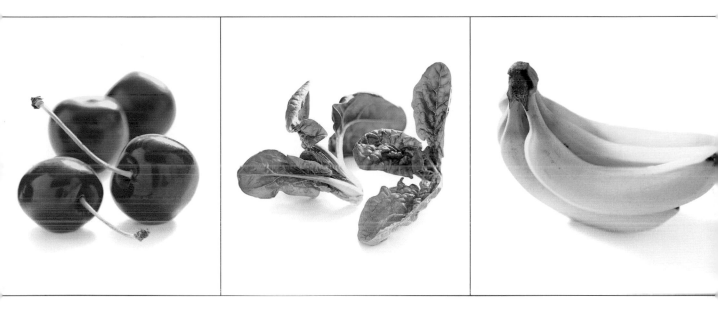

How to Manage or

Prevent Common Ailments

Through Diet

acne

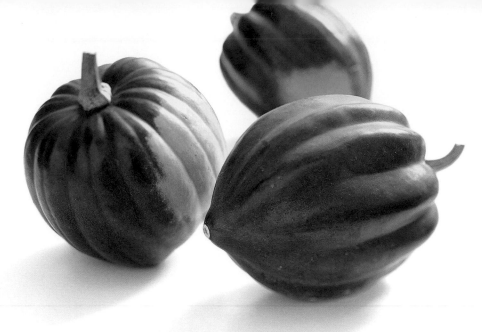

what it is

Acne occurs when an excess amount of sebum (an oily substance produced by glands that lubricates and moistens the skin) blocks the skin's pores at the base of hair follicles, causing small pus-filled eruptions to appear on the face, chest, shoulders, and back.

Pimples, blackheads, and whiteheads are the characteristics of this condition, which can be managed by simple self-care measures, over-the-counter topical medications, or under the supervision of a dermatologist. Though most forms of acne are mild, in its severe form (cystic acne), permanent pits and scars can occur, especially if skin lesions are picked at and squeezed.

One of the most common of all skin problems, acne generally afflicts adolescents, teenagers and young adults, though some older people also suffer from acne. Although it is not a dangerous condition, acne can nonetheless cause distress and discomfort for young people in particular, who may, as a result, suffer from poor self-image, social isolation, depression, and anxiety.

what causes it

Acne is often triggered by hormonal activity, which can increase the production of sebum. Though the hormonal shifts of adolescence make teenagers the primary victims of acne, women who are pregnant, menstruating, or in menopause are also susceptible. Certain medications (such as steroids or oral contraceptives) that affect hormones, as well as stress, can all contribute to the overproduction of sebum and therefore to acne. For some people there may be a genetic component that contributes to the onset of the condition.

how food may help

One of the prevailing beliefs about acne is that certain foods—such as chocolate or pizza—can cause it or make it worse; but this is just a myth. There are, however, certain foods that can help to promote optimal skin health.

Many skin conditions seem to respond to **vitamin A,** which appears to have a beneficial effect on cell growth and maturation. The best dietary sources of vitamin A are found in foods rich in **beta-carotene,** which is converted by the body into vitamin A. Some studies indicate that beta-carotene protects the skin from free-radical stress, and, though research is conflicting, there is also some evidence that it reduces sebum production.

Since inflammation is one of the characteristics of acne, **essential fatty acids** may help alleviate the condition by hindering the body's production of certain inflammatory compounds. **Vitamin E** is also helpful in maintaining healthy skin by teaming up with **selenium** to promote an enzyme called glutathione peroxidase, which may help to reduce inflammation.

The immunity-building mineral **zinc** may help to improve acne, perhaps through its involvement in hormone metabolism as well as the role it plays in healing. And some evidence shows that **vitamin B$_6$** may help to stabilize hormonal fluctuations that can cause acne.

recent research

Misconceptions about diet and acne are still common. A recent Canadian survey investigating beliefs concerning acne found that 32% of patients identify diet as the cause of acne. This is a longstanding myth that just doesn't seem to go away.

your food arsenal

foods	nutrient	health benefits
apricots **asparagus** **sweet potatoes** **winter squash**	beta-carotene	Beta-carotene may reduce sebum production by affecting sebaceous gland activity. Too much sebum is one of the causes of acne.
avocados **bananas** **potatoes** **salmon**	vitamin B$_6$	By helping to regulate levels of hormones implicated in the development of acne lesions, vitamin B$_6$ may reduce outbreaks.
crab **oysters** **tofu** **turkey**	zinc	Zinc has been linked to optimal skin health by enhancing immune function, reducing inflammation, and promoting tissue regeneration and healthy hormone levels.

allergies &
asthma

what it is

Though both allergies and asthma are characterized by an immune response to substances that are triggers only in certain people, the two conditions are not the same. Allergies usually result in watery and itchy eyes, runny nose, excessive sneezing, congestion, difficulty breathing, and sometimes hives. Asthma is a chronic inflammatory respiratory disorder that affects almost 17 million Americans. An asthma "attack" takes place when the bronchial tubes that conduct air to the lungs become constricted, causing difficulty in breathing, shortness of breath, wheezing, and coughing. Inflammation is present in the lungs (bronchial tubes) of people with asthma, even those with mild cases, and this plays a key role in all forms of the disease. Inflammation is also present in some people who suffer from allergies.

what causes it

Allergies or asthma may be linked to a genetically inherited tendency. Preliminary research also suggests that asthma may be *caused* by allergies (it is important to note, however, that while many asthma sufferers also have allergies, not all people with allergies have asthma). The release of a chemical called histamine can cause many of the physical manifestations of both allergies and asthma. Histamine has been linked to inflammation, congestion, and excessive mucus secretion and muscle contraction in the airways, as well as itching accompanied by hives.

Numerous irritants such as dust and dust mites, mold, cockroaches, pollen, and pet dander can set off both allergies and asthma. Other asthma triggers include tobacco smoke, cold air, humidity, exercise, food or drug allergies, as well as respiratory infections such as colds, flu, and bronchitis. (For dietary advice for *Colds & Flu*, see *page 158;* for *Bronchitis*, see *page 146.*)

how food may help

It is prudent to eat a low-fat diet rich in fruits and vegetables, which are linked to respiratory health.

Magnesium may help the lungs to relax and may also reduce inflammation. There is also some research that indicates magnesium may help to usher you into a calm sleep, which is important, since insomnia (usually caused by coughing) tends to occur frequently in people with allergies and asthma.

Believed to be a potent lung protector, the flavonoid **quercetin** is thought to also have the capacity to reduce the release of histamine. Another flavonoid, **luteolin,** may also have this effect. Quercetin also appears to have anti-inflammatory properties.

The antioxidant mineral **selenium** teams up with **vitamin E** to protect cells against free-radical damage, and this protective effect is thought to benefit membranes in airways. Selenium may ensure adequate levels of glutathione peroxidase, which is believed to be a potent free-radical-fighting enzyme.

A diet rich in **omega-3 fatty acids** may help to reduce inflammation, and immune-boosting foods rich in **zinc** may help maintain a strong immune system. **Vitamin C** functions as an antioxidant and helps to shield the lungs from environmental pollutants, which can often exacerbate asthma.

recent research

A recent study showed that eating at least 5 apples a week may strengthen your lungs. The study discovered that men who ate nearly an apple a day had slightly stronger lung function than those who excluded apples from their diets.

Although the researchers were unable to provide a scientific explanation for the protective attributes of apples, a reasonable theory may be that apples are loaded with healthy compounds, including antioxidants and flavonoids, which are thought to fight disease by protecting the body from free-radical damage.

As apples are rich in myriad healthy compounds, it may be the combination of these nutrients that creates the effect. Other research proposes that quercetin, in particular, stands out as a particularly potent flavonoid that helps to maintain lung health.

your food arsenal

foods	nutrient	health benefits
amaranth avocados quinoa sunflower seeds	magnesium	Scientists speculate that magnesium may help relax muscles in the lungs.
apples berries cherries red onions	quercetin	Preliminary studies indicate that the anti-allergenic activity of quercetin may be due to its ability to reduce the release of histamine.
Brazil nuts fish oysters sunflower seeds	selenium	Though the jury is still out regarding selenium's role in asthma, low blood levels of this mineral have been reported in asthmatics.
broccoli citrus fruit peppers strawberries	vitamin C	Vitamin C may help to reduce the harmful effects of environmental oxidants that can worsen allergy and asthma symptoms.

anemia

what it is

Anemia is a fairly common condition that results when the body doesn't have enough iron to produce the hemoglobin (the blood's oxygen-carrying protein) needed to make red blood cells. Proper production of red blood cells helps to supply and transport oxygen to the body's tissues and organs. If your cells don't have a normal supply of oxygen, you feel tired and weak, symptoms associated with iron deficiency anemia (the most prevalent type of anemia), which is a reversible condition. In addition to iron deficiency anemia, there are folate deficiency anemia, pernicious anemia, and more rare types of anemia such as aplastic anemia, hemolytic anemia, thalassemia, and sickle cell anemia.

what causes it

Iron deficiency anemia can result from either an iron-poor diet (more often found in vegetarians), intestinal problems that interfere with proper iron absorption, or blood loss (from an acute incident, such as a hemorrhage; from benign causes, such as hemorrhoids or menstruation; or from gastrointestinal bleeding). Young children and premenopausal women are at highest risk for developing iron deficiency anemia. Pregnancy can also increase the risk for anemia because the iron requirements of the fetus can potentially deplete the mother's stores of the mineral.

how food may help

To produce red blood cells, the body requires, among other nutrients, iron, folate, and vitamin B_{12}. For iron deficiency anemia, you can help build up your iron stores by eating foods rich in either "heme" or "nonheme" **iron.** Heme iron, which is absorbed by the body more effectively than nonheme iron, is available in meat, poultry, fish, and shellfish. Interestingly, heme iron promotes the absorption of nonheme iron from other food when eaten at the same time. It is important for vegetarians to eat ample amounts of nonheme iron (found in certain plant foods) along with foods rich in vitamin C, which improves nonheme iron absorption. To enhance your iron stores, cook in iron pots and pans.

Vitamin C also improves **folate** absorption, which is important in managing folate deficiency anemia. Folate is required for the body's metabolism of amino acids, as well as for the formation of healthy red blood cells. Foods rich in this important B vitamin should be consumed on a regular basis, because folate is water-soluble and the body cannot store a lot of it.

Vegans and vegetarians may be at risk for developing pernicious anemia, which results from a chronic lack of **vitamin B$_{12}$**. It may also be useful to eat foods rich in **beta-carotene,** since this carotenoid is converted in our bodies to **vitamin A,** which may help to mobilize stored iron from the liver. Foods rich in **vitamin B$_6$**, which assists in the formation of hemoglobin, are also beneficial. Make sure you consult a physician before you embark on a nutritional plan to correct your anemia.

foods to avoid

Note that some foods contain substances that may reduce your body's ability to absorb iron: tannic acid in tea, calcium phosphate in dairy products; oxalates in spinach, rhubarb, Swiss chard, and chocolate; and phytates in bran, peas, seeds, and soybeans. All of these may hinder the entry of iron into your digestive system. A high-fiber diet in general may act as an iron inhibitor.

your food arsenal

foods	nutrient	health benefits
asparagus black-eyed peas chicory lentils pinto beans	folate	Folate, along with other nutrients, is important for the manufacture of red blood cells. Adequate intake of this vital B vitamin can also help to prevent development of a type of anemia called folate deficiency anemia. Alcoholics and people with poor diets are at risk for developing this type of anemia.
amaranth clams oysters quinoa tofu	iron	Iron is required for the formation of hemoglobin, which carries oxygen in red blood cells to organs and tissues. Fatigue, weakness, and tiredness associated with iron deficiency anemia are due to insufficient red blood cells and the resulting inadequate distribution of oxygen to the cells.
clams mackerel nonfat plain yogurt sardines trout	vitamin B$_{12}$	Required for the production of red blood cells, this vitamin may help to prevent the onset of a type of anemia that is often found in strict vegans or people whose general diet is poor and lacking in variety.
broccoli citrus fruit peppers strawberries	vitamin C	Folate and iron are best absorbed from plant sources when accompanied by a source of vitamin C.

anxiety & stress

what it is

Anxiety and stress, though slightly different emotional states, are both natural reactions to danger or to an uncomfortable situation. A basic human survival instinct left over from our primordial roots, stress is an automatic protective mechanism that may actually help to alert us to danger.

Stress is a normal part of everyone's life. However, reactions to stress can culminate in anxiety, which, depending upon its severity, can interfere with health. Symptoms of anxiety include a heightened sense of self-awareness and an exaggerated awareness of surroundings, muscle tension, nervousness, insomnia, heart palpitations, intense worry, and feelings of dread and doom. Prolonged feelings of anxiety may signal a more serious anxiety disorder, which can lead to depression. For most people, though, anxiety and stress are all too common hallmarks of living in a fast-paced world that often seems out of our control.

what causes it

Certain factors (the list of potential triggers could be endless) can spur anxiety and stress, including real physical threats, job changes, hormonal changes, medications, financial problems, marital woes, illness, grief, and withdrawal from caffeine, alcohol, tobacco, sedatives, narcotics, or other addictive drugs.

how food may help

Because anxiety and stress can often overstimulate nerves and cause muscles to be tight and tense, it may be helpful to eat foods rich in **calcium** and **magnesium,** two minerals that work together to help regulate nerve conduction and muscle contraction.

Dietary support from **complex carbohydrates,** which are found in most "comfort foods," is another nutritional defense against stress and anxiety. The amino acid **tryptophan** is instrumental in the manufacture of serotonin, a mood-enhancing neurotransmitter that will help you to relax and feel more calm.

Complex carbohydrates not only ensure proper absorption of trypto-phan but they also may dampen the stress response by elevating levels of serotonin.

A number of B vitamins help to release energy from carbohydrates, maintain proper nervous system function, and control glucose lev-els—all of which are useful during stress and anxiety. Specifically, **vitamin B$_6$** assists in the manufacture of brain chemicals—such as serotonin, dopamine, and melatonin—that control mood.

Because stress can create temporary high blood pressure by trig-gering the release of certain hormones, it would be wise to con-sume foods that can combat high blood pressure (see *page 180*). As another side effect of anxiety and stress, the body can experience gastrointestinal woes such as diarrhea (see *page 166*).

Also important are immune-building foods rich in **vitamin C** and **zinc**, whose substances may fight off viruses (the common cold and flu) brought on by the body's weakened state due to stress. Cold sores, too, are frequent companions of stress; see page 156 for some dietary advice that can help you evade and/or manage them.

recent research

A small study recently showed that a vegetarian diet may be linked with reduced anxiety and depression levels. The study participants were divided into two groups, 40 vegetarians and 40 non-vegetarians. Diet analysis of the two groups showed that the vegetarian group consumed more antioxidant-rich foods than did the nonvegetarian group.

Psychological tests were administered to both groups to determine differences in anxiety and depression between both groups. Interestingly, significantly more anxiety and depression were reported in the nonvegetarian group. Authors of the study speculate that the higher level of antioxidants in the vegetarian group may account for this finding.

your food arsenal

foods	nutrient	health benefits
broccoli cooking greens dairy products figs	calcium	Calcium is vital for normal communication between nerve cells and for muscle contraction.
beans potatoes rice whole grains	complex carbohydrates	Eating foods that are high in complex carbohy-drates along with foods high in tryptophan (see below) will help facilitate the proper absorption of the tryptophan.
amaranth avocados sunflower seeds wheat germ	magnesium	Magnesium helps relax muscles.
bananas dairy products peas poultry turnips	tryptophan	The brain uses tryptophan to help produce sero-tonin, a mood-enhancing neurotransmitter.
bananas potatoes salmon	vitamin B$_6$	Vitamin B$_6$ assists in the production of brain chemicals, such as serotonin, which help the body cope with anxiety and stress.

bronchitis

what it is

Bronchitis is swelling and inflammation of the lining of the bronchial tubes of the lungs, caused by an infection or an irritant. This results in narrowed airways, making breathing difficult. Irritation can damage the cells lining the airways. It can also destroy tiny cilia, protective "hairs" that normally trap and sweep away foreign matter; damage to the cilia sets up an environment wherein an accumulation of irritants creates excess mucus, resulting in a heavy, deep cough, shortness of breath, and wheezing.

There are two forms of bronchitis, acute and chronic. Acute bronchitis is more common and it often follows a severe cold or flu (see *Colds & Flu, page 158*), though it can also be triggered by environmental pollutants or a bacterial infection. Though not considered a serious health threat to most people, acute bronchitis may be more dangerous for the very young, the elderly, or for people with a suppressed immune system or who suffer from certain conditions such as heart disease or pulmonary disorders such as asthma.

Bronchitis is termed "chronic bronchitis" when symptoms such as excessive mucus production, coughing, and wheezing are experienced regularly for a long period of time (coughing up phlegm most days for at least three months of the year for at least two years in a row). Chronic bronchitis is principally a disease of smokers, and is a potentially life-threatening disease that causes progressive and permanent damage to the lungs. Pneumonia is another complication associated with chronic bronchitis.

what causes it

Smoking is a primary offender and is believed to be responsible for a majority (80 to 90%) of chronic bronchitis cases. Viral infections such as the flu and the common cold, as well as bacterial infections, can also lead to bronchitis. Other factors that may contribute to bronchitis include exposure to chemical fumes, aerosol products (such as hair sprays, deodorants, and insecticides), dust, smog, and other environmental pollutants.

how food may help

Along with quitting smoking, a diet that includes plenty of fruit, vegetables, and fish may help to protect your lungs from free-radical damage. The inflammatory nature of acute bronchitis may be ameliorated by **omega-3 fatty acids,** which are thought to reduce the production of inflammatory compounds. Though scientific evidence is scarce, alternative practitioners feel that **bromelain,** an enzyme found in pineapples, also reduces inflammation in the airways.

Certain foods contain substances that help to protect your lungs from destructive environmental pollutants. For example, **vitamin C**-rich foods may offer antioxidant protection against free radicals in smog and cigarette smoke.

Fundamental for maintaining optimum health, vitamin C may also maintain a robust immune system to help fight off colds and viruses, which are often implicated in the onset of bronchitis. The mineral **zinc** is also instrumental in maintaining the immune system's defenses.

Preliminary studies indicate that the flavonoid **naringin,** found in white grapefruit, appears to shield the lungs from environmental toxins. Foods rich in **vitamin E** may also prevent oxidative damage to the lungs.

recent research

Numerous studies reveal a beneficial association between fruit and vegetable intake and lung function. Results from a large cross-sectional study carried out in 69 counties in rural China indicate that participants who consume foods rich in vitamin C had better lung function and, consequently, a lower risk for developing pulmonary diseases such as bronchitis than those participants with lower intakes of vitamin C.

Interestingly, study participants consumed about 50% more vitamin C per day than the average American. The authors suggest that the antioxidant properties of vitamin C may protect the lungs from free-radical damage.

your food arsenal

foods	nutrient	health benefits
fatty fish **shellfish**	omega-3 fatty acids	Since bronchitis is an inflammatory disorder, consuming foods rich in omega-3 fatty acids may help to protect lungs by lowering the body's production of inflammatory substances.
citrus fruit **kiwifruit** **pineapple** **strawberries**	vitamin C	The antioxidant properties of vitamin C may help to shield the lungs from free radicals produced by environmental pollutants such as smog and cigarette smoke. Further, vitamin C may help your immune system fight off colds and viruses, which often precede bronchitis.
beans **poultry** **pumpkin seeds** **shellfish**	zinc	The immune-enhancing ability of zinc may protect against viruses that cause colds and flu, which often trigger acute bronchitis.

cancer

what it is

Cancer is a group of more than 100 related diseases caused by an abnormal proliferation of cells that divide continuously. This unregulated cell growth may spread and invade normal tissue, creating malignancy, which can invade surrounding tissues and may spread further. Cancer can strike at any age and can develop in any part of the body. After cardiovascular disease, cancer is the second leading cause of death in the United States.

The good news is that many types of cancer are highly preventable, and with early detection, a great number can be successfully treated. You can reduce your risk for developing cancer through proper medical screening, awareness of symptoms and risk factors, regular self-examination, and a healthy diet and lifestyle. Poor lifestyle decisions may play a substantial role in many cancer cases; the National Cancer Institute estimates that at least 35% of all cancers have a nutritional connection.

what causes it

The development and progression of cancer is a complex, multistep process. Cancer often takes years to develop, and is thought to occur as a result of a combination of factors, including heredity, genetic damage, environment, lifestyle, and diet. The immune system's inability to repair damage caused by outside forces such as cigarette smoke, chemicals, asbestos, radiation (X rays and ultraviolet sunlight), smog and other environmental carcinogens, as well as excessive alcohol consumption, can cause normal cells to mutate into precancerous cells. These cells, in turn, may or may not become cancer cells. Repeated exposure to free radicals can cause basic cellular damage and may induce the onset of cancer.

how food may help

Even if you do have some of the risk factors associated with the development of cancer, you can start to tip the odds in your favor by selecting healthful foods (as well as quitting cigarette smoking and starting an exercise program). First and foremost, you should reduce dietary fat. Studies show a reduced incidence of cancer among people who eat a diet that is low in fat. Replacing saturated fats with **monounsaturated fats** such as olive oil can also protect against cancer and other life-threatening conditions; and preliminary research indicates that **omega-3 fatty acids** may provide protective effects against breast, colon, and prostate cancers by stopping cancer cell growth.

Many other compounds in foods are also under scientific scrutiny for their potential either to prevent the onset of cancer or to prevent cancerous tumors from growing. It is thought that one piece of fruit, for example, could contain *hundreds* of potentially beneficial phytochemicals. Clearly, the best way to ensure that you are benefitting from a diverse array of cancer-fighting nutrients and phytochemicals is simply to consume a large variety of fruits and vegetables.

your food arsenal

foods	nutrient	health benefits
garlic **onion family**	allium compounds	These compounds, also known as sulfur compounds, may stimulate the immune system's natural defenses against cancer, and they may have the potential to reduce tumor growth.
apples **berries** **cherries** **red grapes & wine**	anthocyanins	Anthocyanins, plant pigments classed as flavonoids, may have antioxidant potential to reduce the risk for developing cancer by neutralizing free radicals.
apricots **carrots** **sweet potatoes**	beta-carotene	Studies suggest that this carotenoid may function as a powerful antioxidant and protect cells from free-radical damage.
dark chocolate **green tea** **pomegranates**	catechins	Green tea contains EGCG, a catechin that may help to fight cancer in three ways: It may reduce the formation of carcinogens in the body, increase the body's natural defenses, and suppress cancer promotion.
apples **berries** **broccoli** **citrus fruits** **onion family**	flavonoids	Many flavonoids act as antioxidants, and some have several other biological anticancer effects, mostly related to altering enzymes of metabolism and cell growth. Flavonoids are also thought to prevent DNA damage to cells.
asparagus **beets** **lentils**	folate	This B vitamin is crucial for normal DNA synthesis and repair; low levels of folate are thought to make cells vulnerable to carcinogenesis.

continued on next page

your food arsenal

foods	nutrient	health benefits
broccoli **brussels sprouts** **cabbage**	glucosinolates	Glucosinolates are transformed into a variety of protective substances, which enhance the immune system's defenses and help to block cancer-promoting enzymes.
apricots **pink & red grapefruit** **tomatoes** **watermelon**	lycopene	As an antioxidant, lycopene may detect and destroy harmful free radical molecules. Lycopene is thought to help protect against prostate cancer.
avocados **olives/olive oil** **peanuts/peanut oil** **walnuts**	monounsaturated fat	Monounsaturated fat may protect against breast and colon cancer, though how it works is currently unknown and under review.
apples **berries** **green tea** **pomegranates** **turmeric**	phenolic acids	Phenolic acids are a subgroup of plant polyphenols that may have the ability to destroy free radicals as well as activate cancer-fighting enzymes in the body, which can help to reduce tumors early in the cancer process.
flaxseed **legumes** **pomegranates** **soy foods**	phytoestrogens	Phytoestrogens help to block estrogen by attaching themselves to places (receptor sites) where natural estrogen wants to lodge, thus lowering estrogen levels and reducing the risk of developing hormone-related cancers (breast, uterine, as well as prostate).
peanuts **red & purple grapes** **red wine**	resveratrol	Resveratrol may help fight cancer at three different stages: cancer initiation, promotion, and progression.
Brazil nuts **mackerel** **mushrooms** **shellfish**	selenium	Studies suggest that this mineral may help to prevent lung, prostate, and colon cancer, possibly through its antioxidant abilities, though other actions are under review.
broccoli **cabbage family** **cooking greens**	sulforaphane	This powerful isothiocyanate is thought to activate detoxifying enzymes in the body that fight off cancer, and it also may destroy precancerous cells and block carcinogens.
bell peppers **broccoli** **citrus fruits**	vitamin C	Vitamin C may help to prevent cancer cell division and growth, and it also may inhibit carcinogenic nitrosamines.
nuts **olive oil** **sunflower seeds** **super grains**	vitamin E	Antioxidant protection provided by vitamin E may help to guard cells against free radicals. Vitamin E may also play a role in stimulating the immune system's response to cellular changes.

Antioxidant Vitamins and Trace Minerals: Free-radical molecules are produced in the body by cellular reactions between oxygen and glucose. They can also be generated from environmental sources (cigarette smoke, radiation, and smog) and can cause direct damage to cells. This free-radical damage can set off the initiation of the cancer process. Nutrients that behave as antioxidants neutralize free radicals, thus helping to prevent cells from becoming cancerous. Some of the principal antioxidant nutrients include **vitamin C, vitamin E,** and the trace mineral **selenium.**

Carotenoids: These plant pigments may help the body's immune system defend against harmful free radicals. Carotenoids are also thought to interrupt the process of uncontrolled abnormal division typical of cancer cells. Studies show that some carotenoids may help to stimulate the immune system's natural killer (NK) cell activity. Natural killer cells attack and neutralize cancer cells. Two carotenoids under review for their cancer-fighting abilities include **beta-carotene** and **lycopene.**

Flavonoids: A large class of phytochemicals (there are thousands of flavonoids), flavonoids can be broken down into numerous categories. Each type of flavonoid functions in a different way, with many flavonoids acting as antioxidants. Flavonoids may also improve the absorption of **vitamin C,** an important antioxidant vitamin. Key flavonoid categories that have been studied for their potential to combat cancer include **anthocyanins, citrus flavonoids, quercetin, isoflavones** (in soy), and **catechins** (in tea).

Glucosinolates: Natural chemicals found in cruciferous vegetables, such as broccoli and cabbage, glucosinolates are precursors for some potentially vigorous cancer fighters such as **indoles** and **isothiocyanates.** Glucosinolate derivatives are thought to enhance the body's own defenses against cancer.

Phenolic Acids: These compounds may have the ability to destroy free radicals as well as activate cancer-fighting enzymes in the body, and they may also have the ability to block the formation of carcinogens such as nitrosamines in cigarette smoke and cured meats. Notable phenolic acids that may help to battle cancer are **curcumin** and **caffeic, chlorogenic, ferulic,** and **ellagic acids.**

Phytoestrogens: Often referred to as "plant estrogens," phytoestrogens are plant chemicals that are thought to block estrogens. High levels of estrogen are linked to certain hormone-related types of cancer. There are two main types of phytoestrogens—**isoflavones** such as **genistein** in soy foods and **lignans** in flaxseeds, rye, and sesame seeds.

Sulfur Compounds: Also known as **allium compounds,** sulfur compounds impart pungency to garlic, onions, leeks, chives, and shallots. Sulfur compounds may help to enhance the immune system, inhibit the growth of cancer cells, and may also prevent the formation of nitrosamines, dangerous carcinogens found in cigarette smoke and cured meat.

recent research

Carcinogenic compounds called heterocyclic aromatic amines (HAA) are formed when meat, fish, or chicken are grilled or broiled directly over an open fire.

Animal studies indicate that adding garlic or even cherries to grilled meat, fish, and chicken helps to reduce levels of these carcinogens. Dietary vitamin E as well as the herb rosemary may also help to reduce levels of these cancer-causing substances.

You can also limit the production of HAAs by frequently turning the foods being cooked on the grill. This allows the food enough time to cook through, but reduces the amount of time the surfaces of the food are in direct contact with the grill's open flame.

cataracts

what it is

The leading cause of impaired vision in the United States, cataracts afflict almost 5 million people. The development of cataracts is a gradual, age-related eye disorder that causes the lens of the eye to lose transparency, which impairs vision. When normal proteins in the eye become damaged, they cluster together and become opaque, a process that creates a cloudy area in the lens that over time causes blurry and distorted vision. So common is this condition that it is estimated that more than half of all Americans over age 65 have some degree of cataract formation. The good news is that cataracts are treatable and probably more preventable than previously believed.

what causes it

Researchers feel that chronic free-radical damage may be associated with cataract development. Thought to be the cause of a number of age-related conditions, free-radical damage can result from a lifetime of exposure to sunlight's harmful ultraviolet (UV) rays, cigarette smoke, pollution and other environmental factors. In the case of the eye, free-radical damage can weaken the delicate cell structure in the lens of the eye, which slowly causes development of cataracts. Because most cataracts are age-related, preventive strategies adopted early on may help to delay or avoid them. Diabetes can also cause the development of cataracts.

how food may help

In addition to various lifestyle changes you can make to reduce free-radical damage, such as wearing sunglasses that block UV rays and stopping smoking, certain dietary adjustments can be made that may be beneficial, including consuming a diet rich in fiber and antioxidants. Foods that are high in antioxidants play a significant role in combatting the damage caused by free radicals.

Because **vitamin C** is a potent antioxidant, consuming foods that are high in this nutrient may help protect against cataracts. Studies also show that vitamin C may play a role in preventing the clustering of proteins in the eye, a process associated with cataract formation.

Working hand-in-hand with other important nutrients, such as the mineral selenium, **vitamin E** functions as a powerful antioxidant by shielding cell membranes from harm caused by sunlight. It also protects the vitamin A found in the eye from UV damage.

Although the relationship between **lutein** and cataracts is still under investigation, studies suggest that this carotenoid may act like internal sunglasses by filtering out the sun's harmful ultraviolet rays. Lutein is the yellow substance found inside the macula lutea (the tiny yellow spot in the center of the retina). Lutein absorbs sunlight's harmful waves, thus blocking damage to the delicate structure of the cells in the eyes. A closely related carotenoid compound, **zeaxanthin,** is also thought to defend the lens from free-radical harm incurred from sunlight.

Preliminary research also indicates that **quercetin,** a flavonoid found in a number of foods, may protect against cataracts. Studies suggest that quercetin helps to maintain lens transparency after free-radical damage from sunlight.

Foods rich in **fiber,** such as whole grains, may help prevent onset of diabetes, which can cause cataracts.

recent research

Curcumin, a substance in turmeric (a spice used in Indian curry dishes), may be an effective antioxidant that helps to protect against cataracts. Animal studies show curcumin may protect the lens of the eye from becoming cloudy.

Scientists are still determining the precise mechanisms by which curcumin can protect against cataracts. One theory suggests that curcumin enhances glutathione, a potent antioxidant. Another conjecture is that curcumin's antioxidant power protects the eyes from cell damage caused by sunlight's ultraviolet rays.

your food arsenal

foods	nutrient	health benefits
corn **kale** **kiwifruit** **peas** **spinach**	lutein & zeaxanthin	Lutein may protect the eye from sunlight's dangerous ultraviolet rays by filtering out the light waves that destroy cells in the eye's lens. Zeaxanthin provides antioxidant protection by shielding against free-radical damage.
apples **cherries** **red onions**	quercetin	Quercetin may help to protect eyes even after they have been exposed to sunlight's harmful rays.
bell peppers **broccoli** **citrus fruit** **strawberries**	vitamin C	Vitamin C may play a role in preventing the clumping of proteins in the eye, which is linked to cataract formation.
almonds **avocados** **sardines** **sunflower seeds** **wheat germ**	vitamin E	Some studies suggest that vitamin E's antioxidant activities may help prevent cataract formation.

chronic fatigue syndrome

what it is

This elusive condition is characterized by so many different symptoms that it is often very difficult to diagnose. Many other illnesses have symptoms that mimic those of Chronic Fatigue Syndrome (CFS), and for this reason, your health care practitioner will have to rule out other illnesses and other possible causes of fatigue, such as anemia, depression, fibromyalgia, infection, diabetes, heart disease, thyroid disease, and cancer. Overwhelming and persistent fatigue is the overriding primary symptom of CFS, which is defined as extreme fatigue and malaise not improved with bed rest. Symptoms often last for at least six months and interfere significantly with daily living.

what causes it

The cause of CFS is currently unknown and, as such, is a conundrum to health care practitioners. Numerous medical theories abound, including proposals that CFS is linked with infections such as Epstein-Barr virus (the virus that also causes mononucleosis), allergies, Lyme disease, impaired metabolic function, low blood pressure, adrenal gland dysfunction, immune abnormalities, neurological disturbances, rheumatic diseases, disorders of the central nervous system, autoimmune disorders, hormonal problems, and certain medications. Although no single virus has been implicated, many patients with CFS nonetheless report having had a flulike illness that triggered the symptoms. There is no evidence that CFS is contagious.

how food may help

Although there is no known cure for this ailment, certain nutrients in foods may help to improve symptoms. Some of the symptoms of CFS include swollen glands, inflammation of the joints, and other flulike symptoms, all of which may be relieved temporarily by foods rich in **essential fatty acids (EFAs).** EFAs may help to block release of inflammatory substances in your body. It is thought that there may be an abnormality in essential fatty acid metabolism in some people with chronic fatigue syndrome. Note, too, that a particular type of EFA, **omega-3 fatty acids,** may also help to fight off depression, which often accompanies CFS.

Because **vitamin B$_{12}$** deficiency is associated with fatigue and depression, it's possible that consuming foods rich in this vitamin could help to minimize the fatigue and depression of CFS. Other B vitamins, such as **thiamin, B$_6$,** and **riboflavin,** are instrumental in fighting fatigue by assisting the body in energy production.

For many people, CFS occurs directly after they have fallen ill from a cold, the flu, or an intestinal infection. Therefore, consume foods rich in **vitamin C,** which help to fortify a weakened immune system (believed by many to be a factor in CFS). **Zinc** promotes the destruction of foreign microorganisms and hinders the growth of viruses such as the common cold (see also *Colds & Flu, page 158*), and also helps to enhance and repair the immune system.

Since a number of people with CFS experience headaches and muscle aches, foods rich in **magnesium** are helpful. To combat the accompanying insomnia that plagues many people with CFS, it may be helpful to eat foods rich in the amino acid **tryptophan,** which is converted by your body into the brain chemical serotonin. Note that **carbohydrate**-rich meals often help to increase serotonin levels.

recent research

While people may attribute the onset of CFS to factors such as stress, according to a recent consensus panel meeting at the Centers for Disease Control and Prevention and the Chronic Fatigue and Immune Dysfunction Syndrome (CFIDS) Association of America, stress does not cause Chronic Fatigue Syndrome. It is noteworthy, though, that the panelists stated there is quite a bit of evidence showing that stress can exacerbate existing CFS. Though they also concede that the jury is still out regarding a specific cause, the experts propose that it's probable that an infection could trigger the onset of CFS.

your food arsenal

foods	nutrient	health benefits
amaranth, avocados, quinoa, sunflower seeds	magnesium	Magnesium plays a role in the production and transport of energy and it also assists in the contraction and relaxation of muscles, an important function since people with chronic fatigue syndrome often experience muscle tenderness.
bananas, dairy products, peas, poultry	tryptophan	Though one of the main symptoms of CFS is fatigue, many people suffering from this condition also have trouble sleeping and experience bouts of insomnia. Tryptophan is converted to serotonin, which helps to make you feel relaxed and sleepy. Note that eating foods high in complex carbohydrates will help in the proper absorption of tryptophan.
beans, cashews, clams, poultry, pumpkin seeds	zinc	Foods rich in the mineral zinc may help to keep the immune system working properly. A robust immune system can help to ward off certain viruses, such as the common cold and flu, conditions that may possibly precede the onset of CFS.

cold sores

what it is

Cold sores, also called fever blisters, are painful, sensitive infections that appear on the lips, the outside of the mouth, and occasionally inside or on the nose. Most people have experienced these uncomfortable blisters, and in fact 90% of all people develop at least one cold sore in their lifetime. Often preceded by a burning, pulsating, itching sensation, a small fluid-filled sore will emerge. Within a day or so, the sore ruptures and a scab forms.

Once you have had a cold sore, the virus that causes it remains with you for the rest of your life. It lies dormant in nerve cells and may re-emerge for a variety of reasons, perhaps when the immune system is depressed or when you are under a lot of stress or don't get enough sleep. For most people who have recurrent cold sores, subsequent sores will appear in the same location as the initial sore and will be less painful. Some people are more prone to getting cold sores, and while almost everyone has had the virus, only some people actually experience symptoms. Cold sores generally last for a week to 10 days.

what causes it

Researchers believe that cold sores are most likely caused by the Herpes Simplex Virus Type 1 (not to be confused with Herpes Simplex Virus Type 2, which causes sexually transmitted genital herpes). It is thought that the virus that causes cold sores may be spread by touch from lip sores to other parts of the body, primarily the mucous membranes of the eyes, nose, and, though rare, the genital areas. Careful hand washing, and avoidance of kissing when the sore is in its early stage, are important in preventing its spread. Once it has scabbed over, the cold sore is less contagious.

Certain factors can trigger cold sores, such as being run-down, ultra-violet radiation (too much exposure to the sun), hormonal changes such as menstruation, some medications that reduce your immune system's effectiveness, infections, and emotional stress. Dietary measures can help bolster your immune system's defenses; this is important for the possible prevention and control of cold sores.

how food may help

Some health care providers theorize that a diet high in **lysine** may reduce the recurrence of cold sores. Lysine is an amino acid that is thought to combat the onset of cold sores (or reduce the duration of them) by interfering with the absorption of arginine, an amino acid that is suspected of being necessary for the herpes virus to replicate. So, along with eating foods high in lysine, you should also try to avoid foods that contain arginine (see *Foods to Avoid,* right).

Preliminary studies suggest that antiviral substances found in **garlic** may be effective in preventing cold sores.

Another nutritional strategy to combat and manage cold sores is to regularly eat foods that maintain a strong immune system. Foods rich in **vitamin C** and **zinc** possess antioxidant powers that increase the immune system's ability to help fight off the virus that causes cold sores. Cold sores tend to occur when the body is under stress, which can compromise your immune system (see *Anxiety & Stress, page 144,* for dietary advice).

foods to avoid

Try to stay away from chocolate, peanuts, almonds, seeds, cereal grains, gelatin, carob, beer, and raisins. These foods have an unfavorable arginine-to-lysine ratio, which may make you more susceptible to experiencing a recurrence of cold sores. Some research suggests that arginine-rich foods have specific biochemical actions and proteins that trigger the onset of cold sores.

foods	nutrient	health benefits
chicken dairy eggs turkey	lysine	Lysine is an amino acid that may interfere with the absorption of arginine in the intestine, thus preventing the onset of cold sores.
berries citrus fruits kiwifruit melons	vitamin C	A vital nutrient for the body's healing process, vitamin C is also involved in the production of antibodies and white blood cells, which work to ward off infections and viruses.
beans poultry shellfish whole grains	zinc	Zinc helps to maintain a strong immune system, so that it can destroy viruses, which often opportunistically attempt to strike when the body is run-down.

colds & flu

what it is

The common cold is something that we have all had, and its presence has plagued mankind from the beginning of time. And it has managed, to date, to elude a cure. The common cold is a highly contagious infection that often starts out as throat irritation and a stuffy nose, and culminates in red, watery eyes, sneezing, coughing, sore throat, runny nose, congestion, mild headache, and general fatigue and malaise. Colds rarely cause serious complications, with the exception of ear infections in children. Colds can, however, exacerbate asthma, and also cause lower respiratory tract infections such as bronchitis and pneumonia (especially in the elderly, who are often very susceptible to infection). A cold will generally subside after five to 10 days. Americans develop about two to four colds a year.

With an annual average of 20,000 deaths from complications of the flu (influenza) in this country, the flu virus is certainly more dangerous than the common cold. Flu symptoms include muscle aches, joint pain, high fever, fatigue, headache, sore throat, and sometimes a dry, nonproductive cough. Young children, infants, the elderly, and people with serious medical conditions or who are on immune-suppressing medications, are at increased risk for developing complications such as pneumonia and other respiratory infections.

what causes it

Colds and influenza, which are caused by different types of viruses, are both highly contagious: The viruses can be spread through the air and through contact with things such as telephones and doorknobs. Certain factors can predispose one to contracting either infection, including being run-down (immune defenses aren't working efficiently), having an illness, experiencing prolonged stress, being exposed to cigarette smoke, smog, and other environmental pollutants that can damage the cilia (little hairlike structures that clear the airways) as well as inadequate or infrequent hand-washing.

how food may help

For both the common cold and the flu, drinking plenty of fluids, getting lots of rest, and eating nutritious foods are important keys to hastening recovery. Establishing a nourishing stockpile of protective foods can also be the main line of defense in the difficult task of preventing a cold or flu.

Luteolin, a flavonoid found in rosemary, sage, thyme, and artichokes, may act as a natural antihistamine by interfering with the release of histamine, a chemical pinpointed as one of the causes of congestion and other respiratory symptoms. Studies show that the flavonoid **quercetin** creates a similar result. Quercetin is also linked to optimal lung health.

To fight off viruses that cause these two illnesses, it is helpful to maintain a strong immune system. Folk medicine advocates the use of **garlic** to help prevent common respiratory infections, though there is currently little evidence to support this notion.

The immune-bolstering properties of **vitamin C** and **zinc** may help your body combat both the common cold as well as the flu. Vitamin C may also function as a natural antihistamine. Try to eat foods rich in the antioxidant mineral **selenium:** Preliminary studies indicate that selenium deficiency may prolong symptoms of the flu, including duration of the illness and lung inflammation.

If you already have caught one of these ailments, a bowl of chicken soup can offer some temporary comfort (see *Home Remedy,* right). And the fiery nature of certain foods, such as chili peppers, ginger, horseradish, and mustard, may offer immediate relief from nasal congestion by perking up the nasal passages and alleviating stuffiness.

home remedy

Though nothing will prevent the onset of a cold, rest assured that you can manage its uncomfortable symptoms with a hot, steaming bowl of good old-fashioned chicken soup. Recent research is confirming that chicken soup, a centuries-old home remedy (often dubbed "Jewish penicillin"), may actually have a scientific basis for its ability to offer relief.

Scientists speculate that about 1½ cups of the soup may reduce inflammation in the lungs, a common symptom of many respiratory ailments. Though the actual mechanism by which chicken soup does this has yet to be determined, it may be that chicken soup helps to slow down the activity of neutrophils, white blood cells that can create an accumulation of mucus in the lungs, causing congestion.

Researchers found that both commercial as well as homemade varieties of chicken soup can achieve the same anti-inflammatory effect. Also, inhaling the soothing steam from the soup can help to temporarily open up nasal passages.

your food arsenal		
foods	**nutrient**	**health benefits**
apples **berries** **plums & prunes** **red onions**	quercetin	Some research indicates that this flavonoid may relieve congestion by reducing the release of histamine, which is associated with runny nose, congestion, and watery eyes.
citrus fruit **kiwifruit** **peppers** **strawberries**	vitamin C	Although it will not cure the common cold or influenza, vitamin C, by maintaining a strong immune system, may prevent the onset of these viruses, and it may also reduce the duration of symptoms.
beef **cashews** **chicken**	zinc	There is some evidence that zinc may reduce the severity of symptoms and shorten the duration of the common cold.

constipation

what it is

Constipation is typified by infrequent or difficult bowel movements and hard, dry stools. Hard stools often are a result of excess absorption of water in the intestines. This can happen because the muscle of the colon contracts too slowly, causing the stool to pass through too slowly. Drinking lots of water is important in helping to move stool through the colon. Symptoms of constipation are often accompanied by bloating, abdominal distension, straining, and a feeling of incomplete evacuation. Hemorrhoids can result from the pressure of excessive straining.

The frequency of bowel movements among people varies greatly, ranging from three movements a day to three a week. Generally, fewer than three bowel movements a week indicate constipation. A common misconception about constipation is that a bowel movement every day is necessary. Contrary to common belief, frequency is of less importance than the degree of discomfort associated with bowel movements or the absence of an urge to have one. Constipation and irregularity are common, particularly in older adults and children.

what causes it

Numerous factors are linked to constipation. Excluding causes that are associated with specific diseases, the most common causes of constipation include a hereditary component, lack of exercise, certain types of medication, emotional stress, a diet high in animal fats and processed foods, not eating enough foods high in fiber, and not drinking enough water. Poor bowel habits, such as ignoring the urge to have a bowel movement, can cause constipation. Overuse of enemas as well as laxatives can, over time, interfere with the colon's natural ability to contract. Psychological issues are sometimes the cause of constipation in children. Not surprisingly, constipation is one of the most frequently reported gastrointestinal complaints in this country.

how food may help

There are two types of dietary fiber, insoluble and soluble. Often called "roughage," **insoluble fiber** is particularly effective in promoting regular bowel movements by adding bulk and providing mass to the stool. Insoluble fiber also helps to move the waste through your colon, and eases elimination. **Soluble fiber** can help to soften stools by acting as a gel in the intestine, where it helps to increase water content. Both types of dietary fiber are useful for management of constipation. Dried fruit, such as dried apricots, figs, prunes, and pears, are especially rich in fiber as well as other beneficial nutrients.

High-fat and processed foods are typically fiber-poor. Eating too many of them can contribute to constipation by filling you up without providing the gastrointestinal benefits of fiber. When picking high-fiber foods, choose those that are nutritionally rich in other nourishing compounds: Good choices are dried fruit, peas, beans, lentils, broccoli, and sweet potatoes.

As many high-fiber foods tend to produce bloating and gas, it may be a good idea to increase your consumption of these foods gradually so that your system can adjust to the added fiber. Be sure to drink a lot of water to prevent your digestive system from slowing down.

Foods rich in **magnesium** may also offer some relief. Magnesium is thought to have mild laxative properties.

Prune juice and prunes (and their fresh form, plums) are particularly beneficial in coping with constipation. They are not only rich in both types of fiber but they also contain **sorbitol**—a natural type of sugar that stimulates the digestive system. It may also have a laxative effect.

home remedy

Drinking a hot beverage first thing in the morning is a useful home remedy for constipation. Herbal or decaffeinated tea or hot water with a little lemon juice and honey may be of some help; apparently, the hot liquid stimulates the bowels.

your food arsenal

foods	nutrient	health benefits
broccoli **cabbage family** **flaxseed** **sweet potatoes**	insoluble fiber	Insoluble fiber (often called "roughage") is particularly useful in promoting regular bowel movements by adding bulk and providing mass to the stool, helping to move the waste through the colon, and easing elimination.
apricots **beans** **figs** **plums & prunes**	soluble fiber	Soluble fiber can help to soften stools due to its ability to act as a gel in the intestine, where it helps to increase water content.

depression

recipe rx

what it is

Depression is a common mood disorder that strikes millions of Americans. An all-encompassing illness affecting body, mood, and thought, depression is a treatable condition that often goes untreated. Symptoms of depression include an oppressive feeling of despair and despondency that simply will not go away. Other symptoms that occur are a sense of hopelessness, feelings of guilt, low energy, difficulty concentrating, restlessness, sleep disturbances (such as insomnia or too much sleep), emptiness, negative and sad thoughts, difficulty maintaining normal relationships, as well as a general lack of interest in life. Proper treatment can offer relief for most people who suffer from this potentially debilitating condition.

what causes it

Many factors are linked to depression. They include hereditary, biological, and environmental factors, and significant life events, such as physical illness, the loss of a loved one, or the loss of a job. Also linked to depression are certain medications, alcohol or drug abuse, diet, and having had a baby (as well as other hormonal fluctuations). The biological causes of depression may be attributed to disturbances in neurotransmitters, chemical messengers in the brain, though much about the biochemical causes has yet to be learned.

how food may help

Certain nutrients may have a beneficial effect on the brain chemicals that are responsible for mood. For example, researchers believe that the essential amino acid **tryptophan** may play an important role in normal brain function because it helps produce the neurotransmitter serotonin, which may help to reduce feelings of depression.

Depressed people sometimes turn to foods rich in **complex carbohydrates** (found in "comfort foods"), which are thought to also have a favorable effect on the production of serotonin. Foods high in complex carbohydrates also help the body absorb tryptophan efficiently.

You can also fight the blues by eating foods high in B vitamins. **Folate** is an important B vitamin that is sometimes deficient in people who are depressed. Preliminary research shows that depressed people may have abnormalities in **vitamin B$_{12}$** status as well. A link may exist between low levels of vitamin B$_{12}$ and folate and impaired metabolism of the brain chemicals associated with mood regulation.

Vitamin B$_{12}$ works with folate and **vitamin B$_6$** to help reduce homocysteine, an amino acid linked to depression. Vitamin B$_{12}$ helps to convert homocysteine into other substances, thus preventing a buildup of homocysteine in the bloodstream. Vitamin B$_6$ may also assist in the manufacture of enzymes responsible for the metabolism of certain mood-regulating brain chemicals such as serotonin and dopamine.

Omega-3 fatty acids, which are lacking in most people's diets in the United States, are abundantly present in the brain and are essential for normal brain function. Though little is currently known about how omega-3 fatty acids regulate mood, recent findings show a correlation between low levels of these compounds and depression.

recent research

A recent study indicates that omega-3 fatty acids may help to reduce symptoms of depression. Thirty patients suffering from manic depression (bipolar depression) were administered either a placebo (olive oil) or omega-3 fatty acids (plant or marine sources, such as fish oil), in conjunction with their regular treatment, for four months.

The group receiving omega-3 fatty acids experienced fewer relapses as compared with the group receiving the placebos. Interestingly, the study was brought to a premature conclusion because the benefits of the omega-3 fatty acid treatment were so marked that the researchers felt it was unethical to deny the same benefits to patients taking the placebos.

your food arsenal

foods	nutrient	health benefits
asparagus lentils peas salad greens	folate	There may be a link between folate deficiency and impaired metabolism of brain chemicals associated with mood regulation.
fatty fish shellfish	omega-3 fatty acids	These fats are vital for optimum brain functioning and are linked to a reduced incidence of depression.
bananas dairy products peas poultry	tryptophan	Tryptophan is a precursor of serotonin, a neurotransmitter in the brain that has been shown to be involved in reducing depression.
dairy products fatty fish poultry shellfish	vitamin B$_{12}$	Deficiency in this vitamin has been linked to depression.
bananas peas potatoes	vitamin B$_6$	This B vitamin helps in the manufacture of enzymes responsible for the metabolism of certain mood-regulating nerve chemicals.

diabetes

what it is

Diabetes is characterized by high levels of glucose (a simple sugar that all cells require for energy) in the blood, the result of an impairment in the secretion and/or the action of insulin (the hormone required to utilize glucose). There are two forms of diabetes, Type 1 and Type 2. Type 2 is the more prevalent form of diabetes and is responsible for about 90% of cases. As opposed to Type 1 diabetes, which is usually diagnosed in childhood or adolescence, Type 2 diabetes generally afflicts adults; hence, it is also referred to as adult-onset diabetes. Type 2 diabetes develops gradually and usually affects people over the age of 40 who tend to be obese. Symptoms of diabetes mellitus (the full name of both types of the disease) include frequent and excessive urination, excessive thirst, weight loss, fatigue, and increased hunger, as well as recurring infections, such as urinary tract and vaginal yeast infections. Complications associated with either type of diabetes include cardiovascular disease, nerve damage, vision loss, and kidney disease.

what causes it

Diabetes is a complex disorder, the cause of which is not clearly understood, though genetic factors may play a role in both types of diabetes. In Type 2 diabetes, in addition to a genetic component, metabolic disturbances and obesity have both been implicated in its onset. Numerous studies show that obesity not only promotes the development of diabetes but it also furthers the progression of heart disease. Pregnant women can develop gestational diabetes, placing them at higher risk for developing diabetes later in life. In the less common form of diabetes, Type 1, the immune system mistakenly attacks the body's insulin-producing cells, resulting in insulin deficiency.

how food may help

Before embarking on any type of nutritional plan, people with diabetes need to carefully review any dietary decisions with their health-care provider. Each person's diet needs to be individually tailored to accommodate insulin needs.

Foods high in **complex carbohydrates** tend to be digested at a rate that allows glucose to be released gradually into the bloodstream, which helps in maintaining normal glucose levels.

The importance of **dietary fiber** lies in its ability to slow the absorption of glucose and promote satiety (feeling full), which is helpful for weight loss. **Soluble fiber** also helps to decrease serum cholesterol levels, which is important since many people with diabetes are at an increased risk for developing coronary vascular disease.

Researchers speculate that a low serum **magnesium** level may possibly be a predictor of Type 2 diabetes. Note that foods rich in magnesium, such as rice and whole grains, tend also to be rich in fiber.

Eating heart-healthy foods such as those rich in **monounsaturated fat** is also helpful, particularly when they replace artery-clogging saturated fats.

Because people with diabetes often suffer from vascular problems, a **vitamin C**-rich diet will help to protect veins and connective tissues. Vitamin C also acts as an antioxidant, which is important because some studies show that free-radical oxidation may play a role in the damage to tissues caused by diabetes.

recent research

A recent study shows that dietary fiber may help to lower glucose levels in people with Type 2 diabetes. Researchers studied the effects of two types of diets on 13 patients with Type 2 diabetes. Each participant was administered a diet containing a moderate amount of fiber (8g of soluble fiber and 16g of insoluble) for six weeks, followed by a high-fiber diet (25g of soluble fiber and 25g of insoluble fiber) for another six weeks. The researchers compared the effects of both diets and found that for patients with Type 2 diabetes, a high-fiber diet helps to stabilize blood sugar by slowing the absorption of glucose.

your food arsenal

foods	nutrient	health benefits
beans potatoes rice whole grains	complex carbohydrates	Complex carbohydrates are digested slowly and release glucose gradually into the bloodstream, helping to maintain normal glucose levels.
asparagus beans lentils	dietary fiber	Soluble fiber may help to decrease serum cholesterol levels as well as glucose levels, and it also helps to prevent weight gain.
amaranth brown rice sunflower seeds	magnesium	A low serum magnesium level may possibly be a predictor of Type 2 diabetes. Foods rich in magnesium tend also to be rich in fiber.
avocados canola oil nuts olive oil	monounsaturated fat	These beneficial fats may help to lower blood glucose levels and, when replacing saturated fats, are also helpful in managing heart disease and maintaining weight levels.
bell peppers broccoli citrus fruit	vitamin C	Vitamin C helps to protect connective tissues and veins; many people with diabetes suffer from vascular problems.

diarrhea

what it is

Something that we have all experienced at some time in our lives, diarrhea is typified by the frequent passage of unformed, usually watery stools. Often referred to as a "stomach flu" or "a bug," diarrhea can be extremely distressing, and is sometimes accompanied by abdominal pain and severe cramping. Extreme cases of diarrhea can cause dehydration.

If an infant or child develops diarrhea, a health care provider should be consulted since children are more vulnerable and tend to become weak and dehydrated. Also, the elderly and people with immune system disorders and other serious illnesses should receive professional care to manage diarrhea. For many people, however, most bouts of diarrhea are not dangerous, are self-limiting, and don't last more than three days. If you do experience symptoms of diarrhea for more than three days, you should contact your health care provider to determine if there is a more serious problem.

what causes it

The most common form of diarrhea is generally caused by consuming food or drinking water that has been contaminated with certain viruses, bacteria, or parasites (such as cryptosporidium). Foodborne bacteria (*E. coli*, salmonella, and listeria) are also often found in unpasteurized foods and on improperly cleaned cutting boards and utensils. Wash all cooking surfaces with hot soapy water when handling meat and poultry.

When traveling abroad, particularly in developing countries, be careful to drink carbonated bottled water and avoid unwashed fruit; otherwise you may develop what is known as "traveler's diarrhea," which is linked to consuming local water, ice, or raw foods that may contain bacteria or parasites.

Proper hygiene practices can help to prevent diarrhea linked to viruses and infections. Diarrhea can be caused by fecal contamination of hands or other objects, which can spread rapidly. Therefore, washing hands thoroughly is essential after using the bathroom or changing diapers. Teach and encourage children to maintain proper hygiene, especially before eating meals.

Other factors that can lead to diarrhea include lactose intolerance, stress, eating foods that contain sorbitol, certain medications, megadoses of vitamin C, or antacids containing magnesium. Inflammatory diarrhea (also called chronic diarrhea) is less common and is usually linked to medical conditions such as colitis, irritable bowel syndrome, and other gastrointestinal disorders.

how food may help

One of the most helpful dietary steps to take if you have diarrhea is to replace fluid loss: Drink lots of water. Though you may not feel hungry, try to eat small amounts of food throughout the day. If diarrhea is severe and you simply cannot bear to eat, at the very least, suck on ice chips and try to sip small amounts of clear liquids such as broth and sports drinks (or seltzer mixed with a small amount of sugar and salt).

Some bland **complex carbohydrate**-rich foods (mashed potatoes, dry toast, or rice) tend to be the least aggravating to the digestive system. Be sure to eat white rice and peeled potatoes, as the bran layers of brown rice and the potato skin contain insoluble fiber that can actually worsen diarrhea.

Foods containing the soluble fiber **pectin**, such as applesauce and bananas, are useful in helping to firm stools. These foods also slow down the transit time of waste in the colon. Bananas are a rich source of potassium, which is often lost in the excessive elimination of fluids.

If you are taking antibiotics, foods containing **probiotics** may help to replenish the healthful bacteria in your colon that are destroyed by the medication. The probiotics (healthful bacteria) in yogurt with "active or live cultures" may help to restore a normal balance of bacteria in the intestines.

foods to avoid

During a bout with diarrhea, avoid foods containing caffeine, which can exacerbate symptoms by stimulating colonic activity. Other foods that can make diarrhea worse are prunes, fruit and fruit juices, fatty foods, highly seasoned foods, and alcohol.

Avoid foods high in insoluble fiber (roughage) as they will not absorb excess water in the intestinal tract. Instead, because they are roughage, they will make diarrhea worse by stimulating the colon.

your food arsenal		
foods	nutrient	health benefits
potatoes, peeled white rice	complex carbohydrates	Foods high in complex carbohydrates tend to be bland and easily digested.
applesauce bananas	pectin	A type of soluble fiber that helps to absorb excess fluid in the digestive tract, pectin also slows down transit time in the digestive tract and adds bulk to stools.

eczema

what it is

An inflammatory, noncontagious skin condition, eczema causes itching, flaking, dryness, and often redness. Sometimes small blisters will form and when they burst, the surface of the skin may be left moist and irritated. Persistent scratching of the skin in affected areas can subsequently result in scaly, rough, and thickened patches. There are various forms of eczema, with atopic dermatitis being the most common (it is estimated that more than 15 million adults and children in the United States suffer from it). Eczema often appears in the folds of the skin where your limbs bend, such as elbows and knees, though it can also appear anywhere on the body. Scratching can worsen eczema and cause it to spread.

what causes it

Those with a family history of allergies to foods, pollen, dust mites, and animal dander are more susceptible to eczema. Disturbances in proper immune response (how the body reacts to irritating or infectious substances) may be a contributing factor: Many eczema sufferers have above-normal levels of histamine, a chemical in the body that triggers an allergic defense reaction in the skin (and resulting in inflammation) when it's released. Eczema, particularly atopic dermatitis, has also been associated with asthma and hayfever, though the exact relationship is unclear. Flare-ups of eczema are also linked to anxiety and stress (see *page 144* for dietary advice that may help with the management of stress), as well as extremes in weather. Those with dry skin are also more vulnerable to eczema outbreaks.

how food may help

One of the triggers (as well as a consequence) of eczema is dryness, which may, in part, be ameliorated by foods rich in beta-carotene, vitamin E, and essential fatty acids. **Vitamin A** appears to have a favorable effect upon cell growth and maturation. Preliminary studies indicate that **beta-carotene** (a precursor to vitamin A) may protect the skin from free-radical stress. Foods rich in **essential fatty acids** may decrease swelling by helping to generate hormonelike substances called prostaglandins, which reduce inflammation.

Immune-system abnormalities have been noted in some people who have eczema, and it is sensible for these people (as well as those with a family history of allergies, asthma, and eczema) to eat immune-enriching foods that are high in **zinc, vitamin C,** and **vitamin E.** Vitamin E's antioxidant properties may shield cells from free-radical damage and help to promote skin healing. Vitamin C may also be instrumental in reducing the release of histamine, an inflammatory compound released by the body in response to allergens. As the immune system's response to allergens triggers release of histamine, consuming foods that function as natural antihistamines, such as those rich in vitamin C as well as the flavonoids **quercetin** and **luteolin,** may inhibit this inflammatory reaction. Vitamins C and E operate as robust antioxidants and help to defend against free-radical damage.

recent research

A recent small study suggests that drinking 3 cups of oolong tea daily may relieve symptoms associated with eczema. As eczema is believed to be an allergy-related skin disorder, the study authors speculate that polyphenols in the tea may suppress allergic responses by acting as antioxidants.

your food arsenal

foods	nutrient	health benefits
carrots **mangos** **spinach** **sweet potatoes**	beta-carotene	Beta-carotene acts as an antioxidant by neutralizing harmful elements that could damage skin.
fatty fish **flaxseed** **vegetable oils**	essential fatty acids	Essential fatty acids may facilitate the release of anti-inflammatory substances in the body; this can help to reduce inflammation that often occurs in eczema.
avocados **broccoli** **sunflower seeds** **tomato juice**	vitamin E	Vitamin E is important for maintenance of the immune system. A healthy immune system can help to promote normal responses to allergens, which are linked to eczema.
beans **poultry** **seeds** **whole grains**	zinc	As immune system abnormalities have been noted in some people who have eczema, it may be beneficial to consume foods that are high in zinc, a mineral that enhances immunity.

fibrocystic breasts

what it is

The term "fibrocystic breast disease" is misleading since it is not a disease, but rather a condition that occurs in a large number of women, generally between the ages of 25 to 50. Fibrocystic changes usually mean breast lumpiness.

Characterized by breast tenderness, pain, a dull, heavy feeling, swelling, and lumps (cysts), symptoms of fibrocystic breasts generally are thought to be hormone-related and tend to occur about a week to 10 days before the onset of menstruation. Symptoms most often improve after the menstrual period and, in fact, there appears to be a strong link between fibrocystic breast changes and premenstrual syndrome (see *page 214*). Fibrocystic breast changes usually disappear after menopause (except if you're on hormone replacement therapy), most likely because of the change in hormonal status.

Although fibrocystic breast lumps are benign and do not increase your risk for breast cancer, they can sometimes complicate diagnosing breast cancer (a mammographic image of fibrocystic breasts can sometimes be difficult for radiologists and breast specialists to decipher). Any lump in your breast should be brought to the attention of your health care practitioner.

what causes it

The cause is not completely understood, though fibrocystic breast changes are thought to be caused by an increased estrogen-to-progesterone ratio. Some research suggests that fibrocystic breast changes may be more pronounced in women with higher peak estrogen levels before ovulation and greater declines in progesterone after ovulation. These hormonal fluctuations may lead to a surplus of prolactin, a lactation hormone that can make the breasts swell and feel tender in non-breastfeeding women. More research is required to shed light on fibrocystic breast changes.

how food may help

Although there seems to be little established information about the relationship between diet and fibrocystic breast changes, some research indicates that foods rich in **essential fatty acids** may possibly help to diminish swelling by lowering the body's production of inflammatory substances.

As there is a possible link between elevated estrogen levels and fibrocystic breast symptoms, consuming a diet rich in soy **isoflavones** and other **phytoestrogens** such as **lignans** (in flaxseeds) may help to reduce estrogen. Phytoestrogens are mildly estrogenic phytochemicals that block estrogen by attaching to areas in the body (so-called receptor sites) that would otherwise be claimed by estrogen.

Preliminary studies suggest that the soy isoflavone **genistein** in particular may have an effect on menstrual cycle patterns and increase cycle length, thus reducing estrogen exposure. This, in turn, may reduce fibrocystic breast changes.

A low-fat, high-fiber diet may be helpful for women with fibrocystic breast disease. Eating foods rich in **fiber** and decreasing the intake of foods high in saturated fat may reduce circulating estrogen, though more studies are required to determine how estrogen levels are affected by a high-fiber diet.

Caffeine does not cause fibrocystic breast changes; however, some women do feel that caffeine (found in coffee, tea, colas and some other soft drinks, and chocolate) exacerbates breast tenderness and discomfort. If your symptoms seem to be reduced by eliminating caffeinated foods from your diet, then it may be prudent to do so. (The same is true for eliminating foods high in salt.)

recent research

Though scientific evidence is scant regarding vitamin E and fibrocystic breast changes, many women nevertheless continue to attest to vitamin E's benefits, such as reduced pain, tenderness, and cyst size.

The problem, however, with dietary vitamin E is that a large segment of the population isn't consuming enough foods rich in this important vitamin. Recent findings from a government survey of approximately 16,300 Americans indicate that almost 30% of adults in the United States don't get enough vitamin E.

Good sources of this antioxidant vitamin include wheat germ, almonds and other nuts, vegetable oils, olive oil, and green leafy vegetables. However, because the top food sources of vitamin E tend to be high in fat, it may be a good idea to consult your health care provider to determine if you should take a vitamin E supplement.

your food arsenal

foods	nutrient	health benefits
fatty fish **flaxseed** **nuts** **seeds**	essential fatty acids	Essential fatty acids may reduce swelling associated with fibrocystic breasts by lowering the body's production of inflammatory substances.
apples **kidney beans** **lentils** **whole grains**	dietary fiber	Fibrocystic disease may be linked to excess estrogen, and some studies show that when women with fibrocystic breasts are placed on a high-fiber, low-fat diet they experience a decrease in estrogen levels.

gout

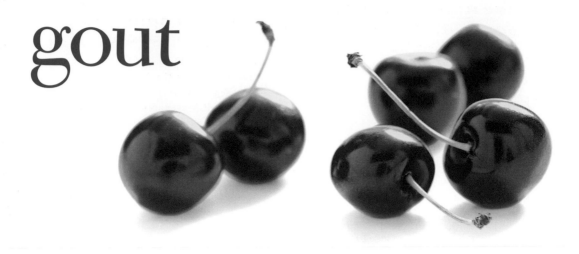

what it is

Often first characterized by sudden, extreme pain and inflammation in a single joint (generally the big toe), gout is a type of rheumatic disorder (an inflammation or pain in the joints or muscles) that usually strikes men. (The likelihood of women suffering from gout tends to increase after menopause.) Persistent episodes of gout, which occur for years, can potentially affect joints in the knees, elbows, wrists, hands, and feet, as well as other parts of the body.

Elevated blood levels of uric acid, one of the body's waste products, can lead to the accumulation of tiny, painful needlelike crystals in the joints. As a natural reaction to this accumulation, the immune system releases compounds in the body that produce inflammation, causing the joints to become sensitive, inflamed, red, and warm to the touch.

Though gout seems to appear out of nowhere, chances are that a symptom-free buildup of uric acid in the blood has been going on for years. The first attack of gout is usually followed by a complete remission of symptoms; but in untreated cases, many people can expect a recurrence. In fact, if left untreated, gout can lead to other serious conditions, such as kidney stones or other kidney problems, as well as destruction of the affected joint. Considered an intermittent disease, gout may be asymptomatic for years, but then produce a painful attack without warning.

what causes it

Gout occurs when there is either an increased production of uric acid or failure of the body to eliminate it efficiently. Being overweight (see *page 208* for advice on losing weight) and/or having high blood pressure (see *page 180* for dietary advice) or high cholesterol (see *page 182* for dietary advice) are also risk factors for gout. There is also a possible association with kidney disease, as well as with certain medications that tend to decrease uric acid excretion from the body—e.g., diuretics ("water pills"), immuno-suppressive drugs, or low doses of aspirin—thus raising uric acid levels in the blood. Alcohol consumption as well as fasting can also raise uric acid levels. Alcohol not only contains purines (see *Foods to Avoid*, right), but it also intensifies the body's production of uric acid, interferes with the kidneys' ability to excrete uric acid, and dehydrates the body, which can increase uric acid levels.

how food may help

Although gout can't be prevented, there are dietary steps you can take to lessen the symptoms to some extent, starting, clearly, by avoiding purine-rich foods (see *Foods to Avoid*, right). Maintaining a normal weight is very important for people who are susceptible to gout. But note that crash dieting or fasting can increase uric acid levels and can cause an acute gout attack. Be sure to drink an ample amount of water to help remove uric acid crystals from the body.

Home remedies for gout that many people swear by include eating **celery** (and/or celery seeds) and/or a half pound of **black cherries** every day. Though no current research offers evidence to support a connection between these foods and the relief of gout, it is possible that they reduce inflammation.

Also, **bromelain,** an enzyme found in pineapples, may reduce inflammation. Eating foods rich in **essential fatty acids** may also help to reduce inflammation.

There is also some preliminary evidence that eating **tofu,** which is derived from soy and is a good source of protein, may be a better choice than meat-based protein for people suffering from gout.

foods to avoid

Certain foods are high in purines, compounds that are thought to exacerbate an attack of gout in people already with the condition. To play it safe, if you feel that you are predisposed to gout or if you have had gout in the past, try to avoid purine-rich foods, such as anchovies, herring, organ meats, and sardines.

your food arsenal

foods	nutrient	health benefits
celery	unidentified	There is no scientific evidence to support claims that celery (and celery seeds) can help with gout management, but folk remedies suggest that they help lower uric acid levels and alleviate pain.
dark cherries	unidentified	Anecdotal information suggests that black cherries may be helpful in reducing inflammation and pain associated with gout. Folk wisdom suggests that beneficial effects similar to those of black cherries may be attributed to blueberries, raspberries, and strawberries.

heart disease

what it is

The leading cause of death in developed countries, heart disease is actually atherosclerosis—an accumulation of fatty plaque deposits along the inside of artery walls. The plaques impede blood flow throughout the body's blood vessels, and when a delicate artery in the heart clogs and deprives the organ of oxygen and nutrients, a heart attack occurs.

what causes it

Heart disease is typically caused by factors related to lifestyle, such as high blood pressure, high cholesterol, obesity, inactivity, stress, and smoking. Declining estrogen levels, diabetes, family history, elevated levels of blood lipids called triglycerides, oxidative damage from free radicals, and increased age also contribute to heart disease.

how food may help

Consuming a low-fat diet with unsaturated fat from olive oil, nuts, and fatty fish can significantly improve cholesterol levels. Fatty fish are also rich in **omega-3 fatty acids,** which have shown promise in reducing the risk of death from certain types of heart attack. Olive oil and nuts are especially good sources of **vitamin E,** which may inhibit the oxidation of LDL cholesterol, a critical factor in the formation of artery-clogging plaque. **Monounsaturated fat** is also beneficial to heart health.

Consuming plenty of **vitamin C** may protect against heart disease by scavenging harmful free radicals, strengthening blood vessels, and possibly regulating blood pressure. **Flavonoid** phytochemicals are thought to enhance the antioxidant actions of vitamin C, and numerous studies link flavonoids in fruit, vegetables, tea, and red wine to protection against heart attacks. The actions of these powerful antioxidants may delay the breakdown of artery-clogging cholesterol that contributes to heart disease. Researchers believe a unique flavonoid in tomatoes, called **lycopene,** may prevent atherosclerosis by preventing harmful LDL cholesterol from being oxidized. One study of over 1,000 middle-aged men from 10 European countries found those who had the most lycopene in their diet reduced their risk for heart attack by half.

Potent **sulfur phytochemicals** in garlic and the onion family may protect against cardiovascular disease. Research suggests that regular garlic consumption may inhibit, and even shrink, fatty plaques in the arteries. Some experts recommend a half to 1 clove per day.

Mounting data link elevated levels of the amino acid homocysteine to clogged arteries and heart disease. **Folate,** a key B vitamin, appears to team up with **vitamins B$_6$** and **B$_{12}$** to lower homocysteine levels. According to one study, when participants adopted a diet high in folate, average homocysteine levels dropped by an impressive 7%. Tuna, avocados, and potatoes provide generous amounts of vitamin B$_6$; poultry and seafood are rich in vitamin B$_{12}$.

A diet rich in soy foods and soluble fiber has been shown to improve heart health by reducing harmful LDL cholesterol. **Soy protein** (25g per day), the **soluble fiber** in oats (beta-glucan), beans, and soluble fiber from psyllium seed husk and flaxseed are especially beneficial.

Because high cholesterol is a major cause of atherosclerosis, and high blood pressure contributes to heart disease, refer to *pages 180–183* for dietary advice on managing these conditions.

recent research

In a small clinical trial, researchers found that eating a bowl of oatmeal after a meal high in saturated fat significantly protected blood vessels from the harmful effects of the fat. The oatmeal prevented the restricted blood flow in arteries that is typical after a high-fat meal and is a symptom of heart disease. The soluble fiber in oats is believed to slow the absorption of fat into the bloodstream, as well as suppress cholesterol absorption in the digestive tract.

your food arsenal

foods	nutrient	health benefits
beans **carrots** **oats**	soluble fiber	Soluble fiber is especially beneficial for improving cholesterol levels, which lowers the risk for developing atherosclerosis.
asparagus **lentils**	folate	Folate helps reduce levels of homocysteine, an amino acid linked to heart disease.
avocados **olive oil**	monounsaturated fat	Because they are not easily damaged by oxidation, these fats are less likely to promote clogged arteries and should replace saturated and trans fat whenever possible.
fatty fish **flaxseed** **shellfish**	omega-3 fatty acids	These heart-healthy fats may reduce the risk for heart attack by reducing blood clotting, lowering levels of harmful triglycerides, and decreasing the risk for irregular heartbeat.
soy foods	soy protein	Numerous studies have confirmed that 25g of soy protein per day can improve cholesterol levels, lowering the risk for cardiovascular disease.

heartburn

what it is

The burning discomfort of heartburn, or acid reflux, is familiar to more than one-third of Americans, some on a daily basis. Heartburn is usually triggered by eating and occurs when stomach acid washes up into the digestive tube (esophagus), burning the back of the throat. The fiery pain may radiate across the chest, traveling from behind the breastbone to the neck. Belching, flatulence, or nausea may accompany acid reflux, and the burning distress may last from one to four hours.

Recurring indigestion (occurring at least twice a week) is medically termed gastroesophageal reflux disease, or GERD, and may be quite severe. Symptoms include painful heartburn, increased salivation, a chronic hoarse voice, and regurgitation. Left untreated, corrosive stomach acid may gradually erode the delicate lining of the esophagus, a process that is linked to esophageal cancer. Fortunately, consuming healing foods and altering eating habits can help quell fiery heartburn.

what causes it

A muscular valve at the bottom of the esophagus, the lower esophageal sphincter (LES), serves as a gatekeeper to the stomach and seals off its contents, blocking backwash into the esophagus. Numerous factors, however, may weaken the LES, or cause it to relax, resulting in heartburn. (Hiatal hernia is another cause of GERD.) Smoking and excess abdominal pressure from pregnancy or obesity may weaken the LES, preventing this valve from closing tightly. Certain foods and medications may relax and open the LES, allowing stomach acid to splash into the esophagus. Additional heartburn triggers include acidic foods (tomatoes and citrus fruits and juices), which may promote excess stomach acid and irritate a damaged esophageal lining; and overeating, tight-fitting clothes, and lying down or bending over after eating, all of which may push stomach contents upward.

how food may help

Several dietary changes are recommended to help prevent heartburn flare-ups and to minimize irritation to the esophagus.

Though scientific data are scant, simple alterations to eating habits, such as eliminating trigger foods, may prevent reflux. Common heartburn triggers include coffee (both decaffeinated and regular), alcohol, peppermint, chocolate, onions, and tomato products. In general, spicy, fatty, or acidic foods frequently lead to heartburn. If irritating foods and beverages must be part of the menu, eat them in very small portions. Drink beverages between meals, instead of with them, to suppress reflux. In addition, remain upright for up to an hour after eating and don't eat for two to three hours before going to bed.

Many experts recommend eating small, low-fat meals each day. Large meals distend the stomach, increasing the chance of reflux. Smaller portions, consumed more frequently throughout the day, may be easier to digest, preventing heartburn distress. Eating slowly is important as well, because eating too fast (and too much) can overload the LES muscle, pressuring the valve to open and propel acidic juices into the esophagus. A low-fat diet is thought to prevent heartburn, since high-fat foods may exacerbate acid reflux by prolonging digestion and weakening the LES valve.

Some experts believe soothing, mild **ginger** tea may help protect against heartburn. Though quite spicy on its own, ginger is thought to strengthen the LES valve, preventing acid backwash into the esophagus.

Studies have linked obesity with an increased incidence of heartburn, so maintaining a healthy weight is important for heartburn prevention. Too much weight around the abdomen appears to stress the LES valve, allowing stomach contents to seep out. **Fiber**-rich foods may assist weight loss by improving feelings of fullness without encouraging overindulgence in extra calories.

Eating a diet rich in high-fiber **complex carbohydrates** may ease digestion and help prevent heartburn. Experts suggest centering meals around such low-fat complex carbohydrates as beans, vegetables, and whole grains.

home remedy

Chewing gum, preferably sugarless, after meals may ease heartburn. Some research suggests that the saliva produced by gum chewing may help neutralize and sweep away acidic stomach juices. (Note, however, that excessive gum chewing is not recommended since it increases swallowed air and belching, which can lead to reflux.)

your food arsenal

foods	nutrient	health benefits
beans **potatoes** **rice** **whole grains**	complex carbohydrates	Complex carbohydrates may ease heartburn because they are generally bland and gentle on stomach digestion.
beets **lentils** **pomegranates**	dietary fiber	By improving satiety, dietary fiber may promote weight loss, which may significantly improve heartburn symptoms.

hemorrhoids

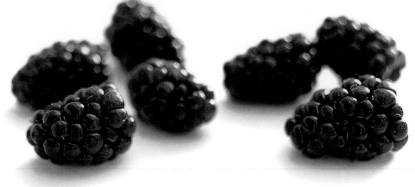

what it is

Varying in symptoms and severity, hemorrhoids are extremely common, affecting most adults at least once in their lifetime. Hemorrhoids, also known as piles, are really varicose veins, or weakened swollen veins, in the anus or rectum. Veins—vessels that transport blood to the heart—are delicate, and veins in the rectum and anus are fragile. Hemorrhoid symptoms include itching, pain, and bleeding. Hemorrhoids are classified as either internal or external and tend to worsen over time if not treated.

what causes it

Pregnancy, obesity, or frequent heavy lifting may lead to hemorrhoids by creating excess pressure on veins, weakening them. Because straining during bowel movements stresses veins, constipation may aggravate hemorrhoids. Bouts of diarrhea and prolonged sitting or standing may also contribute to the condition. A predisposition toward frail veins and poor muscle tone around veins tends to run in families.

how food may help

Regular exercise, a high-fiber diet, and plenty of fluids are key to managing hemorrhoids. Frequent physical activity may help tone muscles around veins, enhancing their ability to propel blood.

Dietary fiber eases elimination and prevents constipation. **Insoluble fiber** promotes regularity and **soluble fiber** softens waste and stimulates intestinal contractions, making stools easier to pass. Research has shown that a high-fiber diet can significantly improve hemorrhoid symptoms, including soreness and bleeding. It is essential to drink at least 8 glasses of water each day when eating a high-fiber diet.

Vitamin C may help fortify vessel walls and reduce swollen veins. Flavonoids are thought to enhance the actions of vitamin C. Preliminary human studies suggest **flavonoids** may improve blood vessel function, possibly strengthening vein tissue. These phyto-chemicals are potent antioxidants that may combat free-radical damage and reduce blood vessel breakage. The citrus flavonoid **hesperidin** is thought to enhance the actions of vitamin C and may improve blood vessel function. **Diosmin,** a related flavonoid found in rosemary and citrus fruit, may strengthen blood vessels as well. Experimental studies suggest that **rutin,** a flavonoid present in apples and buckwheat, may fortify support cells and connective tissue in blood vessels. The grapefruit flavonoid **naringin** (related to rutin and hesperidin) is thought to bolster blood vessel structure and function.

Laboratory research indicates that **quercetin,** a flavonoid found in red onions, apples, and blueberries, may have powerful anti-inflammatory properties that protect against faulty veins. In addition, scientists believe **tannin compounds** (also known as proanthocyanidins) in blackberries may benefit veins by protecting against damaging free radicals.

The infection-fighting mineral **zinc** is important for the healing process and may help to minimize irritation while hemorrhoid tissue mends.

recent research

A matched case-control study of 47 patients, with and without hemorrhoids, found that people who routinely skipped breakfast had as much as seven times the risk for developing hemorrhoids. Experts believe that breakfast may provide a unique opportunity for bulking up on dietary fiber.

your food arsenal

foods	nutrient	health benefits
flaxseed prunes salad greens whole grains	insoluble fiber	Fiber promotes regularity and minimizes straining during bowel movements, which otherwise pressures veins, contributing to hemorrhoids. Fiber may also help tone muscles around veins.
apples beans carrots plums	soluble fiber	Soluble fiber eases elimination by bulking up the stool and stimulating contractions of the digestive tract.
apples berries citrus fruits grapes	flavonoids	Experimental research suggests flavonoids may bolster blood vessels by reducing fragility and permeability. Preliminary human studies indicate flavonoids may improve blood vessel function and relieve hemorrhoid symptoms.
citrus fruits kiwifruit peppers strawberries	vitamin C	Vitamin C may help fortify blood vessel walls and may protect against free radicals that can undermine blood vessel strength.
poultry seeds shellfish wheat germ	zinc	Zinc may enhance the healing of hemorrhoids.

high blood pressure

what it is

Blood pressure is technically the force of blood as it pushes against artery walls during circulation. High blood pressure, or hypertension, is labeled "the silent killer," because symptoms don't emerge until damage has already been done. Statistically, high blood pressure is defined as at least 140 (systolic)/90 (diastolic), recorded at two separate times.

what causes it

For the majority of high blood pressure cases, the cause is unknown, and this is referred to as essential or primary hypertension. Factors that increase the risk for hypertension include obesity, smoking, gender (male), race (African American), family history, stress, and a high-sodium diet.

how food may help

To control blood pressure, experts recommend consuming a diet low in saturated fat and rich in a variety of produce, whole grains, and low-fat dairy. An array of healing nutrients, including **calcium, dietary fiber, magnesium, potassium,** and **vitamin C,** are plentiful in many of these delicious, nourishing foods and can substantially lower blood pressure.

Foods containing at least 350mg of potassium (10% of the DV) and less than 140mg of sodium per serving can carry an FDA-approved label stating the food may reduce risk associated with hypertension and stroke.

Heart-healthy fats, **monounsaturated** and **omega-3s,** may lower blood pressure and are recommended in place of harmful saturated and trans fats. These unhealthy fats are found primarily in animal-based foods and commercially prepared foods, and can clog arteries, raising blood pressure.

Observational studies indicate that moderate amounts of **protein,** particularly from plants, are linked to healthy blood pressure. Legumes, soy foods, and grains such as amaranth and quinoa, offer ample protein without saturated fat.

Arginine, a protein building block, is thought to benefit hypertension by increasing amounts of nitric oxide, a substance involved in blood vessel dilation. Nuts, fish, and dairy products provide generous amounts of arginine.

A wealth of disease-fighting phytochemicals has been suggested for blood pressure control. Epidemiological data link a flavonoid-rich diet (plenty of fruits and vegetables) with healthy blood pressure; scientists believe **flavonoids** may relax blood vessels, lowering pressure.

Pungent, robust **sulfur compounds** in garlic and onions may assist in blood vessel dilation and help reduce both diastolic and systolic blood pressure, as suggested by preliminary clinical evidence.

A phytochemical found in celery, **phthalide (3-n-butyl phthalide),** has shown promise in reducing blood pressure as well, possibly by reducing levels of stress hormones, which constrict blood vessels.

Though research is scant, **rutin,** a phytonutrient abundant in apples and buckwheat, is thought to lower blood pressure by stabilizing blood vessels and preventing excess fluid accumulation in the body.

foods to avoid

Most researchers advise a sodium-restricted diet to help lower blood pressure. A portion of the population, including African Americans, older people, and individuals suffering from diabetes, appears to be particularly sensitive to sodium, and may benefit significantly from eating low-sodium foods. Many experts recommend no more than 2,400mg of sodium each day for healthy individuals. The best way to reduce sodium intake is to avoid adding salt to food at the table, to omit salt when cooking, and avoid most processed foods, which are usually loaded with sodium.

your food arsenal

foods	nutrient	health benefits
broccoli, cooking greens, dairy products, figs	calcium	According to population studies, low levels of calcium are related to a higher risk for elevated blood pressure, particularly in sodium-sensitive individuals, the elderly, and African Americans.
asparagus, lentils, pomegranates	dietary fiber	Observational studies demonstrate a beneficial association between generous fiber intake and reduced blood pressure.
amaranth, quinoa, seeds	magnesium	Observational dietary studies, such as the extensive Honolulu Heart Study, link high magnesium intake with reduced blood pressure.
fatty fish, flaxseed, shellfish	omega-3 fatty acids	Research indicates that these cardioprotective fats may help blood to circulate more freely, lowering blood pressure.
avocados, bananas, potatoes, quinoa	potassium	Findings from the Dietary Approaches to Stop Hypertension (DASH) study support previous research that indicates a potassium-rich diet may improve blood pressure, and may be just as important as a low-sodium diet.
berries, broccoli, citrus fruits, peppers	vitamin C	Population-based and preliminary clinical studies suggest that vitamin C may have a benefit by widening blood vessels and promoting excretion of environmental toxins, such as lead, which can contribute to high blood pressure.

high cholesterol

what it is

Cholesterol, a fatlike substance, circulates in the blood primarily in two forms. LDL cholesterol (the "bad" cholesterol) can clog arteries and contribute to cardiovascular disease. HDL, the "good" cholesterol, sweeps harmful cholesterol out of the arteries. Medical experts recommend that total cholesterol levels be no higher than 200mg/dl and that HDL levels be no lower than 40mg/dl.

what causes it

A diet high in cholesterol and particularly saturated fat and trans fatty acids is associated with high cholesterol levels. Genetic factors, smoking, inactivity, and obesity raise your risk of having unhealthy cholesterol levels.

how food may help

Eating plant-based meals is an excellent strategy for reducing cholesterol, as animal products and processed foods contain cholesterol-raising saturated fat, trans fatty acids, and dietary cholesterol. Substitute heart-healthy **monounsaturated** for cholesterol-raising fat (saturated and trans fat) as often as possible.

Long maligned as a fatty food, **nuts** are rich in unsaturated fat that benefits the heart, according to numerous studies. One large-scale study found that women who ate 5 ounces of nuts per week reduced their risk for heart disease by one-third. In another study, people who consumed 8 to 11 walnuts each day in place of other fats significantly cut their LDL ("bad") cholesterol.

Foods high in **soluble fiber** are useful for lowering LDL cholesterol. Studies show that soluble fiber in oats, carrots, and psyllium (available in health food stores) is particularly beneficial. Research has found that 3g of **beta-glucan** (a soluble fiber in oats) can lower cholesterol by 5% when consumed regularly.

Foods high in **flavonoids,** including **lycopene,** may help moderate cholesterol levels, according to research. Some evidence suggests that drinking orange juice, which is brimming with flavonoids, can improve cholesterol levels.

Scientists believe that **sulfur compounds** in garlic and onions may have cholesterol-lowering properties. An analysis of clinical studies found that regularly eating about ½ to 1 garlic clove may reduce cholesterol by almost 10%.

A small study of healthy women found that those participants who ate about 3 ounces (or ⅔ cup) of **fresh shiitake mushrooms** daily for a week experienced a 9 to 12% reduction in cholesterol. Shiitakes are rich in several heart-healthy phytochemicals, including **eritadenine.**

Evidence is accumulating that plant protein, such as **soy protein,** may help reduce cholesterol. An FDA-approved health claim for soy foods states that daily consumption of as little as 25g of soy protein per day (e.g., ⅓ cup soy nuts or 3½ cups soy milk) can help lower cholesterol in people with high cholesterol levels. Phytoestrogens in soy (**isoflavones**) are thought to enhance the cholesterol-lowering effect of soy protein. **Flaxseed**—rich in vegetable protein, lignans (phytoestrogens), heart-healthy fat, and soluble fiber—has demonstrated impressive cholesterol-lowering effects in clinical research.

> ### recent research
>
> Soluble calcium pectate fiber in carrots helps lower cholesterol, as evidenced by a government study that showed a significant drop in blood cholesterol among individuals who ate 1 cup of carrots per day. On average, participants experienced an 11% decrease in their blood cholesterol after only three weeks.

your food arsenal

foods	nutrient	health benefits
apples **citrus fruits** **onions**	flavonoids	Though the mechanism is as yet unclear, there is growing evidence that flavonoid-rich foods contribute to healthy cholesterol levels.
apricots **tomatoes** **watermelon**	lycopene	Preliminary evidence indicates that this carotenoid may help lower LDL cholesterol by interfering with cholesterol synthesis in the body.
avocados **olive oil**	monounsaturated fat	Replacing harmful saturated and trans fats with monounsaturated fats helps lower dangerous LDL cholesterol.
beans **carrots** **flaxseed** **oats**	soluble fiber	By forming a gel-like mass around food particles in the digestive tract, soluble fiber helps prevent cholesterol from being absorbed and promotes its excretion from the body.
soy foods	soy protein	Numerous clinical studies have confirmed that consuming 25g to 50g of soy protein each day can significantly lower LDL cholesterol.
garlic **onions**	sulfur compounds	Some studies suggest that individuals who consume diets rich in onions and garlic have lower cholesterol levels.

hyperthyroidism

what it is

Rapid heartbeat, insomnia, weight loss, and sweating are hallmarks of an overactive thyroid. The condition occurs when excess thyroid hormone is manufactured and released by the butterfly-shaped thyroid gland, which surrounds part of the windpipe. This vital gland maintains a delicate balance of energy-regulating thyroid hormone in the blood that influences metabolism. A surplus of hormone accelerates energy metabolism, speeding up body processes. Women are far more likely to suffer from hyperthyroidism than men. With proper treatment (including prescription drugs) the condition is quite manageable.

what causes it

An overactive thyroid may have one of several origins. In Grave's disease (a form of hyperthyroidism), an autoimmune disorder leads to an overproduction of thyroid hormone. Excess thyroid hormone may also be caused by abnormal nodules present in the thyroid gland or by inflammation of the gland. In rare instances, a cancerous growth or a dysfunctional pituitary gland, which influences thyroid hormone synthesis, may lead to hyperthyroidism.

how food may help

To maintain adequate energy and weight, an individual with hyperthyroidism may need to consume 15 to 20% more calories than a healthy person. Once prescription drugs take effect, this additional caloric requirement may diminish. Protein and nutrient-dense foods are recommended to protect body muscle stores from being depleted by an accelerated metabolism.

Goitrogens, substances that interfere with iodine absorption, may benefit hyperthyroidism. They are found in raw (cooking deactivates them) cruciferous vegetables, such as cabbage. Research is scant, but some anecdotal prescriptions call for half a head of raw cabbage each day to help manage the condition.

Iodine is an essential component of thyroid hormone, and limiting this mineral is believed to suppress the synthesis and secretion of thyroid hormone.

Experimental research suggests that the antioxidant **vitamins E** and **C** may possibly combat oxidative damage linked to hyperthyroidism. An accelerated metabolism may speed up the generation of destructive free radicals. In addition, foods high in the healing nutrient **beta-carotene,** such as carrots, pumpkin, and sweet potatoes, may benefit individuals with an overactive thyroid; beta-carotene is converted to vitamin A, which is believed to modify iodine utilization in the body.

Evidence is accumulating that an overactive thyroid may alter calcium metabolism in the skeleton. An always-changing tissue, bone is in a constant state of being remodeled, and excess thyroid hormone appears to reduce bone mass through this process, raising the risk for bone-thinning osteoporosis. A **calcium**-rich diet may help combat this risk by improving bone density. And **vitamin D** promotes bone strength by enhancing calcium absorption.

Other nutrients important for bone strength include **vitamin K** (in leafy greens such as kale); **omega-3 fatty acids** (in fatty fish and walnuts); and minerals such as **magnesium, manganese,** and **potassium** (in fruits and vegetables). **Vitamin C,** in addition to improving bone density, is essential for the connective tissue (collagen) matrix that holds bones together. Researchers believe that estrogenlike plant compounds, **isoflavones** (in soy) and **lignans** (in flaxseed), promote bone strength as well, staving off fractures.

Digestive disturbances, particularly diarrhea, often accompany an overactive thyroid. (For advice on managing *Diarrhea*, see *page 166*.)

(For advice on managing *Diarrhea*, see *page 166*.)

> ## recent research
>
> New research suggests that excess thyroid hormone may increase the risk for bone-thinning osteoporosis. In a preliminary study, women with a history of an overactive thyroid had double the risk for hip fracture, compared with healthy women. Scientists believe elevated thyroid hormone hastens bone turnover, thus weakening bones. (For dietary advice on *Osteoporosis*, see *page 206*.)

your food arsenal

foods	nutrient	health benefits
broccoli **cooking greens** **dairy products** **figs**	calcium	A calcium-rich diet is important, because hyperthyroidism often spurs calcium loss from bones.
berries **citrus fruits** **melons** **peppers**	vitamin C	Experimental research links hyperthyroidism with reduced blood levels of vitamin C, which is thought to improve symptoms of the condition.
avocados **nuts** **seeds** **whole grains**	vitamin E	Animal research indicates that this antioxidant vitamin may protect against oxidative damage associated with hyperthyroidism.

hypothyroidism

what it is

A healthy thyroid gland successfully regulates energy metabolism by synthesizing and releasing sufficient amounts of thyroid hormone. In hypothyroidism, too little thyroid hormone is manufactured or released, causing a slowdown in body processes. The drop in thyroid hormone depresses energy levels, compromises nutrient absorption, and promotes weight gain. Constipation, depression, goiter (enlargement of the thyroid), dry skin, fatigue, and sensitivity to cold frequently accompany an inactive thyroid. Research indicates that people who suffer from the disorder have an elevated risk for heart disease because they can develop high levels of artery-clogging cholesterol.

Experts estimate that from 10 to 25% of the U.S. adult population may be afflicted with some form of hypothyroidism; the condition is most prevalent among the elderly and, for unknown reasons, women are up to 10 times more likely than men to have an underactive thyroid.

what causes it

The most common cause of hypothyroidism in the United States is an autoimmune disease called Hashimoto's thyroiditis in which immune cells accumulate in thyroid tissue and reduce thyroid hormone synthesis. Treatment for *hyper*thyroidism, surgery on the thyroid gland, radiation, a hormonal imbalance elsewhere in the body, medication, or genetic factors may also lead to an inactive thyroid. In some instances, insufficient amounts of the mineral iodine—a major constituent of thyroid hormone—can cause hypothyroidism.

Note that iodine deficiency is rare in developed countries because iodine is abundant in the food supply, particularly in iodized salt. Substances that interfere with iodine absorption, called goitrogens, are found in some foods and are believed to possibly contribute to hypothyroidism (see *Foods to Avoid,* right).

how food may help

Because of their sluggish metabolism, people with hypothyroidism may require only half the calories of a healthy adult, at least until their prescription medication becomes effective, normalizing metabolism. Opting for fiber-rich, nutrient-dense foods cuts calories and satisfies the appetite, helping to stave off the weight gain frequently associated with hypothyroidism. A plant-based diet high in **complex carbohydrates** may ease depression symptoms linked with hypothyroidism and supports weight loss (when eaten in moderation).

Though iodine deficiency is rare in the United States and other developed nations, a deficiency of the mineral may result in hypothyroidism. The thyroid gland uses **iodine** to create thyroid hormone, and when the mineral is lacking, the thyroid gland swells to what is known as a goiter, to more effectively capture iodine. Note that the human requirement for iodine is very small, but extremely important since thyroid hormone regulates energy production.

Several vitamins and minerals are essential for normal thyroid function, including **zinc,** which teams up with **vitamin E** to assist in the synthesis of thyroid hormone. Research suggests that low levels of zinc may possibly be linked to an elevated risk for hypothyroidism, particularly in the elderly. Important dietary sources of zinc include poultry and shellfish, and vitamin E is found in sunflower seeds and wheat germ. **Vitamin B$_6$,** plentiful in bananas and salmon, is also required for thyroid hormone synthesis and proper iodine absorption. The mineral **selenium,** present in nuts and whole grains, is thought to activate thyroid hormone.

Cholesterol levels are often elevated among people with hypothyroidism. Substituting healthy fats for harmful fats is a key to managing cholesterol, but there are other dietary measures that help. (See *High Cholesterol, page 182.*)

To combat constipation, which typically accompanies hypothyroidism, drink plenty of water and eat a diet plentiful in both insoluble and soluble fiber. (For more information, see *Constipation, page 160.*)

foods to avoid

Because raw goitrogens may interfere with the body's absorption of iodine and synthesis of thyroid hormone, it may be advisable for people with hypothyroidism to avoid certain foods containing goitrogens, including raw cruciferous vegetables, peanuts, pine nuts, and soybeans. Heat inactivates goitrogens.

your food arsenal

foods	nutrient	health benefits
beans **beets** **lentils** **pomegranates**	dietary fiber	Both insoluble and soluble fiber help alleviate constipation, which often accompanies hypothyroidism. In addition, fiber may protect against high cholesterol and weight gain, both of which are frequently associated with hypothyroidism.
iodized salt **saltwater fish** **seaweed**	iodine	This mineral is essential for the manufacture of thyroid hormone. Note that excess iodine can be detrimental.

immune deficiency

what it is

Each day our bodies face an endless barrage of infectious agents, and the immune system mounts an aggressive defense against these foreign invaders. Its army includes macrophages, killer T-cells, and B-cells. An overburdened immune system or a deficiency in its arsenal may compromise the body's ability to fend off illness.

what causes it

A depressed immune system may stem from poor diet, stress, genetic factors, age, insufficient rest, obesity, medications, chemotherapy, short-term infections, or chronic illness. Oxidative damage from free radicals may undermine immune cell potency as well.

how food may help

Researchers are uncovering powerful links between a nourishing diet and strong immunity. Adequate **protein** and calories are vital for maintaining the immune system, since all immune cells are composed of protein. A low-fat diet with little saturated fat is thought to limit destructive free radicals that can progressively damage and compromise immune cells. Healthful **essential fatty acids** are believed to enhance immunity.

A wealth of nutrients, including **iron, zinc,** and **vitamins C** and **E,** strengthen infection-fighting cells and may revitalize an aging immune system. (Note that excessive intake of iron and zinc can reduce immunity.) **B vitamins**—found in complex carbohydrates, shellfish, lean poultry, and leafy greens—help maintain immunity, including antibody production.

Studies indicate that healthful **probiotic bacteria** in "active-culture" yogurt may combat pathogens by crowding them out of the body; beneficial bacteria may also manufacture infection-fighting compounds.

Garlic and onions may stimulate the fighting power of macrophages and T-cells because of their powerful **sulfur compounds,** which may also block enzymes that allow organisms to invade healthy tissue.

Eating **shiitake mushrooms** may enhance immunity because researchers believe healing compounds, including **lentinan,** may stimulate the body's production of immune cells.

Preliminary research indicates that **CAY-1,** a substance in cayenne, may ward off microbes that cause pneumonia and yeast infections.

Experts believe **flavonoid** phytochemicals abundant in whole grains and produce, such as pomegranates, may elevate the potency of immune cells and may damage the genetic machinery in germs that allows them to multiply.

Studies suggest that a diet low in **carotenoids,** such as lycopene and beta-carotene, may weaken resistance. Carrots and sweet potatoes are rich in **beta-carotene,** and tomato products contain abundant amounts of **lycopene,** which has shown promise in protecting lymphocytes from oxidative stress that can compromise their infection-fighting power. According to one laboratory study, a three-week tomato-rich diet consisting of ¼ cup of tomato puree (with 16.5mg of lycopene) improved immune cell resistance to oxidative damage.

recent research

In a small six-week clinical study, researchers found that volunteers (age 60 or older) who twice a day drank 6 ounces of milk supplemented with yogurt-derived bacteria showed improved immune activity. The immune enhancement could possibly protect against viruses and the development of cancer cells.

your food arsenal

foods	nutrient	health benefits
carrots **sweet potatoes** **tomatoes**	carotenoids	Research suggests that the antioxidant properties of carotenoids may protect immune cells from destructive free radicals.
fatty fish **seeds**	essential fatty acids	These fats are vital for wound healing and optimal functioning of T-cells.
fatty fish **lentils** **poultry**	iron	Adequate amounts of this mineral are required for the manufacture of B-cells and T-cells.
yogurt	probiotics	Evidence is accumulating that these friendly bacteria improve immune responses against viruses and cancer cells.
berries **citrus fruits** **peppers**	vitamin C	In addition to protecting against oxidative damage, this vitamin may enhance the function of immune cells.
avocados **olive oil** **seeds**	vitamin E	According to studies, vitamin E may enhance T-cell activity and assist in the production of antibodies.
poultry **shellfish** **whole grains**	zinc	This mineral works with enzymes to heal wounds and may possibly bolster the body's resistance against cold viruses.

infertility & impotence

what it is

Infertility—an inability to conceive a child after at least one year of regular unprotected intercourse—affects an estimated 15% of couples in the United States. Repeated miscarriages are considered to be a form of infertility as well. Impotence (also called erectile dysfunction, or ED) is the persistent inability to attain or maintain an erection, and is particularly prevalent in males over age 50.

what causes it

A woman's inability to conceive may result from hormonal imbalances, ovulation problems, weight fluctuations, intense exercise, stress, thyroid disease, or possibly smoking. Male infertility is attributed to defective or an insufficient number of sperm, or impaired reproductive glands. The most common cause of impotence is restricted blood flow to the penis.

how food may help

The B vitamin **folate,** typically recommended for women before preconception and during pregnancy, may be vital for male reproduction as well. According to new research, deficient sperm counts are significantly associated with low folate in healthy men. The vitamin's reproductive role in men is unclear, but scientists believe normalizing folate levels through a diet rich in this B vitamin may possibly offset diminished sperm levels.

The antioxidant mineral **selenium** may team up with **vitamin E** to defend against oxidative damage in reproductive organs. Selenium helps ensure normal sperm function, and low levels of this mineral in women have been associated with miscarriages.

Vitamin B$_{12}$ and **iron** may protect against infertility as well. Some evidence suggests vitamin B$_{12}$ may improve sperm count and motility, even in men who are not B$_{12}$ deficient. In rare instances, men and women may be B$_{12}$ deficient (suffering from pernicious anemia), which hinders fertility and can lead to sterility. Low levels of the blood-nourishing mineral iron may impede conception in women.

Since atherosclerosis is a frequent underlying cause of impotence, reducing fat buildup in the arteries may improve blood flow to the penis, thus preventing impotence. **Vitamin C** is important for blood vessel health and may promote uninhibited circulation that allows blood vessels in the penis to enlarge and accommodate blood. **Flavonoids** are believed to enhance vitamin C actions and may fortify blood vessel structure, as well as prevent hardening of the arteries. Instead of saturated and trans fats, eat unsaturated fat, particularly the monounsaturated type, to prevent the buildup of fatty plaques in arteries.

your food arsenal

foods	nutrient	health benefits
asparagus beans salad greens spinach	folate	Preliminary research links low folate levels in healthy men with reduced sperm count. In addition, low levels of folate may be associated with repeated miscarriages and diminished fertility in women.
guava tomatoes watermelon	lycopene	Preliminary studies suggest that this carotenoid, which is concentrated in the testes, may improve sperm count and motility, particularly in men with low blood levels of lycopene.
Brazil nuts seeds shellfish whole grains	selenium	Deficiencies in this antioxidant mineral have been associated with fertility problems, including miscarriages. Scientists believe this mineral is also part of an important structural component in sperm.
berries broccoli citrus fruits peppers	vitamin C	This antioxidant vitamin may shield against oxidative damage, which can reduce sperm count and quality. Vitamin C is also thought to help maintain blood vessels and improve blood flow diminished by atherosclerosis, a frequent underlying cause of impotence.
avocado nuts olive oil seeds	vitamin E	Animal research suggests this vitamin may delay age-associated infertility in women. Vitamin E may protect sperm membranes against oxidative damage and, according to lab research, may facilitate fertilization.
beans poultry shellfish	zinc	This vital mineral is essential for ovulation, development and maturity of sperm, and fertilization.

insomnia

what it is

Insomnia is one of the most widespread health complaints today; sleepless, restless nights are common to more than one-third of the adult population worldwide. Insomnia is waking earlier than planned or having difficulty falling asleep or remaining asleep, and is not a disease itself, but rather a symptom of an underlying health or emotional problem. Daytime fatigue and irritability are consequences of sleep deprivation. For many of us, insomnia is only a temporary annoyance, but chronic sleep debt may mortgage health, since sufficient rest is vital for physical and mental well-being. A variety of diet and lifestyle factors may improve sleep habits, diminishing insomnia and its impact.

what causes it

Like a nagging cough or a fever, insomnia stems from an underlying condition. Stress, anxiety, and depression are the leading causes of temporary sleeplessness. Brief bouts of insomnia commonly result from an erratic sleep schedule, short-term illness (such as bronchitis cough), pain, or environmental factors such as noise. Medications and serious chronic health conditions can disrupt sleep as well. Also as you age, sleep patterns change. Additional insomnia triggers include vigorous night-time exercise, pregnancy, heartburn, alcohol, and too much caffeine.

how food may help

A nutritional formula to induce sleep has not yet been discovered, but a variety of nutrients are important for sleep and may help remedy insomnia.

When eaten along with starchy foods, the amino acid **tryptophan,** found in many high-protein foods, may promote drowsiness by fueling the production of serotonin, a brain chemical that fosters relaxation and feelings of well-being (or calm). **Vitamin B$_6$** and the mineral **magnesium** help convert tryptophan to serotonin. Vitamin B$_6$ assists in the production of additional brain chemicals that regulate sleep and mood, including melatonin and dopamine. Bananas and potatoes are good sources of vitamin B_6 and magnesium. Though the mechanism is unclear, mild **calcium** deficiencies may be associated with sleep disturbances as well.

Complex carbohydrates may promote restful sleep because they enhance the brain's absorption of sleep-inducing tryptophan. Complex carbohydrates may also ease heartburn-related insomnia. Eating too much or too close to bedtime frequently causes heartburn, an underlying cause of sleep disturbances for millions of Americans. Eating plenty of bland carbohydrates may prevent heartburn. **Thiamin** (vitamin B_1) helps transform complex carbohydrates into useful energy for the body and is essential for healthy nerve function. Low levels of this B vitamin are thought to interfere with a good night's sleep.

Eating foods rich in B vitamins may help fight the blues, a common cause of insomnia. B vitamins foster the production of the brain's neurotransmitters, essential for restful sleep and a peaceful mood. A deficiency of **folate** and **vitamin B_{12}** is sometimes found in people who are depressed. Folate is abundant in lentils and asparagus, and vitamin B_{12} can be found in seafood and lean poultry. In addition, there is growing evidence that folate and vitamin B_{12} team up with vitamin B_6 to lower levels of the amino acid homocysteine, which may be associated with depression. **Niacin,** present in poultry and fish, is thought to be useful for relieving depression-related insomnia as well, though clinical evidence is lacking.

Evidence is emerging that **omega-3 fatty acids,** such as those present in fatty fish, flaxseed, and walnuts, play a key role in optimal mental activity, which may influence mood and insomnia. Some findings suggest depression may be related to inadequate intake of these healthful fats.

Easing the symptoms of menopause may relieve insomnia, as declining hormone levels are frequently connected to sleep disturbances. Studies suggest that consuming foods high in **phytoestrogens,** plantlike estrogen compounds, helps relieve the severity of menopause symptoms, including hot flashes. Findings from population studies indicate that women who regularly consume isoflavones (phytoestrogens in soy foods) tend to suffer far less from unpleasant menopause symptoms.

home remedy

A glass of warm milk with honey is a traditional home remedy for insomnia. Milk is a good source of tryptophan and calcium, while carbohydrate-rich honey may enhance the bioavailability of tryptophan.

your food arsenal

foods	nutrient	health benefits
beans **potatoes** **whole grains**	complex carbohydrates	Foods high in complex carbohydrates may promote drowsiness by enhancing tryptophan absorption.
dairy products **poultry**	tryptophan	The body converts this amino acid into the sleep-inducing brain chemical serotonin.

irritable bowel syndrome

what it is

At some point in their lives, nearly 20% of adults experience alternating bouts of constipation and diarrhea characteristic of irritable bowel syndrome (IBS). The most common gastrointestinal disorder in the United States, IBS occurs when the muscles of the intestinal tract contract in abnormal, uncoordinated spasms. Abdominal pain, bloating, flatulence, and mucus in the stool frequently accompany IBS. Some people have either constipation or diarrhea predominantly, while others suffer from both. Symptoms of the disorder range from mild to debilitating, but IBS is not life-threatening, nor does it lead to or signal more serious conditions such as colon cancer.

what causes it

A single cause for IBS has not yet been established, though experts have proposed many potential triggers. Possible offenders that may overstimulate the nervous and digestive system include stress and overuse of antibiotics. Researchers believe stress aggravates symptoms, regardless of the underlying reason for the disorder. Because it may have a variety of causes and symptoms, IBS is usually diagnosed by eliminating ailments with similar symptoms, and then devising a strategy to alleviate IBS discomfort. This may include stress management techniques, prescription drugs, and diet modifications.

how food may help

To relieve IBS symptoms, experts recommend eating small, frequent meals since large volumes of food distend the stomach and may lead to gastrointestinal distress. It is equally important to eat slowly; eating too quickly may increase swallowed air, which promotes irritating intestinal gas. Chew foods thoroughly to slow eating and to ensure optimal nutrient absorption in the digestive tract. Drinking peppermint or ginger tea may help settle an uneasy digestive system. Low-fat, high-fiber meals are generally suggested since fatty, greasy food may encourage uncomfortable bowel contractions. Note that IBS sufferers with diarrhea may experience increased symptoms with foods high in insoluble fiber.

Dietary fiber enhances digestive function, promoting regular, rhythmic intestinal contractions. In particular, **insoluble fiber** helps to bulk up feces and ease elimination, relieving IBS-associated constipation. Foods high in **soluble fiber,** on the other hand, absorb water and are especially beneficial for bouts of diarrhea. Clinical studies indicate that psyllium, a type of dietary fiber, may ameliorate IBS for some people. Psyllium bulks up the stool and absorbs water in the digestive tract, alleviating intestinal spasms and promoting regular bowel movements without increasing abdominal cramping or flatulence. To reduce intestinal discomfort, gradually increase fiber in your diet and drink at least 8 glasses of water each day.

Because a bout of IBS-related diarrhea may diminish beneficial bacteria in the colon, **probiotic bacteria** may be useful by replenishing friendly flora. Preliminary research suggests that **fructooligosaccharides (FOS)**, sugar molecules in foods such as bananas, may foster the growth of beneficial bacteria. While other foods may contain FOS, bananas appear to be one of the least irritating to the digestive tract.

To quell flatulence associated with IBS, soak gassy foods, including broccoli and cauliflower, before cooking. Drain and rinse foods such as beans and then cook in fresh water. Steaming gassy vegetables may also reduce flatulence.

Food intolerances, particularly lactose intolerance, commonly trigger IBS symptoms, so determining such food sensitivities may ease symptoms. It is important to keep a food diary and be aware of foods that may trigger symptoms. To evaluate lactose intolerance, first avoid lactose-containing foods and beverages for several days (a wash-out period). Then drink 2 glasses of nonfat milk on an empty stomach. Monitor symptoms for four hours and repeat the test with lactase-treated milk.

foods to avoid

Alcohol, caffeine, fat, and sorbitol (a type of sugar present in high amounts in prunes and some commercially prepared foods) can irritate the intestines, exacerbating IBS symptoms. In addition, to minimize IBS discomfort, experts advise testing for intolerances to the milk sugar lactose and possibly fructose sugars (found in fruits and fruit-based foods). Some gas-producing foods, such as broccoli, cauliflower, and onions, may also aggravate IBS symptoms.

your food arsenal

foods	nutrient	health benefits
yogurt	probiotics	Research suggests these healthful bacteria enhance the growth of friendly flora in the intestines that may be reduced in individuals suffering from irritable bowel syndrome.
bulgur salad greens sweet potatoes	insoluble fiber	Increasing insoluble fiber intake is useful for combatting constipation associated with irritable bowel syndrome.
beans carrots	soluble fiber	This type of fiber may relieve bouts of diarrhea, associated with irritable bowel syndrome.

kidney stones

what it is

Millions of Americans are plagued by kidney stones (or renal calculi), which occur when stone-forming compounds from the urine accumulate in the kidney and start to crystallize. The stones are typically composed of calcium, combined with phosphate or oxalate. (Less common are so-called struvite stones, which can result from kidney or chronic urinary tract infection; and even less frequently, gout-related uric acid stones may form.) Passing one kidney stone dramatically increases the chance of having another stone, but experts believe these odds can be improved through exercise and diet alterations.

what causes it

Heredity and chronic dehydration seem to contribute to kidney stone formation, but the specific cause is unknown. Certain factors and conditions may predispose individuals to kidney stones, including a sedentary lifestyle and being Caucasian or Asian. For undetermined reasons, possibly genetics, some people tend to have higher concentrations of calcium in their urine, which promotes crystal formation and accounts for the majority of stones. Additional risk factors include kidney disease, chronic bowel inflammation, intestinal surgery, and medications such as diuretics. Scientists do not believe that eating any specific food causes stones to form in people who are *not* susceptible. Research suggests, however, that for those who *are* susceptible, oxalates and purines (naturally occurring compounds in some foods) may fuel stone formation.

how food may help

Drinking plenty of fluids, especially water, is perhaps the most important dietary advice for the prevention and management of kidney stones. Water dilutes the urine, making it difficult for salts to crystallize and stones to form. Note that diluted urine should not be darker than pale yellow, and fluid intake should be adjusted accordingly. Experts recommend twelve 8-ounce glasses of water a day to avoid kidney stones.

Research suggests that drinking orange juice and lemonade may effectively help prevent kidney stones. In addition to the beneficial water content of lemonade and orange juice, alkaline substances called **citrates** in these juices may help neutralize stone-forming acids, inhibiting the formation of certain calcium-based kidney stones. Incidentally, the valuable mineral **potassium,** also found in orange juice and lemonade, may be useful since potassium is linked to a reduced risk for kidney stones. To help prevent struvite kidney stones, eat **tannin**-rich blueberries. (Although cranberries have tannins, they should be avoided because they are high in oxalates.)

Because animal protein may lower the concentration of beneficial citrates in the body, people prone to developing kidney stones may benefit from eating less animal protein and more plant protein. Animal protein is also thought to elevate the concentration of stone-forming calcium and oxalates in the urine.

Because urinary calcium and oxalates contribute to kidney stones, foods high in **insoluble fiber** (but low in oxalates) may help by binding excess oxalates and calcium in the digestive tract, preventing their accumulation in the urine. **Magnesium** may be beneficial as well, because it may bind oxalates in the intestines. It is important to check with your doctor before substantially increasing fiber consumption, because reducing calcium levels may raise the risk for bone-thinning osteoporosis.

Despite the evidence that dietary calcium raises urinary calcium, and urinary calcium encourages kidney stones, two powerful observational studies found that people who ate the most calcium-rich foods were significantly less likely to suffer from calcium-based kidney stones. Researchers surmise that dietary calcium may block the body's absorption of harmful oxalates. (Note that the study subjects who consumed the most dietary calcium also consumed the most fluids, potassium, magnesium, and phosphate.) However, calcium consumed in supplement form may actually increase the risk for stones.

foods to avoid

Because they may increase the chance of kidney stones, certain foods should be limited or completely avoided by people at risk for the condition. These foods include refined carbohydrates, salty foods, alcohol, foods high in animal protein, purine-rich foods, and oxalate-rich foods. Purine-rich foods include organ meats, anchovies, sardines, and herring. Foods high in oxalates include beets and beet greens, chocolate, chard, cranberries, dandelion greens, nuts, parsley, rhubarb, spinach, strawberries, tea, and wheat bran.

your food arsenal

foods	nutrient	health benefits
broccoli peas	insoluble fiber	Generous amounts of insoluble fiber are thought to bind stone-forming oxalates and calcium.
avocados quinoa	magnesium	This valuable mineral may lower levels of harmful oxalates, a major component of many kidney stones.
bananas potatoes	potassium	Research links high potassium intake with a reduced risk for kidney stones.
blueberries	tannins	By protecting against urinary tract infections, tannins may prevent struvite kidney stones, which are associated with chronic UTIs.

macular degeneration

what it is

The leading cause of blindness in the elderly, macular degeneration affects one out of three people over the age of 75. The disease impairs the macula, which is the central part of the retina and is important for clear, sharp vision. As the disease progresses, blank spots gradually appear in the central field of vision. Approximately 90% of macular degeneration sufferers have the "dry" form, and the more serious "wet" form accounts for the remainder of macular degeneration cases.

what causes it

Experts believe that harmful free radicals—unstable oxygen molecules—cause damage to the retina, leading to macular degeneration. It's thought that age-related changes and genetics contribute to the condition as well. Sunlight exposure, pollution, cigarette smoke, and a high-fat diet can increase the amount of destructive free radicals in the eye. Having cardiovascular disease or diabetes may elevate the risk for the disease as well by restricting blood flow to the eye.

how food may help

A natural protective pigment in the macula helps filter out the damaging light rays that contribute to macular degeneration. **Lutein** and **zeaxanthin,** carotenoids abundant in vegetable pigments, are highly concentrated in macular pigment and in the retina. Studies link diets rich in lutein and zeaxanthin with a reduced risk for macular degeneration, and the progression of the disease may even be slowed by this pair. Consumption of dark green, carotenoid-rich, leafy vegetables, particularly spinach and collard greens, has been associated with a reduced risk for macular degeneration, suggesting that carotenoids such as lutein and zeaxanthin (as well as **beta-carotene**) are protective agents.

Another carotenoid, **lycopene,** may protect against macular degeneration because its unique structure and biochemistry make it especially adept at combatting harmful oxidative damage. Preliminary human studies have found that low levels of lycopene are associated with an elevated risk for macular degeneration.

Scientists believe a diet rich in antioxidant vitamins and minerals, such as **vitamins C** and **E, selenium,** and **zinc,** may also defend against macular degeneration by scavenging free radicals in the retina. Vitamin C is particularly concentrated in the eye. Evidence is accumulating that these nutrients are essential for eye health, and deficiencies may increase the risk for macular degeneration.

recent research

One large observational study of men and women between the ages of 55 and 80 found that participants who consumed the most carotenoids in their diets had about a 40% lower risk for macular degeneration. The effect was particularly strong in people who ate the most spinach and collard greens.

your food arsenal

foods	nutrient	health benefits
carrots spinach winter squash	beta-carotene	Carotenoids such as beta-carotene, found in orange vegetables and dark leafy greens, are linked to a reduced risk for macular degeneration.
collard greens peppers spinach sweet potatoes	lutein & zeaxanthin	These antioxidant pigments are concentrated in the macula and retina, which suggests they may protect vision cells from oxidative damage. Observational studies associate a lower risk for macular degeneration with diets rich in lutein and zeaxanthin.
apricots tomatoes watermelon	lycopene	According to preliminary research, people with low levels of this antioxidant carotenoid may have as much as twice the risk for macular degeneration.
barley Brazil nuts poultry shrimp	selenium	Some observational studies indicate that individuals who consume a diet abundant in antioxidant minerals, such as selenium, may be less likely to develop macular degeneration.
berries broccoli citrus fruits peppers	vitamin C	Epidemiologic evidence suggests that a diet plentiful in vitamin C may help stave off macular degeneration. Vitamin C is thought to combat free-radical damage in the eye, which can lead to macular degeneration.
avocado nuts olive oil	vitamin E	High blood levels of tocopherols (vitamin E compounds) may be related to a reduced risk for early-onset macular degeneration.
beans poultry shellfish whole grains	zinc	According to preliminary evidence, depressed levels of zinc may be tied to macular degeneration. Zinc is critical to the metabolic function of enzymes important to the retina.

memory loss

what it is

Mild lapses in memory—forgetting names and misplacing objects—are common with age as elements of the cognitive network may falter. Some forgetfulness is to be expected with age and is relatively benign. Profound memory loss is a universal symptom of dementia, and Alzheimer's disease is one form of dementia.

what causes it

Benign age-related memory loss may result from shrinkage of the brain's nerves, diminished production of brain chemicals, or restricted blood flow to brain tissue. Genetic factors, head injuries, viruses, and cardiovascular disease may contribute to Alzheimer's disease.

how food may help

Exercise and a sound diet are instrumental in preserving brain longevity and sustaining memory. Protective brain nutrients include **complex carbohydrates** and **B vitamins,** which help ensure healthy nerve transmission and sufficient quantities of neurotransmitters. In a study of healthy elderly people, memory significantly improved after consuming 50g (about 1½ ounces) of either potatoes or barley, both complex carbohydrates. B vitamins help convert food, such as complex carbohydrates, into brain fuel. In addition, some epidemiological evidence associates low levels of **vitamins B$_6$, B$_{12}$,** and **folate** with Alzheimer's disease.

Scientists believe the blood-nourishing mineral **iron** may be important for neurotransmitter activity, and some research suggests depressed levels of iron can impair memory function. In one study of nonanemic adolescent girls, mild iron deficiency was associated with slightly impaired short-term memory and poorer performance on a test of verbal learning, compared to girls with adequate iron intake. Fish, poultry, and lean meats are excellent sources of iron.

Blueberries show promise in fighting age-related memory decline; preliminary studies link blueberries with improved cognitive function. The exact mechanism has not yet been clearly established, but the antioxidant actions of **flavonoids** in blueberries are thought to reverse some parameters of age-related memory loss by defending against harmful free radicals, which can accumulate in brain cells and compromise memory function. Flavonoids may enhance blood flow to brain tissue involved with memory as well. Additional antioxidant nutrients, including **beta-carotene, isoflavones,** and **vitamins E** and **C,** may also help preserve memory.

Unobstructed blood flow to the brain is essential for mental fitness, since brain cells require continuous nourishment and accessible communication with supporting systems in the body. Fatty deposits in the arteries frequently impede blood flow to the brain, impairing memory. The risk for arterial plaques may be reduced by consuming **monounsaturated fat** in place of trans fatty acids and saturated fat; population research has found that a diet high in monounsaturated fat protects against age-related cognitive decline. Additional cardioprotective nutrients, such as **soluble fiber,** maintain unclogged blood vessels. Another heart-healthy fat, **DHA,** is a building block for brain tissue, and low levels have been associated with age-related dementia, including Alzheimer's disease.

recent research

There is growing evidence that high levels of beta-carotene and vitamin C are associated with superior memory performance in people age 65 or older. Researchers believe these antioxidants may delay brain aging and enhance mental longevity and fitness by combatting destructive free radicals in the brain. Carrots, sweet potatoes, and pumpkin are excellent sources of beta-carotene; and citrus fruits, kiwifruits, and peppers provide generous amounts of vitamin C.

your food arsenal

foods	nutrient	health benefits
beans potatoes rice whole grains	complex carbohydrates	Through glucose metabolism, complex carbohydrates may elevate production of neurotransmitters or influence proteins in the digestive tract, which signal brain cells and enhance memory.
blueberries strawberries	flavonoids	Experimental research suggests that flavonoids in blueberries (and possibly strawberries) may slow age-related decline in mental function, including neuron deterioration.
soy products	isoflavones	According to preliminary evidence, soy isoflavones may protect against Alzheimer's by hindering protein changes that contribute to the disease.
avocados olive oil	monounsaturated fat	Scientists hypothesize that cardioprotective nutrients such as monounsaturated fat may preserve memory by maintaining blood flow to the brain.
avocados seeds	vitamin E	This powerful antioxidant is under review for its potential to enhance memory and slow the progression of Alzheimer's disease.

migraine

what it is

The classic manifestation of a migraine is a throbbing, acutely painful headache, beginning usually near one eye or temple (the word migraine is derived from the Greek word *hemikrania*, meaning "half of the head"). Pain can extend throughout one or both sides of the head, and, if the migraine is untreated, it can sometimes last for up to three days. Pain is usually worsened by physical activity. Early warning signs of an impending migraine may include an aura (seeing a bright light) and other visual disturbances such as blind spots and temporary loss of peripheral vision. Other warning signs include temporary nausea, weakness, and sensitivity to noise and bright or flashing lights.

what causes it

Though the exact cause of migraines is currently unknown, there are certain factors that are associated with this type of headache. During a migraine attack, blood vessels in the brain undergo spasms, which cause constriction and then rapid dilation. This triggers the release of brain chemicals that cause inflammation and throbbing pain. A strong hereditary factor is also a component of this affliction, which occurs more often in women than in men.

Caffeine withdrawal, exposure to bright or flashing lights, oral contraceptives, vasodilating medication, dehydration, changes in sleep patterns, stress, hormonal changes, and consumption of foods that contain certain chemicals can trigger migraines. Preliminary research suggests that an imbalance of the brain neurotransmitter serotonin may also play a role in the onset of this debilitating type of headache.

how food may help

Generally speaking, there is some evidence that low blood sugar can contribute to the onset of migraines. Eating regularly, without skipping meals, is important to prevent low blood sugar.

A drop in magnesium levels before or during a migraine attack has been noted in some people with migraines; it's also been noted that migraine sufferers are lacking in this mineral. Therefore, foods rich in **magnesium** may help diminish the severity of migraine pain.

Some migraine sufferers are thought to have low energy, and **riboflavin** helps to increase energy reserves by releasing energy from carbohydrates and producing red blood cells.

Some studies indicate that migraine sufferers have reduced levels of the mood-regulating neurotransmitter serotonin. Foods rich in **tryptophan,** an amino acid that boosts serotonin levels in the brain, may offer some relief of symptoms. Make sure to eat foods rich in complex carbohydrates to increase absorption of tryptophan.

To help reduce inflammation, a diet rich in **omega-3 fatty acids** may aid in migraine management. If you are experiencing nausea, consume foods seasoned with **ginger,** a spice thought to help alleviate stomach distress.

Because certain substances in food may induce a migraine attack, some people find it helpful to maintain a daily record of food and beverage intake, as well as a specific record of any migraine attacks, to help identify and avoid suspected migraine triggers (see *Foods to Avoid,* right). Maintaining a daily food record helps isolate and identify specific foods that might play a role in provoking a migraine. It may be useful to eliminate the suspected food from your diet for a few weeks, then reintroduce it, to determine if a migraine attack correlates with intake of the targeted food. Although most of the information on dietary migraine triggers is based on anecdotal reports rather than hard science, it is noteworthy to mention that if you feel that a certain food or foods are migraine triggers, it is advisable to eliminate that food from your diet.

foods to avoid

There are several compounds implicated in the onset of migraines. They are: nitrites (found in bacon, hot dogs, and cured meats), tyramine (found in pepperoni, red wine, chicken livers, active yeast preparations, and aged cheeses), tannins (found in nuts, apple juice, grapes, berries, coffee, red wine, and tea), and sulfites (used as preservatives in wine and dried fruits).

Monosodium glutamate (MSG)—a common ingredient in food served in Chinese restaurants and also contained in many commercial products including seasonings (read labels carefully)—might also be a migraine trigger. The artificial sweetener aspartame is also a likely suspect.

Though chocolate is a possible trigger food, research is conflicting, and some studies show that chocolate is more benign than previously believed.

your food arsenal

foods	nutrient	health benefits
amaranth grain **avocados** **rice** **winter squash**	magnesium	People with migraines tend to have impaired magnesium metabolism as well as low levels of this important mineral. Note that although nuts are a good source of magnesium, it is not advisable to eat them, since they contain tannins, which could trigger migraines.
mushrooms **poultry** **quinoa**	riboflavin	Riboflavin has the potential to increase energy reserves in brain cells, which are often reduced in some people who suffer from migraines.

osteoarthritis

what it is

Decades of use stress cartilage, the spongy, protective cushions located at the ends of bones. With age, damaged cartilage does not repair itself as effectively as it once did and may progressively deteriorate into osteoarthritis, or degenerative joint disease. The initial symptoms of the condition, joint stiffness and discomfort, are usually mild; but, eventually, once-cushioned bones begin to rub together, creating friction, tenderness, and gnarled joints.

Any joint is vulnerable to osteoarthritis, but it usually occurs in the ankles, feet, fingers, hips, knees, neck, or spine. The pain and stiffness of osteoarthritis most frequently affect the weight-bearing joints, and diseased joints may become knobby and deformed. If joint stiffness restricts movement, nearby muscles may become weaker, which contributes to even greater joint pain and stiffness. A very common age-related ailment, osteoarthritis affects an estimated 75% of people over the age of 50 and the condition is most prevalent among the elderly.

what causes it

Years of use gradually break down cartilage and its supporting structural tissue. Cartilage and related tissue-repair mechanisms gradually become deficient as a person ages, contributing to osteoarthritis. In addition, excess body weight, a genetic predisposition, defects in joints or cartilage, joint injuries, or repetitive joint motions associated with physical activity can lead to osteoarthritis.

how food may help

Several nutrients may benefit osteoarthritis, alleviating joint pain and inflammation as well as promoting cartilage repair. Research suggests that **vitamin C** may minimize cartilage loss and slow the progression of osteoarthritis. Another powerful antioxidant, **vitamin E,** may relieve osteoarthritis symptoms, according to preliminary clinical research.

Population studies link low levels of **vitamin D** with an elevated risk for osteoarthritis. Vitamin D's partner, **calcium,** may help bolster weight-bearing joints damaged by osteoarthritis and also stave off osteoporosis.

Some clinical evidence suggests that consuming **omega-3 fatty acids** and **shogaols** and **gingerols** (healing substances in ginger) may help relieve the tenderness and swelling of osteoarthritis. These compounds exhibit potent anti-inflammatory properties.

Though scientific data are limited, some experts believe consuming pineapple may defend against osteoarthritis and possibly improve symptoms. The pineapple enzyme **bromelain** is thought to alleviate swelling associated with osteoarthritis, because this compound has demonstrated anti-inflammatory activity in laboratory research.

Because osteoarthritis is more prevalent among women, some experimental evidence suggests that certain forms of estrogen may worsen the disease. So, scientists believe that **phytoestrogens** (estrogenlike plant compounds) may block the possible influence of natural estrogen on osteoarthritis. Phyto-estrogens are plentiful in soy foods.

recent research

Observational research has found that older people who consumed inadequate amounts of vitamin D, and who had low levels of this bone-strengthening vitamin in their blood, had a substantially higher risk for progressively worsening osteo-arthritis of the knee. Another study suggests that elderly women with low blood levels of vitamin D may have an elevated risk for osteoarthritis in the hip.

your food arsenal

foods	nutrient	health benefits
fatty fish **shellfish**	omega-3 fatty acids	According to clinical research, these anti-inflammatory fats may improve the symptoms of arthritis, including morning stiffness, joint tenderness, and fatigue.
ginger	shogaols & gingerols	Phytonutrients in ginger may ameliorate the pain and swelling of arthritis by interfering with the synthesis of inflammatory compounds.
berries **broccoli** **cantaloupe** **peppers**	vitamin C	Research suggests that this nutrient may minimize cartilage loss and slow the progression of osteoarthritis. Vitamin C seems to squelch harmful free radicals and enhance tissue repair.
fatty fish **milk**	vitamin D	This vitamin has been shown to hinder the breakdown of bone and the progression of osteoarthritis. Population studies link low levels of vitamin D with an elevated risk for osteoarthritis.
avocados **nuts** **olive oil** **seeds**	vitamin E	Experimental data suggest that vitamin E may foster the growth of healthy cartilage. Vitamin E has demonstrated a benefit in preliminary clinical research involving osteoarthritis patients.

osteoporosis

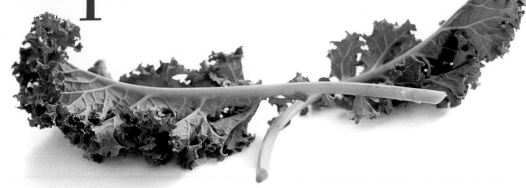

recipe rx

what it is

Aptly named for the Latin phrase "porous bones," osteoporosis is a debilitating, progressive skeletal disease that silently robs bones of their mineral density and strength. More than 25 million Americans, mostly women, are afflicted with or are at high risk for this bone-thinning disease, which leads to fractures and collapsed vertebrae.

what causes it

A lack of hormones (usually estrogen), exercise, and/or calcium may deplete bone mass and impair bone structure, weakening bones. Estrogen levels decline after menopause, leaving women, particularly those who are small-boned or underweight, with a heightened risk for the disease. An unbalanced diet, genetic predisposition, steroid use, cigarette smoking, and low testosterone levels (in men) may also contribute to the disease.

how food may help

A lifelong, high-quality diet rich in **calcium** nourishes and strengthens bones. Most of the body's calcium is stored in the skeleton, where this mineral provides a sturdy foundation for bone tissue. Consuming plenty of calcium throughout childhood and early adulthood helps build peak bone mass, which may offset bone loss later in life. During adulthood, daily calcium intake may bolster bone density.

A variety of nutrients in foods—including **isoflavone** and **lignan** phyto-estrogens, and **vitamins C, D,** and **K**—help promote bone strength as well, staving off fractures. The trace mineral **manganese,** plentiful in pineapple, is thought to improve the body's absorption of other bone-building minerals. Animal research suggests that **omega-3 fatty acids,** especially those found in fatty fish—such as salmon, herring, and tuna—may stimulate the growth of new bone protein, an important structural element in bone tissue.

Because elevated levels of homocysteine have been implicated in osteoporosis, the B vitamins **folate, B$_6$,** and **B$_{12}$** may be useful by converting this amino acid to a less harmful substance. Lentils and greens are high in folate, bananas and rice contain vitamin B$_6$, and fish and poultry are good sources of vitamin B$_{12}$.

Evidence is accumulating that a diet rich in fruits and vegetables may protect against osteoporosis. Observational studies indicate that men and women who consume the most fruits and vegetables have higher bone-mineral density, an important defense against fractures. Well-known bone-building vitamins and minerals are plentiful in produce, and even **potassium** and **magnesium** in fruits and vegetables may preserve bone strength. Research links these minerals to a slower decline in bone-mineral density. Foods rich in potassium may also help reduce high blood pressure, which scientists believe promotes calcium excretion, thus raising the risk for the bone-thinning disease.

Eating **plant protein** (in vegetables, soy foods, and grains such as quinoa) instead of animal protein, and consuming a diet that is not excessive in protein, is recommended because preliminary research suggests that animal protein and an overabundance of protein in general may raise the risk for osteoporosis-related fractures.

recent research

A large-scale, 10-year study of middle-aged women found that participants with the highest vitamin K consumption from foods had a 30% reduced risk for hip fracture. The richest sources of dietary vitamin K include kale, brussels sprouts, lettuce, broccoli, and spinach. Kale is a leading source of the bone-strengthening vitamin, providing about 550mcg in just 1 cup of raw greens.

your food arsenal

foods	nutrient	health benefits
cooking greens **dairy products**	calcium	The cornerstone of healthy bones, calcium raises bone density, an important measure of how well bones resist fractures.
lentils **soy foods**	isoflavones	Researchers believe these estrogenlike compounds promote bone density. Studies indicate isoflavones may conserve bone mass, particularly during perimenopause and menopause.
flaxseed	lignans	A study of healthy postmenopausal women (not on hormone replacement therapy) suggests that flaxseed, which is high in lignans, may retain bone mass, elevate antioxidant status, and help prevent urinary loss of calcium.
berries **citrus fruits** **peppers**	vitamin C	In addition to enhancing bone density, vitamin C helps form the connective tissue (collagen) matrix that holds bones together.
dairy products **fatty fish**	vitamin D	Necessary for optimal calcium absorption, vitamin D enhances bone strength.
kale **spinach**	vitamin K	This vitamin may strengthen bone by stimulating osteocalcin, a protein essential for bone strength.

overweight

what it is

Health experts warn that being overweight—defined as weighing more than 20% over the recommended ideal for your height—is a medical concern. Adults and children who are obese—defined roughly as 30 to 40 pounds over a healthy weight range (which is significantly more than 20% overweight)—are particularly susceptible to disease. Virtually every population group is becoming increasingly heavier and scientific evidence links the epidemic of excessive weight to a higher risk for diabetes, certain cancers, high blood pressure, heart disease, and various chronic conditions, including varicose veins and arthritis.

what causes it

Consuming too many calories and not expending enough energy lead to weight gain. A sedentary lifestyle, a calorie-dense diet, and genetics are major contributors to obesity.

how food may help

Adopting a healthy eating style and increasing physical activity are critical for balancing energy expenditure. For permanent weight loss, most experts agree that a gradual, realistic weight loss, without mortgaging overall health, is most successful. In addition to learning to cook delicious, healthful food, it's important to listen to hunger cues, learn to limit portions, and avoid calorie-laden convenience foods. Swapping spice for salt and limiting alcohol may improve weight loss efforts as well. Since there is a tendency to overeat when eating fast, slow down—it takes about 20 minutes for the stomach to signal the brain that it is full. Counting total calories is important, but note that there is some evidence that the body stores dietary fat more readily than it does protein or carbohydrate, which can contribute to weight gain.

Preliminary evidence suggests that **calcium** may stimulate fat loss by suppressing hormones that cause us to store, rather than burn, excess fat. Some research among significantly overweight men found that a high-calcium diet assisted weight loss. **Vitamin D** is essential for proper calcium absorption and research findings suggest that it may be particularly important for obese people to consume foods high in this vitamin. Scientists believe obese individuals may have reduced levels of bioavailable vitamin D. Excess body fat stores this fat-soluble vitamin, making it unavailable for its healthful activities, including strengthening the skeleton.

Several studies suggest that diets centered around low-fat **complex carbohydrates**—fruits, vegetables, and whole grains—help maintain healthy weight loss and prevent weight gain. Complex carbohydrates are rich in fiber and nutrients. Experts recommend at least five servings of fruits and vegetables each day to stave off extra pounds. Fruits and vegetables provide an abundance of nourishment and volume for their calorie content. A 5-ounce baked potato (with skin) has about 60% fewer calories and far more fiber than a medium (3½-ounce) serving of french fries.

Because they satisfy the appetite sooner and usually take longer to eat, foods high in **dietary fiber** are believed to aid in weight loss. Dietary fiber may slow the rate of digestion in the stomach as well. Filling up on high-fiber foods leaves less room for high-fat, calorie-dense foods. Some evidence suggests **soluble fiber** may assist in regulating blood sugar levels, thus controlling hunger pangs. In addition, research suggests that a high-fiber diet may slow fat absorption, helping you to feel fuller more quickly, while acquiring fewer fat calories. In one study, individuals consumed as much as 36g of fiber each day and absorbed up to 130 fewer calories, translating to a potentially significant weight loss.

According to preliminary research, green tea **catechins** may benefit energy expenditure and weight loss. Data from animal studies suggest that these green tea polyphenols may foster weight loss by stimulating fat oxidation.

your food arsenal

foods	nutrient	health benefits
broccoli **cooking greens** **dairy products** **figs**	calcium	Experimental research indicates that this indispensable mineral may promote the burning of calories rather than their storage as body fat.
beans **rice** **whole grains**	complex carbohydrates	Diets rich in low-fat complex carbohydrates have been associated with healthy body weight.
asparagus **beets** **lentils**	dietary fiber	High-fiber foods may prompt feelings of fullness with fewer calories.

perimenopause & menopause

what it is

Well before menstruation ceases (menopause), a woman's hormone levels may fluctuate for up to 10 years, during a phase known as perimenopause. A woman in perimenopause still menstruates, but experiences symptoms of diminished hormone levels. During menopause, a woman's body produces fewer reproductive hormones and no longer releases eggs or menstruates. Perimenopause and menopause symptoms include hot flashes, mood swings, night sweats, insomnia, and vaginal dryness.

what causes it

Perimenopause occurs as the ovaries gradually produce smaller quantities of the female hormones estrogen and progesterone. A lack of ovarian hormones during menopause, or as a result of surgical removal of the uterus and ovaries, halts ovulation (the release of an egg for fertilization) and ends menstruation. A woman has completed menopause after not having a period for 6 to 12 consecutive months.

how food may help

Consuming foods high in **phytoestrogens** (natural estrogenlike compounds in plant foods) may ease both perimenopause and menopause symptoms. Phytoestrogens are similar in structure to human estrogen but have milder estrogenic properties. Some evidence suggests that **isoflavones,** a type of phytoestrogen in soy foods, may relieve hot flashes and vaginal dryness associated with menopause. Epidemiological data indicate that women who consume soy phytoestrogens as a part of their daily diet—for example in such countries as China and Japan—tend to suffer far less from unpleasant menopause symptoms. In one recent six-year study of about 1,000 Japanese women between the ages of 35 and 54, researchers found that women who consumed the most soy products experienced significantly fewer hot flashes.

Researchers believe soy isoflavones may also help reduce the risk for heart disease, a major killer among postmenopausal women. After menopause, a woman's risk for heart attack increases tenfold because of declining estrogen levels. To combat this increased risk, a heart-healthy diet is recommended, which emphasizes plant-based meals full of cholesterol-lowering **soluble fiber,** monounsaturated fats, and omega-3 fatty acids. Replacing saturated and trans fats with **monounsaturated fat** helps reduce cholesterol levels and protect against clogged arteries. Several studies have found that eating **omega-3 fatty acids,** which are plentiful in fatty fish and walnuts, may help prevent heart attacks and stroke as well.

Diminishing estrogen levels during perimenopause and menopause predispose women to osteoporosis. To protect against this bone-thinning disease, consume plenty of bone-building **calcium** and **vitamin D,** the cornerstones of sturdy bones. Studies show that postmenopausal women with the highest intakes of calcium and vitamin D have the lowest risk for osteoporosis-related bone loss and fractures.

To ease the feelings of insomnia and mild depression that frequently accompany menopause, consume foods high in **tryptophan,** such as milk, poultry, and nuts. This amino acid is converted into the brain chemical serotonin, which promotes relaxation and rest. Tryptophan may also help reduce feelings of mild depression. **Complex carbohydrates,** such as beans, potatoes, and grains, may be helpful as well because they are believed to enhance the bioavailability of tryptophan in the brain.

Eating foods rich in **B vitamins** may help fight the blues; low levels of these vitamins may be linked to depression. B vitamins also foster the production of certain brain neurotransmitters required for restful sleep and a peaceful mood.

your food arsenal

foods	nutrient	health benefits
broccoli dairy products	calcium	Postmenopausal women are particularly vulnerable to bone-thinning osteoporosis, which calcium helps to prevent.
fatty fish flaxseed shellfish	omega-3 fatty acids	Because a woman's risk for cardiovascular disease dramatically increases after menopause, these healthful fats are recommended to help prevent heart disease and stroke.
flaxseed soy foods	phytoestrogens	These estrogenlike plant compounds may ease symptoms of perimenopause and menopause.
dairy products fatty fish	vitamin D	By improving calcium absorption, this fat-soluble vitamin helps to strengthen bones.

pregnancy

how food may help

Certain lifestyle decisions (such as eating healthful foods) can help improve pregnancy outcome. While it is important to maintain a healthy diet throughout pregnancy (the fetus requires essential nutrients at every stage of development), good nutrition during the first trimester of pregnancy is particularly vital because rapid growth of the spinal cord, heart, brain, and most fetal tissues occurs during this period.

In fact, improving diet *before* conception will help to build up nutritional reserves of vitamins and minerals (folate, iron, calcium, and vitamin B_{12}, for example) and other compounds in foods required by the fetus for proper growth. Accumulating nutrients prior to pregnancy will allow the fetus to draw upon them without depleting the mother's supply.

The changing physiological demands of pregnancy require a wide range of nutrients that will help the body to prepare for and sustain a healthy full-term pregnancy, labor, delivery, and breastfeeding. Daily food choices should include ample amounts of whole grains, vegetables, legumes, fruit, dairy foods, low-fat sources of protein, about six to eight 8-ounce glasses of water, and a minimum of sweets and saturated fats. Generally, most pregnant women need to increase their daily caloric intake by only 300 calories.

Calcium is particularly important because the fetus uses it for tooth, bone, and skeletal development. If a woman doesn't consume enough calcium, the fetus will take what is needed from her supply, so plentiful amounts of calcium are important to help preserve the mother's bone density. And for women who are planning on breastfeeding, calcium is vital for lactation.

Pregnant women need **iron** to replenish their red blood cell supply and to accommodate the demand created by increased blood volume. A pregnant woman's blood supply increases in order to provide nutrition to the growing fetus; adequate iron is required to help both the mother and baby transport oxygen through the body. The fetus also accumulates iron for use during early life. Foods high in **vitamin C** will facilitate iron absorption, and these foods are also rich in other beneficial substances. To achieve adequate iron levels, iron supplements may be recommended by a health care provider.

Folate is a B vitamin that is instrumental in preventing birth defects such as spina bifida and brain malformations, which can develop within the first month after conception. To ensure optimal levels of this important vitamin, experts recommend women take folic acid (the synthetic form of folate) supplements three months prior to conception. And because about half of all pregnancies are unplanned, a daily intake of folate is suggested for all women of childbearing age.

Protein is needed for the placenta and for the cellular development of the fetus. Lean poultry as a protein source also brings with it **vitamin B$_{12}$** and **zinc,** both critical to a healthy pregnancy. Exact protein needs should be discussed with a health care provider.

Complex carbohydrates can help the woman meet energy demands, and they will also supply glucose needed by the fetus for proper nervous system development. These foods are also chock-full of nourishing vitamins, minerals, and fiber.

Eating small meals and avoiding long periods without food may alleviate nausea that is caused by hormonal changes within the first trimester. In addition, try eating soda crackers or dry toast upon waking and at bedtime. Snack on nutrient-dense, high-protein foods and avoid foods high in salt or fat. **Ginger,** as well as foods rich in **vitamin B$_6$,** can serve as natural antinausea agents. To prevent constipation (a common problem in pregnancy), select nourishing fiber-rich foods such as broccoli, lentils, whole grains, dried fruits, and flaxseeds.

foods to avoid

Studies on the effects of caffeine on the unborn child have been contradictory; however, common sense dictates that caffeinated foods should be limited, as caffeine is a stimulant. All alcoholic beverages should be eliminated entirely, and smoking should be stopped altogether.

Although fish contain healthy oils, it is not advisable for pregnant women to eat large amounts of fish because a form of mercury called methylmercury can damage an unborn child's developing nervous system.

In addition, don't eat unpasteurized dairy products as they may harbor listeria (a type of bacteria), which could harm the unborn fetus. To avoid other foodborne illnesses, it is important to wash fruit and vegetables carefully, and not to drink unpasteurized cider.

your food arsenal

foods	nutrient	health benefits
broccoli **cooking greens** **nonfat milk** **nonfat plain yogurt**	calcium	Optimal intake of calcium is vital since a woman's body will "rob" calcium from its own bones to give it to the fetus if the mineral is in short supply. The fetus requires this bone-nourishing mineral for skeletal development.
asparagus **beets** **lentils**	folate	This important B vitamin helps to prevent neural tube defects that can develop within the first four weeks after conception.
amaranth **clams** **quinoa** **tofu**	iron	Pregnant women require extra iron to replenish their red blood supply and to accommodate the demand created by increased blood volume. The fetus accumulates iron for use during early life.

premenstrual syndrome

what it is

As many as 75% of menstruating women can identify with the physical and emotional symptoms of premenstrual syndrome (PMS). A highly individualized experience, PMS is characterized by a constellation of symptoms including moodiness, tearfulness, irritability, bloating (water retention), insomnia, fatigue, food cravings, headaches (sometimes migraines), breast tenderness, and depression. Symptoms generally start a week or a few days before menstruation and continue into the first few days. If symptoms become disruptive and impair daily life, it would be prudent to seek medical treatment.

what causes it

The exact cause of PMS is currently unknown, though theories suggest that PMS may result from an imbalance of hormones. This imbalance can cause mood fluctuations and food cravings. Preliminary studies indicate a possible link between PMS and abnormal metabolism of prostaglandins (hormonelike substances) or the hormone progesterone. Also, PMS may be associated with decreased levels of the brain chemical serotonin, which is instrumental in the regulation of mood, appetite, and feelings of well-being.

how food may help

Although food doesn't prevent PMS, certain substances in food may offer relief from some of the distressing symptoms of PMS.

Calcium may help to reduce mood disturbances, abdominal cramping, bloating, and muscular contractions resulting from PMS. Calcium may help regulate brain chemicals and hormones that affect mood.

Foods high in **complex carbohydrates** can be helpful in that they increase the production of serotonin, a brain chemical that regulates mood and appetite. Foods rich in complex carbohydrates also help to regulate glucose levels, which are thought to fluctuate in women with PMS.

Women who experience PMS often have low **magnesium** levels, which may predispose them to PMS-induced headaches.

Though research has been conflicting, some studies show that foods rich in **vitamin B₆** may help to stimulate production of serotonin and reduce anxiety and depression caused by PMS. Also, vitamin B₆ may help to increase the accumulation of magnesium in the body's cells.

One of the reasons that PMS is less common in Asian countries may be the high consumption of soy foods in those cultures. Soy isoflavones such as **genistein** (as well as **lignans** in flaxseeds) are phytoestrogens that may help to balance hormonal fluctuations by reducing high estrogen levels, believed to play a role in PMS.

Eating foods that are rich in **omega-3 fatty acids,** such as fish and shellfish, may decrease menstrual pain by promoting the production of anti-inflammatory prostaglandins. Omega-3 fatty acids may also reduce depression (see *page 162*), which is one of the many symptoms of PMS.

In addition to adding foods to the diet to help manage PMS, there are also some foods to be avoided. Reducing caffeine intake as well as sodium may help to reduce PMS symptoms.

recent research

A recent study indicates that a meat-free diet may be helpful in relieving symptoms of PMS. Researchers asked 33 women to adhere to a meat-free diet for two months, then go back to their normal diet for the following two months.

The researchers discovered that when the women adhered to the meat-free diet, they had fewer symptoms of PMS, fewer menstrual cramps, less water retention, and lower cholesterol levels. As a bonus, they lost weight.

The study participants who went back to their normal diets experienced PMS, cramps, and weight gain. Study authors suggest that the reduction of dietary fat and the adoption of a vegetarian diet alter estrogen levels.

your food arsenal

foods	nutrient	health benefits
nonfat plain yogurt skim milk tofu	calcium	Studies indicate that this mineral may help to reduce mood disturbances, cramping, and bloating resulting from PMS.
beans potatoes rice turnips whole grains	complex carbohydrates	By lowering the rate at which glucose enters the bloodstream, foods high in complex carbohydrates may offer satisfaction for those women plagued by PMS-induced food cravings. Further, complex carbohydrates are thought to increase levels of the brain chemical serotonin, which helps to regulate mood.
amaranth avocados quinoa sunflower seeds	magnesium	Some studies show that women suffering from PMS have low levels of magnesium.
avocados bananas potatoes salmon	vitamin B₆	This vitamin is believed to reduce anxiety and depression by increasing serotonin and other brain chemicals involved with mood.

prostate problems

what it is

"Prostate problems" generally translate into either benign prostatic hyperplasia (BPH) or prostate cancer. Though there are other types of prostate problems, such as prostatitis, BPH and prostate cancer are the most prevalent. Since these prostate problems have similar symptoms, it is vital to consult with a health care provider to seek proper testing and care.

Benign prostatic hyperplasia, also known as enlarged prostate, is one of the most common health problems facing men over the age of 60. In BPH the prostate gland enlarges and eventually places pressure on the urethra. Symptoms of BPH include difficulty with urination (stopping and starting), bladder irritation, a frequent urge to urinate (particularly during the night), dribbling, and a sensation of not emptying the bladder.

Prostate cancer is the most commonly diagnosed male cancer and the second leading cause of male cancer deaths in the United States. Checkups are advisable, particularly for men who experience painful or difficult urination, blood in the urine, painful ejaculation, impotence, or pain in the lower back.

what causes it

A common part of aging, BPH develops slowly over time. It is possible that a hormonal component may be associated with BPH. Prostate cancer may be linked to a hormonal cause, though research is still in the early stages. There is a genetic component, with men who have a family history of the disease being at higher risk compared with men who have no relatives with prostate cancer. Environmental factors also play a role in prostate cancer.

how food may help

Although more research is required in this area, some evidence does show a relationship between nutritional factors and prostate health.

Studies indicate that the antioxidant mineral **selenium** may protect against BPH, and it also may reduce the risk for developing prostate cancer, possibly by preventing oxidative damage to cells in the prostate gland. Selenium may protect against prostate cancer initiation, and it also may play a role in reducing prostate tumor growth by inducing apoptosis (cancer cell death).

Vitamin E teams up with selenium to confer antioxidant protection against free-radical damage to the prostate. Preliminary research also shows that vitamin E may decrease serum androgen concentrations, which are believed to be hormonal factors associated with prostate cancer.

The isoflavone **genistein,** found in soy foods, may help to protect against prostate cancer as well as possibly reducing tumor growth.

Preliminary research suggests that **lycopene** may help to decrease DNA damage to cells in prostate tissue, and it may play a role in initiating cancer cell death.

Laboratory research also shows that the flavonoid **quercetin** may help to prevent and treat prostate cancer. Quercetin may block the hormonal activity in androgen-response receptors in prostate cells, preventing the growth of cancer cells. Further research is required to see if these laboratory findings can extend into the realm of human research. Studies indicate that quercetin may also reduce symptoms of prostatitis.

recent research

A study conducted by Harvard scientists found a compelling link between lycopene and prostate cancer prevention. The study examined other carotenoids but only lycopene emerged as having protective effects.

The study participants who consumed the greatest amounts of lycopene showed a 21% decreased risk for prostate cancer.

Men who ate more than 10 servings of lycopene-rich tomato-based foods showed a 35% decreased risk for developing prostate cancer compared with those who ate fewer than 1.5 servings of tomato-based foods per week.

Studies, however, do not show that lycopene has a protective effect against BPH or prostatitis. In fact, tomato products may aggravate those conditions due to the acidic nature of tomatoes.

your food arsenal

foods	nutrient	health benefits
soy foods	genistein	Studies show that this isoflavone may reduce prostate cancer cell growth, possibly through hormonal actions.
apricots tomatoes watermelon	lycopene	Lycopene has been linked to the prevention of prostate cancer, possibly through its antioxidant properties.
Brazil nuts shrimp whole grains	selenium	This mineral may slow down the course of prostate cancer by inducing cancer cell death without harming healthy cells.
sardines sunflower seeds wheat germ	vitamin E	Vitamin E may protect the prostate gland, possibly through its antioxidant abilities.

psoriasis

what it is

Healthy skin cells gradually divide and migrate to the top layer of skin, replacing old cells. In psoriasis, however, skin growth is accelerated; skin cells multiply too quickly and, instead of being shed from the skin's surface, accumulate in thick patches. The plaques of raised pink skin typically occur in small areas on the scalp, elbows, knees, or lower back. The rash is not contagious and is typically not painful or very itchy.

About 15% of psoriasis sufferers have a widespread rash that interferes with daily activities. Debilitating joint pain and inflammation, similar to arthritis symptoms, affect at least 5% of people with the disorder. Psoriasis is chronic and commonly emerges between the ages of 10 and 30, affecting men and women equally.

what causes it

Experts are unsure of the exact cause of psoriasis, but they suspect a number of factors, including an inherited predisposition. The condition tends to run in families, particularly among fair-skinned people, and several genetic determinants have been discovered that make some people more susceptible.

Evidence is accumulating that many of the steps leading to the condition originate from an overzealous immune response—an army of infection-fighting cells invades healthy skin tissue, triggering inflammation. Researchers believe there may be a genetic basis for this immune reaction, and they have found an unusually high number of immune cells in psoriasis plaques. Emotional stress and certain drugs, such as ibuprofen, may precipitate psoriasis flare-ups. Additional triggers include poor diet, skin injuries, sunburn, hormones, illness, alcohol, and cold dry weather.

how food may help

Although research on how nutrition can help this complex skin disorder has not yielded a wealth of information, what we do know is that an overall healthy diet that emphasizes **antioxidant**-rich fruit and vegetables is beneficial for general skin health, as the antioxidants neutralize harmful elements that could damage skin. Foods high in **vitamin C** have antioxidant properties that protect against free-radical damage to the skin caused by environmental toxins.

Low levels of **selenium, zinc,** and **vitamin A** have been reported in people with psoriasis. Foods rich in these substances may have a general beneficial effect upon skin health. **Beta-carotene** is converted by the body to vitamin A, which is vital for maximum skin health. The beta-carotene and selenium act as antioxidants. Dietary zinc not only builds the immune system but it is also important for speeding up the healing of the skin.

Consuming foods rich in **omega-3 fatty acids** may reduce the inflammatory aspect of psoriasis. Some studies show that people with psoriasis may have abnormal levels of inflammatory agents called leukotrienes, which are thought to be involved in the development and progression of psoriasis.

In addition, some food sources of omega-3 fatty acids, such as salmon, mackerel, and sardines, are also good natural sources of the sunshine vitamin, **vitamin D;** low serum levels of this vitamin have been associated with psoriasis.

Preliminary studies suggest that some psoriasis patients may benefit from a gluten-free diet, though it would be wise to consult a nutritionist or a dermatologist before altering your diet. Total caloric intake may be important as well; some studies show a correlation between being overweight and the incidence of psoriasis.

recent research

A study (conducted in Italy) that examined the relationship between nutrition and psoriasis suggests that a diet rich in carrots, tomatoes, and fresh fruits seem to have a beneficial effect upon study participants with psoriasis.

The authors of the study speculate that the protective substances in the foods may be carotenoids, as well as vitamins that have antioxidant properties. Note that foods containing high levels of antioxidants tend to contain phytochemicals that offer a wide range of benefits.

your food arsenal

foods	nutrient	health benefits
broccoli **carrots** **sweet potatoes** **tomatoes**	antioxidants	Antioxidants such as beta-carotene, vitamins C and E, and the mineral selenium are important defenders against free radicals that may harm the skin.
fatty fish **shellfish**	omega-3 fatty acids	It is believed that omega-3 fatty acids help to counteract the formation of inflammatory agents called leukotrienes.

rheumatoid arthritis

what it is

This chronic inflammatory disease of the joints is the most serious form of arthritis and can affect the entire body. Fever, loss of appetite, and a general ill feeling frequently accompany inflamed, stiff joints.

what causes it

A type of autoimmune disease, rheumatoid arthritis stems from an abnormal immune response in which the body's own immune cells attack and invade the protective linings of joints and sometimes internal organs, causing inflammation. Researchers suspect viruses and hormonal, genetic, and dietary factors as causes of the condition.

how food may help

Anecdotal evidence suggests that consuming a diet high in unprocessed foods—fruits, vegetables, and whole grains—lowers the risk for debilitating rheumatoid arthritis; and a plant-based diet has been linked with pain relief among sufferers. Decreasing both total fat and calories is believed to further ameliorate symptoms.

A diet rich in healing vitamins and minerals, most notably **vitamins C** and **E,** may help prevent and manage rheumatoid arthritis. **Selenium** may enhance the antioxidant actions of vitamin E and helps support an important inflammation-fighting enzyme, glutathione peroxidase. Low levels of selenium, as well as zinc and beta-carotene, have been associated with rheumatoid arthritis.

Some preliminary evidence suggests that **zinc** may help alleviate symptoms of rheumatoid arthritis. Along with its own antioxidant properties, zinc is integral to the body's attack on free radicals.

Because some drugs prescribed for rheumatoid arthritis deplete the important B vitamin **folate,** some experts advise consuming folate-rich foods.

Several studies link low antioxidant status with an increased risk for the disorder, so a diet filled with antioxidant flavonoids, including those found in **green tea,** may be helpful. Epidemiological data link high green tea consumption with reduced rates of rheumatoid arthritis, and preliminary animal research using the equivalent of 4 cups of green tea supports this finding. Protection is attributed to the powerful antioxidant polyphenols in green tea.

Some evidence suggests that powerful antioxidants in **turmeric** (the spice responsible for the bright yellow color of curry powder) may modify inflammatory compounds and activate the body's own anti-inflammatory actions.

The anti-inflammatory actions of **bromelain, omega-3 fatty acids,** and **ginger** may ameliorate the condition as well. Researchers believe omega-3s may inhibit the production of inflammatory compounds called prostaglandins and leukotrienes, both of which contribute to joint inflammation. One small clinical study found that 5g of fresh ginger per day provided significant relief from rheumatoid arthritis symptoms.

> ### recent research
>
> Observational data suggest that women who consume at least one serving of fish each week may have a significantly lower risk for rheumatoid arthritis. Omega-3 fatty acids may be a protective factor, since fatty fish such as salmon and tuna are excellent sources of these healthful fats.

your food arsenal

foods	nutrient	health benefits
pineapple	bromelain	The pineapple enzyme bromelain has been reported to decrease inflammation associated with rheumatoid arthritis, possibly by blocking the formation of inflammatory compounds.
apples berries citrus fruits onions	flavonoids	Because they may support connective tissue and quell inflammation, flavonoids may help relieve symptoms of rheumatoid arthritis.
salmon mackerel tuna	omega-3 fatty acids	Clinical studies demonstrate a beneficial effect of these fats on arthritis symptoms, including joint stiffness, tenderness, and fatigue.
ginger	shogaols & gingerols	Ginger exhibits potent antioxidant activity and is thought to suppress the development of inflammatory compounds.
citrus fruits peppers strawberries	vitamin C	This healing nutrient supports connective tissue in the joints, provides valuable antioxidant activity, and may inhibit inflammation.
avocados nuts seeds whole grains	vitamin E	Preliminary clinical findings suggest this potent antioxidant may help relieve the pain and stiffness of rheumatoid arthritis.

rosacea

what it is

Rosacea is a chronic, inflammatory, vascular skin condition that affects approximately 13 million people in the United States. The disorder is typified by prolonged redness and the occurrence of acnelike bumps on the cheeks, forehead, nose, chin, or eyes. Rosacea is most common among fair-skinned women between the ages of 30 and 60.

In the early stages of rosacea, sporadic occurrences of blushing, flushing, and redness of the face take place, and are often mistaken for simple blushing. If left untreated, tiny blood vessels swell and become larger, and facial redness can become permanent. If untreated, men with rosacea often develop rhinophyma, which causes the nose to become enlarged, red, and bulbous. Because of the redness (as well as the rhinophyma), rosacea is sometimes unfairly attributed to alcoholism.

If you suspect that you may have rosacea, it is important to seek treatment as soon as possible, because proper treatment can reduce symptoms and help to prevent the disorder from getting worse.

what causes it

Though a single cause has not yet been identified, certain people may have a hereditary tendency to develop rosacea. Some scientists suspect that rosacea may result from an abundance of microscopic mites that live in human skin. These tiny organisms may block the sebaceous gland openings, thus promoting inflammation.

Other potential causes include immune system abnormalities. Also, anecdotal reports show a connection between stress and the exacerbation of rosacea. Hormonal changes caused by menopause may also be a factor in its onset.

Histamines, chemicals released by the body as a natural response to allergens, cause inflammation and may also trigger rosacea. A common rosacea trigger, facial flushing may be brought on by blushing, stress, heat, sun, wind, cold, spicy foods, or certain medications. More research is required to identify the causes of this skin disorder.

how food may help

Although research on how diet may help rosacea is currently lacking, certain foods may help to promote general optimal skin health. Foods rich in **beta-carotene** and **vitamin E** may be helpful for general skin health because they act as antioxidants by neutralizing harmful elements that could damage skin.

To offset stress that may trigger or aggravate rosacea, it may be helpful to eat foods that are rich in **vitamin B$_6$,** which assists in the production of certain brain chemicals that help to regulate mood.

Rosacea is believed to be a disorder linked to swollen blood vessels, so it may be useful to eat foods high in **essential fatty acids,** which are thought to have anti-inflammatory properties.

Eating foods high in antioxidant-rich, immune-building **vitamin C** may help to protect the skin from free-radical damage as well as inflammation caused by histamines. Foods containing vitamin C are also useful for protecting veins. Foods rich in **zinc** help to promote healing and enhance the functioning of the immune system.

foods to avoid

Although the exact cause of rosacea is currently unknown, we do know that certain foods may cause the characteristic flushing and redness. For example, people with rosacea should try to avoid spicy foods, hot drinks, and alcoholic beverages. You may not have to give up hot coffee or tea altogether—just allow them to cool a little bit before drinking them. There is no common ingredient at the root of these triggers.

It might be helpful to keep a diary of foods and episodes of flushing and redness to try to determine which foods may be triggers for the condition.

your food arsenal

foods	nutrient	health benefits
fatty fish **flaxseed** **pumpkin seeds**	essential fatty acids	As inflammation of the skin occurs in rosacea, it may be useful to eat foods rich in essential fatty acids, which help to reduce swelling by generating substances in the body that can reduce inflammation.
berries **broccoli** **citrus fruits** **kiwifruit**	vitamin C	The antioxidant properties of vitamin C may help to protect the skin from free-radical damage caused by pollution and the sun's harmful rays. Vitamin C may inhibit the release of histamine, a substance that is thought to cause inflammation as the immune system's response to allergens.

sinusitis

what it is

One of the most common ailments in the United States, sinusitis is an infection of the lining of one or more of the sinus cavities, causing inflammation. There are two types of sinusitis: acute, which lasts for three weeks or less, and chronic, which often lasts for three to eight weeks but can continue even longer. Some 37 million Americans are affected by sinusitis every year. Both types of sinusitis are extremely uncomfortable and symptoms can range from intense pain to a general malaise.

In sinusitis, tissues swell and cells produce thick mucus, which is unable to drain properly through the small sinus channels and openings. What results is a heavy pressure that builds up, causing a sinus headache, congestion, persistent cough, fatigue, tender cheekbones, and pain around the sinus areas. A typical sinus headache tends to be mild in the morning and gets worse during the day. It is also sometimes accompanied by fever, runny nose, congestion, irritation, and general fatigue and weakness.

what causes it

Both acute and chronic sinusitis often develop after an upper-respiratory infection (a cold or flu) spreads to the sinus cavities. Blockage of the sinus passages caused by allergies, the flu, or the common cold may lead to the development of bacterial infections that can lead to acute sinusitis. It is thought that some forms of chronic sinusitis result from an immune system response to naturally occurring fungi in the nose. Studies suggest an association between asthma and sinusitis.

Other potential causes of sinusitis may include allergies; bacteria that cause infections of mouth, gums, or teeth; exposure to airborne or environmental irritants such as tobacco smoke, smog, mold spores, or dust; and polyps inside the nasal cavities.

how food may help

Sinusitis often follows a cold or the flu, so it is important to maintain a strong immune system to avoid these infections. Foods containing the antioxidant **vitamin C** can help to bolster your immune system by stimulating the activity of antibodies and immune system cells. Dietary **zinc** is also an important defender against invading viruses and infections, and it may also have anti-inflammatory properties.

One of the symptoms of sinusitis is inflammation along the nasal passages caused by allergens. These allergens initiate an immune response, which releases histamines and other chemicals that are thought to cause congestion. The anti-inflammatory actions of certain flavonoids such as **luteolin** and **quercetin** may decrease congestion by reducing the body's release of histamine.

It may also be useful to eat pineapple, which contains the enzyme **bromelain.** Preliminary studies indicate that this substance may have anti-inflammatory properties. Note that pineapple is also a good source of vitamin C, which may also dampen inflammation.

A hot cup of tea soothes the soul and may also help to reduce congestion. Not only does the steam help to temporarily open up the nasal passages, but tea also contains **theophylline,** a compound believed to ease breathing by relaxing the smooth muscles in the walls of the airways.

Eating spicy foods, such as horseradish, mustard, and ginger, can provide temporary relief by reducing congestion. **Allyl isothiocyanate,** a pungent substance in horseradish and mustard, helps to thin mucus. Be sure to also drink plenty of water and fluids to keep mucus thin.

home remedy

For temporary relief of congestion from sinusitis, try eating some chili peppers. Chili peppers as well as cayenne pepper contain capsaicin, a powerful and fiery compound that acts as a mucolytic agent by breaking up mucus and promoting mucus flow, offering temporary relief from pressure in the sinuses.

your food arsenal

foods	nutrient	health benefits
berries **citrus fruits** **peppers** **pineapple**	vitamin C	Vitamin C helps to maintain a strong immune system, and it works to fight off colds—a common antecedent to sinusitis. Vitamin C may also help to minimize the inflammation and swelling of mucous membranes lining the sinuses by preventing the release of histamine.
beans **crab** **poultry** **wheat germ**	zinc	The immune-fortifying capability of zinc may help to ward off viruses that are often implicated in the onset of sinus problems.

sprains & strains

what it is

Sprains and strains can afflict young and old, couch potatoes and professional athletes. A sprain is an injury to a ligament, which links bone to bone and supports a joint. It is usually the result of a ligament being stretched too far or being torn. A strain, on the other hand, is an injury to a tendon (which connects muscle to bone) or a muscle. The time it takes sprains and strains to heal depends on their severity, but relatively speaking a strain usually takes longer since the damaged fibers in muscles require more time to mend.

Both sprains and strains vary in severity and levels of discomfort, and, depending upon how serious the damage is, both types of injury can cause sharp pain as well as impairment of power and movement. Ankles are the joints most vulnerable to sprains, while the back and hamstring muscle (back of the thigh) are the most common strains. Swelling occurs in both sprains and strains.

what causes it

Often the result of a sudden force, typically a twisting motion, sprains and strains sometimes occur during jogging, running, or playing basketball. Lifting a heavy object or weight, or extending and stretching muscles and tendons too far (for example, when swinging a golf club or a tennis racket) can all cause injury. Overweight people and sedentary people are especially vulnerable to sprains or strains.

how food may help

Clearly, what you eat will not prevent a sprain or a strain; however, diet certainly has an effect on overall health and weight. Maintaining a healthy weight is key, as excess pounds place stress on joints and increase the risk for injuries to muscles and ligaments.

Muscles require glycogen (derived from glucose) for optimum exertion for athletic events. To ensure that muscles receive enough fuel, you should eat foods rich in **complex carbohydrates.** Glucose from complex carbohydrates is metabolized slowly, and supplies the required energy for a sustained level of exertion.

Protein is required for muscle and joint health. Low-fat sources of protein, such as soy foods and certain grains such as amaranth and quinoa, are excellent plant-based alternatives to meat protein.

Vitamin C is helpful in keeping ligaments and tendons strong. It also helps to repair tissue.

Omega-3 fatty acids are particularly beneficial in that they may help to accelerate the healing of ligaments injured by sprains. Also, omega-3s may have an anti-inflammatory effect, which can relieve discomfort from swelling in joints.

Though scientific evidence is scarce, anecdotal reports indicate that **bromelain** may also reduce swelling. Bromelain is an anti-inflammatory enzyme found in pineapple (pineapples are also a good source of vitamin C, which is important for collagen).

Certain minerals are needed for bone, ligament, and muscle health. For example, **magnesium, calcium,** and **phosphorus** form bones; and **manganese** is required for the formation of cartilage and connective tissue. **Zinc** promotes tissue repair and growth.

The "sunshine vitamin," **vitamin D** assists in regulating blood levels of calcium and phosphorus and is essential for the maintenance of healthy cartilage and bones. The body also needs vitamin D to help properly absorb calcium from food. Vitamin D is found in fortified milk and salmon (which coincidentally is a good source of omega-3 fatty acids).

recent research

Results of a laboratory study on the effect of omega-3 fatty acids suggest that they speed up the healing of ligament cells. The experimental study compared arachidonic acid (an omega-6 fatty acid), eicosapentaenoic acid (an omega-3 fatty acid), and a third substance that served as a control. The researchers compared the cells of the ligaments treated with each compound and examined the rate at which the ligament cells healed over a 72-hour period.

While both the arachidonic acid and the eicosapentaenoic acid revealed the ability to heal the cells, the omega-3 showed a significantly greater ability to enhance the entry of new cells into the wound area and to speed up collagen synthesis. This experiment indicates that omega-3 fatty acid in foods may have the ability to speed up the healing of ligament injuries that occur in sprains.

your food arsenal

foods	nutrient	health benefits
beans potatoes rice whole grains	complex carbohydrates	Complex carbohydrates provide fuel and, as they take longer to digest than simple carbohydrates, are useful for sustained energy.
amaranth fish nonfat dairy soy foods	protein	Important for muscle and joint health as well as tissue repair, protein can be found in numerous low-fat foods that also confer a wide range of other nutritional benefits.
berries citrus fruits kiwifruit pineapple	vitamin C	This vitamin helps to build and maintain collagen, the fibers that make up the tissue between tendons, ligaments, bones, and cartilage.

stroke

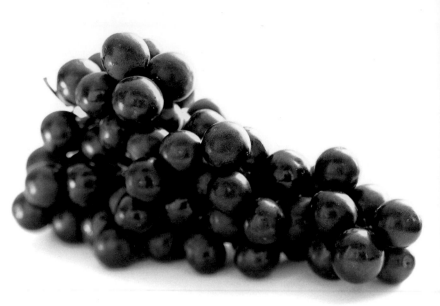

what it is

A stroke occurs when a blocked or ruptured artery suddenly deprives the brain of oxygen-rich blood, potentially leading to permanent detrimental effects on physical and emotional well-being. Speech, vision, movement, and sensation are most commonly compromised by a stroke.

what causes it

The most common type of stroke, ischemic stroke, is caused by a blood clot that blocks blood flow to the brain. A clot usually forms as a result of fatty plaque buildup that narrows arteries near or in the brain and impedes circulation. A clot may also form in another part of the body, travel, and lodge in a blood vessel that nourishes the brain. Hemorrhagic strokes, caused by a ruptured, bleeding artery in the brain, are less common.

how food may help

Numerous studies indicate that eating a low-fat diet rich in fruits and vegetables significantly protects against stroke. One study found that people who ate vegetables six to seven days per week cut their risk for stroke by over 50%. Eating plenty of whole grains is important for stroke protection as well since data suggest a whole-grain diet may reduce risk for the condition. Several nutrients and phytochemicals plentiful in produce and whole grains—**calcium, flavonoids, fiber, magnesium, omega-3 fatty acids, potassium, resveratrol,** and **vitamin C**—have shown promise in protecting against the condition.

Scientific evidence is accumulating that free-radical-fighting antioxidants, such as resveratrol and **selenium,** may protect against ischemic stroke. Researchers believe **vitamin E** may protect against stroke by squelching free radicals and inhibiting oxidation of LDL ("bad") cholesterol, which can clog arteries and contribute to stroke.

There is growing evidence that elevated levels of the amino acid homocysteine, long linked to heart attacks, may also up the risk for stroke: As levels of homocysteine increase, stroke risk tends to increase as well. The B vitamins **folate, vitamin B$_6$,** and **vitamin B$_{12}$** appear to team up to lower homocysteine levels. According to one study, when participants adopted a high-folate diet, average homocysteine levels dropped by an impressive 7%. Citrus fruit and lentils are excellent sources of folate, and seafood is high in B$_6$ and B$_{12}$.

Since elevated blood pressure and high cholesterol increase the risk for stroke, see pages 180–183 for advice on managing blood pressure and cholesterol.

recent research

A 14-year study of almost 80,000 women between the ages of 34 and 59 found that participants who ate 4 ounces of fish two to four times each week cut their risk for clot-related stroke by nearly half. The effect was particularly strong in women who consumed fatty fish, such as salmon and tuna, which are rich in omega-3s.

your food arsenal

foods	nutrient	health benefits
broccoli dairy products figs	calcium	A meta-analysis of 42 studies found that calcium has a small but significant benefit on blood pressure. Calcium is thought to inhibit blood clots that lead to a stroke.
asparagus beets lentils	dietary fiber	Studies link a high fiber intake from fruits and vegetables with a reduced risk for stroke. Soluble fiber in particular is believed to interfere with atherosclerosis and blood clots, which can lead to an ischemic stroke.
apples berries onions	flavonoids	Population-based studies suggest that dietary flavonoids, particularly quercetin, may reduce fat deposits in arteries that can block blood flow to the brain.
fatty fish shellfish	omega-3 fatty acids	Eating two or more servings of fatty fish, such as salmon, each week may lower the risk for certain types of stroke by 50%, according to studies. Scientists surmise that the omega-3 fatty acids abundant in fatty fish impede formation of blood clots, protecting against stroke.
bananas orange juice potatoes	potassium	By contributing to lower blood pressure and possibly diminishing blood clots, potassium may decrease stroke risk.
peanuts red grapes red wine	resveratrol	Preliminary evidence suggests this phytochemical may inhibit blood clots and also help to relax blood vessels.
citrus fruits kiwifruit melons	vitamin C	A population-based study found that individuals with the lowest levels of vitamin C in their blood had a 70% increased risk for stroke. The protective effects of vitamin C may extend beyond its antioxidant properties, according to researchers.

tooth & mouth conditions

what it is

Gum disease, dental caries (cavities), canker sores, and bad breath (halitosis) all fall into the category of tooth and mouth conditions. Gum disease (gingivitis) develops when bacteria infect the crevices between gums and teeth. Gums typically become red and swollen and, when left untreated, could lead to tooth loss.

One of the major causes of tooth loss is dental caries, which can be traced to tooth-coating plaque. Bacteria, food debris, saliva, and acid combine to form plaque. Gradually, the corrosive acids dissolve tooth enamel, creating pits in the grooved surfaces on teeth. Canker sores are small shallow white ulcers that can suddenly flare up on the gums, tongue, soft palate, or inside the cheeks. Bad breath is a frequent consequence of poor dental hygiene, dry mouth, infrequent eating or drinking, or lingering food smells (e.g., garlic or onions).

what causes it

Poor dental hygiene—a lack of brushing, flossing, or rinsing—frequently leads to gum disease, cavities, or bad breath. Increasing age and a genetic predisposition may leave some people more prone to poor dental health as well. A multitude of additional factors, including odor-causing and infectious bacteria, stress, smoking, a poor or high-sugar diet, and chronic illness, may contribute to tooth and mouth conditions.

how food may help

Population studies have found that a high consumption of sweet, sticky ("cariogenic") foods—such as juice, soda, and candy—increases risk for dental decay. To reduce risk, experts advise limiting sugar intake and minimizing the amount of time that teeth are exposed to sugary and sticky foods and drinks.

On the other hand, there is a wealth of foods that can improve dental health. For example, there are several anticariogenic foods that are believed to inhibit plaque formation (thus protecting against cavities and gum disease). Nuts, cheese, popcorn, tea, and fibrous vegetables, such as celery, may help prevent tooth decay, because cavity-inducing bacteria do not easily ferment them.

Preliminary research on green tea suggests that its powerful **catechin, EGCG,** may prevent *Streptococcus mutans*, a major culprit in tooth decay, from sticking to tooth enamel and initiating cavities.

Some evidence suggests a carbohydrate-like component in **shiitake mushrooms** may reduce plaque formation, though research is very preliminary. Chewing sugar-free, xylitol-sweetened gum may prevent cavities by inhibiting growth of decay-causing bacteria and reduce the amount of plaque.

Calcium is the cornerstone of solid, sturdy teeth and may protect against gum disease. Research has found that adults, particularly between the ages of 20 and 40, with the lowest calcium intakes (below 500mg daily) have twice the risk for gum disease. Scientists believe that one way in which calcium may improve resistance against infection is by strengthening the jawbone and maintaining tooth structure.

Foods high in **insoluble fiber** may help by removing food particles from between teeth and in gum pockets. Crunchy, fibrous foods, such as carrot sticks, may cleanse teeth, as well as stimulate gum tissue.

Vitamin C is essential for healthy gums and may enhance the healing of cuts and sores in the mouth. Some experts believe low levels of the amino acid **lysine** contribute to canker sores.

home remedy

To freshen bad breath, create a homemade herbal mouthwash with parsley and cloves. In a heatproof bowl, combine several sprigs of coarsely chopped parsley with 2 cups of boiling water. Next add ¼ teaspoon of cloves or 2 whole cloves. Let cool to room temperature (with occasional stirring), strain, and use as a mouthwash, gargling several times a day. (Store it in the refrigerator.) Parsley's chlorophyll content and the eugenol (a type of phytochemical) in cloves are thought to neutralize bad breath.

your food arsenal

foods	nutrient	health benefits
almonds broccoli cooking greens dairy products	calcium	This bone-building mineral is essential for sturdy teeth, and research suggests that adults with low calcium intakes have a significantly increased risk for gum disease.
green tea pomegranates	catechins	These powerful green tea polyphenols, particularly EGCG, may prevent cavity-causing bacteria from adhering to teeth.
broccoli celery salad greens	insoluble fiber	This type of dietary fiber may dislodge food particles from between teeth and gums.
beans dairy & eggs	lysine	Canker sores have been associated with a deficiency in this amino acid.
berries citrus fruits peppers	vitamin C	In addition to promoting healing in the mouth, this vitamin is a vital component of connective tissue of teeth and bones.

urinary tract infection

what it is

Urinary tract infections (UTIs) are among the most common bacterial infections and are characterized by a frequent urge to urinate and a painful burning sensation during urination. Symptoms may also include mild fever, back pain, abdominal cramps, and blood in the urine. The infection typically affects the bladder or the urethra, the tube that carries urine away from the bladder out of the body. Because of a shorter urethra (which makes it easier for bacteria to migrate up to the bladder), women are far more likely to suffer from a UTI than men. UTIs often recur, and if an infection is left untreated, it can lead to a serious kidney infection.

what causes it

UTIs are caused by bacteria that migrate into the urethra. Urine is usually free of germs, but bacteria from the genital area or rectal area may travel into the urinary tract through the urethra and, most commonly, up to the bladder, where they attach to the bladder lining, multiply, and cause an infection. Ignoring the urge to urinate increases the risk for a UTI. Other causes include not drinking enough fluids, improper hygiene (wiping should be front to back), pregnancy, and sexual activity.

how food may help

Because a UTI may rapidly progress into a dangerous infection, it is best to immediately consult a physician if you are suffering from the condition.

To improve urine flow during an infection, drink at least one 8-ounce glass of water each hour to wash harmful germs out of the urinary tract. Regularly consuming plenty of water may help prevent infectious bacteria from taking hold in the urinary tract in the first place. Folk healers often recommend parsley to help flush out a UTI. Compounds in parsley, such as **myristicin** and **apide,** may act as diuretics, increasing urine flow.

Conventional science has begun to confirm another traditional folk remedy for urinary tract infections—drinking **cranberry juice.** A clinical trial of 153 elderly women found that women who drank 10 ounces of low-calorie cranberry juice each day had 50% fewer bacteria in their urine. The cranberry drinkers were also 25% less likely to have infected urine from month to month.

Researchers have isolated tannin compounds in cranberry juice and have found that these substances may be highly protective against UTIs. It's thought that the tannin compounds may combat UTIs by preventing bacteria from attaching to the bladder and kidney walls, multiplying unrestrained, and causing an infection. The bacteria are instead flushed out in the urine.

Cranberries are also thought to acidify urine, making the urinary tract a less hospitable environment for harmful bacteria to thrive. And **vitamin C** (in addition to fortifying the body's immune defenses) may also acidify urine, making it more difficult for infectious bacteria to colonize.

If infectious bacteria in the genital area are allowed to multiply unrestrained, they may travel from the genitals into the urethra, causing a UTI. But consuming **probiotics** (beneficial bacteria) can be helpful, since this promotes the growth of healthy bacteria in the body. These bacteria crowd out harmful microbes and may even secrete anti-infective substances. Our bodies house over 400 species of healthful bacteria, which feed on nondigestible carbohydrates, such as **fructooligosaccharides (FOS).** Consuming FOS (in onions and artichokes, for example) may help friendly flora to flourish.

recent research

Like cranberry juice, blueberry juice may wash harmful bacteria out of the urinary tract, because blueberries have protective tannin compounds similar to those found in cranberries.

your food arsenal

foods	nutrient	health benefits
yogurt	probiotics	Though clinical data are scant, the beneficial bacteria in "active culture" yogurt may inhibit the growth of microorganisms that can cause UTIs. These beneficial bacteria are also thought to foster the growth of friendly flora in the body, which may be reduced by antibiotic therapy.
blueberries cranberries	tannins	Research suggests that these phytonutrients, plentiful in berries, inhibit bacteria from sticking to the lining of the urinary tract, thus preventing infection.
berries broccoli citrus fruits peppers	vitamin C	This indispensable vitamin reinforces the body's immune defenses against infection.

varicose veins

what it is

Typically an unsightly cosmetic problem in the legs and feet, varicose veins look like swollen bluish cords just beneath the skin's surface. Sore, achy legs may accompany varicose veins, though pain and tenderness are usually mild. Lumpy skin frequently surrounds bulging veins and small patches of flooded capillaries—superficial spider veins—may cluster in the area or appear on the ankles and thighs. Blood clots may occasionally develop in varicose veins, but clots in these superficial veins are generally not considered life-threatening. Women are at least twice as likely as men to have varicose veins, and diet and lifestyle factors may play an important role in preventing and managing the condition.

what causes it

Weak vessel walls or faulty valves inside veins may hamper circulation, causing blood to pool and distend veins. Less frequently, phlebitis (inflammation of a vein) or inherited abnormal vein structure may result in varicose and spider veins. The condition tends to run in families, and hormones, obesity, pregnancy, lack of exercise, increasing age, and heavy lifting may also lead to varicose veins. Constipation, tight clothing, leg crossing, and prolonged sitting and standing may increase the risk for the disorder by unduly pressuring veins.

how food may help

Insoluble fiber promotes regularity and reduces straining during bowel movements. This is important, because straining contributes to varicose veins by increasing abdominal pressure and blocking blood flow from the legs. **Soluble fibers** such as pectin, gum, and psyllium are particularly useful in easing elimination by bulking up waste and promoting contractions of the digestive tract.

Vitamin C is thought to benefit varicose veins by teaming up with antioxidant flavonoids to fortify vessel walls and fend off oxidative damage, which may compromise vein strength. A host of **flavonoids,** especially those abundant in citrus fruit, may bolster vein structure by reducing blood vessel frailty and leakiness. The citrus flavonoid **hesperidin** is thought to enhance the actions of vitamin C and may be required for optimal capillary function. **Diosmin,** a flavonoid found in rosemary and citrus fruit, may prevent blood vessel fragility, which can lead to varicose veins. A flavonoid in white grapefruit called **naringin** may also enhance blood vessel health. According to preliminary research, **rutin,** a flavonoid present in apples and buckwheat, may promote blood vessel health by bolstering cell membrane support cells and structural tissue. In laboratory studies, the highly active flavonoid **quercetin** (closely related to rutin, hesperidin, and diosmin and found in red onions and blueberries) has exhibited potent anti-inflammatory properties, which may protect against varicose veins.

Additional antioxidants are under review for their benefit to vein health, including **green tea** polyphenols and **vitamin E** (a potent antioxidant found in avocados and olive oil), which may be important for blood vessel health by improving vessel function and strengthening capillaries. And finally, researchers believe **tannin compounds** (also known as proanthocyanidins) may benefit varicose veins because these antioxidants are incorporated into cell membranes where they are thought to protect against damaging free radicals.

home remedy

Eating pineapple may improve unsightly varicose veins. Though clinical evidence is lacking, a protein-digesting pineapple enzyme, bromelain, is thought to reduce proteinlike fibrin deposits that build up around varicose veins and give a lumpy appearance to the tender skin.

your food arsenal

foods	nutrient	health benefits
asparagus **beets** **lentils** **pomegranates**	dietary fiber	Dietary fiber decreases pressure on blood vessels in the legs by promoting regular bowel movements and reducing strain during bowel movements.
apples **berries** **citrus fruits** **grapes** **whole grains**	flavonoids	Experimental research suggests flavonoids may team up with vitamin C to fortify blood vessel membranes and to enhance vessel function by reducing breakage, free-radical damage, and permeability.
berries	tannins	These antioxidant compounds (also known as proanthocyanidins) may help reduce blood vessel leakage and protect vessels against free-radical damage.
berries **broccoli** **citrus fruits** **peppers**	vitamin C	This vitamin may strengthen blood vessels and defend membranes against damaging free radicals. A deficiency in vitamin C leads to blood vessel frailty.

yeast infection

what it is

The irritating discharge and uncomfortable burning of a vaginal yeast infection afflicts most women at some point in their lives. Infrequently, men may develop a genital yeast infection, though they may not display any apparent symptoms.

Normally, small numbers of harmless microorganisms live harmoniously in the linings of the vagina, digestive tract, and skin. These friendly germs assist with digestion, combat invading pathogens, and help manufacture essential nutrients. The vagina is an ideal warm, moist environment for many fungi, especially yeast, to thrive. So when the balance of vaginal flora is upset, an infectious overgrowth of yeast organisms, usually *Candida albicans*, may occur. As yeast multiplies unrestrained, an unpleasant white, lumpy, cottage cheese-like discharge is secreted and the external genital area frequently becomes inflamed and itchy and may cause burning or pain during intercourse.

what causes it

Benign vaginal yeast may grow unchecked when pH (acid/base) levels or the balance of bacteria and yeast in the vagina are disturbed. Hormonal changes from pregnancy or birth control pills frequently change vaginal pH levels, leading to yeast infections. Antibiotic therapy for any condition commonly causes yeast infections by depleting the friendly bacteria that usually prevent vaginal yeast from multiplying out of control.

A yeast infection may also be symptomatic of a depressed immune system overburdened from stress, sleep deprivation, chemotherapy, or illness, including HIV and diabetes. In addition, wearing nylon underwear, tight jeans, or using spermicides, deodorant tampons, or douches may increase risk for infection.

how food may help

Increasing the body's levels of healthful **probiotic bacteria** may prevent overgrowth of infectious vaginal yeast. These friendly flora help crowd out infectious yeast and maintain an acidic environment that prevents these irritating fungi from multiplying unchecked. Confirming the folk medicine belief in these healthful microbes, some clinical evidence suggests that consuming sufficient quantities of yogurt with live bacteria cultures, including *Lactobacillus acidophilus*, may alleviate symptoms of a yeast infection and lower the risk for repeated infections.

Since probiotic bacteria thrive on nondigested sugars known as **fructooligosaccharides (FOS),** consuming more FOS compounds may foster the growth of beneficial bacteria. These compounds are believed to nourish friendly flora, enhancing and sustaining their growth in the body.

Garlic may be a natural anti-yeast agent, because animal and test-tube studies have demonstrated this bulb's ability to inhibit the growth of *Candida albicans*, the organism commonly responsible for vaginal yeast infections. The highly active substance **allicin,** which gives garlic its pungent odor and bite, is thought to be responsible for garlic's antifungal activity.

By enhancing immunity, **vitamin C** may protect against yeast infections. This vitamin, abundant in citrus fruit and peppers, is believed to galvanize infection-fighting white blood cells, which may fortify immune defenses.

According to test-tube studies, a compound isolated from cayenne pepper, **CAY-1,** has shown promise in fighting a range of microbes, including the fungus that leads to yeast infections. CAY-1 is a natural protective agent in cayenne pepper, defending the plant against invading fungi native to its tropical habitat. The compound does not seem to have toxic effects against human cells and appears to effectively knock out yeast.

home remedy

Some anecdotal evidence suggests that eating 1 clove of chopped fresh garlic (about 4g) each day may suppress chronic yeast infections.

your food arsenal		
foods	**nutrient**	**health benefits**
garlic	allicin	Laboratory experiments have demonstrated garlic's antifungal activities, attributed to the pungent phytochemical allicin.
yogurt	probiotics	Some research suggests that these healthful bacteria may suppress the growth of *Candida albicans*, the fungus responsible for yeast infections.
artichokes onion family	fructooligosaccharides (FOS)	These indigestible carbohydrate compounds may promote the growth of friendly vaginal bacteria, which protect against the growth of yeast.

recipe rx

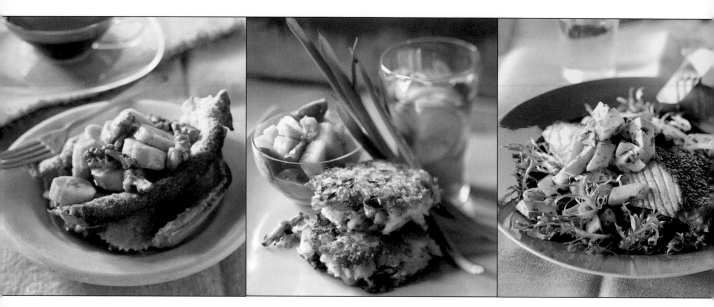

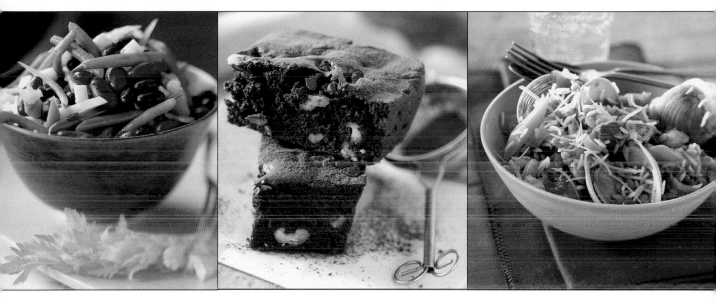

Delicious Dishes

That Maximize the

Fighting Power of Food

mango-berry shake

If you purchase an unsweetened soy milk, you may need to increase the honey.

- 1   LARGE MANGO, PEELED, PITTED, AND CUT INTO WEDGES (2 CUPS)
- 2   CUPS CANTALOUPE CHUNKS
- 1   PACKAGE (12 OUNCES) FROZEN UNSWEETENED RASPBERRIES
- 1½   CUPS SOY MILK
- 2   TABLESPOONS FRESH LIME JUICE
- 2   TABLESPOONS HONEY
- 1   TEASPOON VANILLA EXTRACT
- 1   TEASPOON GROUND GINGER

Working in 2 batches, combine the mango, cantaloupe, raspberries, soy milk, lime juice, honey, vanilla, and ginger in a blender. Blend until smooth.

Makes 4 servings. Per serving: 217 calories, 2.7g total fat (0% saturated), 6g protein, 47g carbohydrate, 1.5g fiber, 0mg cholesterol, 52mg sodium

warm pineapple-ginger punch

This hot and spicy punch is a nice change from mulled cider. It's also a good source of bromelain.

- 4   CUPS PINEAPPLE JUICE
- 1   CUP SLICED FRESH GINGER (NO NEED TO PEEL)
- 1   TABLESPOON HONEY
- 1   CINNAMON STICK, SPLIT LENGTHWISE
- 8   WHOLE CLOVES
- ¼   TEASPOON PEPPER

In a medium saucepan, combine the pineapple juice, ginger, honey, cinnamon, cloves, and pepper; bring to a boil. Reduce to a simmer and cook for 10 minutes. Strain and serve warm.

Makes 4 servings. Per serving: 152 calories, 0.2g total fat (0% saturated), 1g protein, 38g carbohydrate, 0g fiber, 0mg cholesterol, 4mg sodium

mexican-spiced hot cocoa

Spiced with cinnamon and nutmeg, this Mexican-style cocoa is rich in calcium and magnesium.

- 1   TABLESPOON UNSWEETENED COCOA POWDER
- 2   TEASPOONS DARK BROWN SUGAR
- ¼   TEASPOON CINNAMON
- ⅛   TEASPOON NUTMEG
- 1   TABLESPOON BOILING WATER
- 1   CUP LOW-FAT (1%) MILK
- ½   TEASPOON VANILLA EXTRACT
- ⅛   TEASPOON ALMOND EXTRACT

1 In a large mug, stir together the cocoa powder, brown sugar, cinnamon, and nutmeg until well combined. Add the boiling water, and stir until completely moistened and smooth.

2 In a small saucepan, heat the milk for 3 minutes over low heat, or until hot. Stir the milk into the cocoa mixture until well combined. Stir in the vanilla and almond extracts and serve.

Makes 1 serving. Per serving: 160 calories, 3.4g total fat (62% saturated), 9g protein, 24g carbohydrate, 1.6g fiber, 10mg cholesterol, 127mg sodium

banana-peanut smoothie

The soy milk provides isoflavones while the banana contributes a healthy amount of potassium.

- 1   CUP SOY MILK
- 1   MEDIUM BANANA
- 2   TEASPOONS CREAMY PEANUT BUTTER
- 2   TEASPOONS HONEY
- 2   ICE CUBES

In a blender, combine the soy milk, banana, peanut butter, honey, and ice cubes. Blend for 1 minute, or until thick and smooth.

Makes 1 serving. Per serving: 341 calories, 9.8g total fat (11% saturated), 14g protein, 53g carbohydrate, 2.4g fiber, 0mg cholesterol, 166mg sodium

warm pineapple-ginger punch ▶

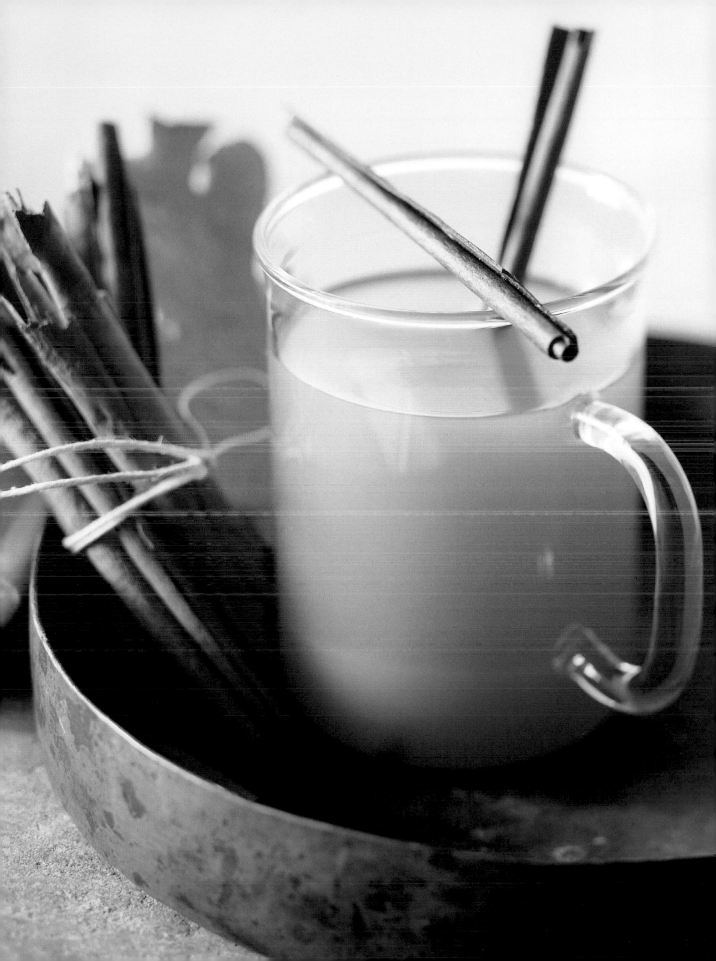

hot & spicy tomato-apple gazpacho

Tomato juice, packed full of lycopene, provides the base for this take-off on a traditional gazpacho. Both spicy and sweet, this is a refreshing summer soup.

- 3 CUPS TOMATO JUICE
- 3 TABLESPOONS TOMATO PASTE
- 1 LARGE APPLE (UNPEELED), CUT INTO CHUNKS
- ¾ CUP FINELY CHOPPED RED ONION (ABOUT 1 MEDIUM)
- 2 CLOVES GARLIC, PEELED
- ⅓ CUP NATURAL (UNBLANCHED) ALMONDS
- ¼ CUP RED WINE VINEGAR
- 2 TEASPOONS LOUISIANA-STYLE RED PEPPER SAUCE
- 1 TEASPOON CHILI POWDER
- ¾ TEASPOON GROUND CORIANDER
- ¼ TEASPOON SALT
- 4 PLUM TOMATOES, CUT INTO ½-INCH CHUNKS
- 1 HASS AVOCADO, CUT INTO ½-INCH CHUNKS

1 In a blender, combine the tomato juice, tomato paste, apple, ½ cup of the onion, the garlic, almonds, vinegar, red pepper sauce, chili powder, coriander, and salt; process until blended but not pureed (it should still have a chunky texture).

2 Pour the gazpacho into a serving bowl and stir in ½ cup of water and the tomato chunks; chill.

3 Serve the soup topped with the remaining ¼ cup onion and the avocado.

Makes 4 servings. Per serving: 213 calories, 12g total fat (12% saturated), 6g protein, 26g carbohydrate, 5.4g fiber, 0mg cholesterol, 985mg sodium

spiced cream of butternut squash soup

Curry powder and ginger lend a decidedly Indian feel to this nutrient-packed soup. Not only is it soothing, but it also provides a hefty amount of beta-carotene as well as potassium, calcium, and magnesium.

- 2 TEASPOONS OLIVE OIL
- 1 LARGE ONION, FINELY CHOPPED
- 4 RED APPLES
- 2 POUNDS BUTTERNUT SQUASH, PEELED AND THINLY SLICED (ABOUT 6 CUPS)
- 1 LARGE BAKING POTATO, PEELED AND THINLY SLICED
- 2 TEASPOONS CURRY POWDER
- 1 TEASPOON GROUND GINGER
- 1 TEASPOON SALT
- ½ TEASPOON CINNAMON
- 1 CUP LOW-FAT (1%) MILK
- ¼ CUP ROASTED CASHEWS, COARSELY CHOPPED

1 In a large saucepan, heat the oil over medium heat. Add the onion, and cook, stirring frequently for 5 minutes, or until golden brown.

2 Peel, core, and slice 3½ of the apples. Add to the pan along with the butternut squash, potato, curry powder, ginger, salt, and cinnamon, and stir to combine. Add 3 cups of water; cover and simmer for 30 minutes, or until the squash is tender.

3 Transfer to a food processor and process until smooth. Return the mixture to the pan, add the milk, and whisk to combine. Cook over low heat until heated through.

4 Meanwhile, thinly slice the remaining ½ apple (unpeeled). Spoon the soup into 4 mugs or soup bowls and top with the cashews and apple slices.

Makes 4 servings. Per serving: 314 calories, 7.7g total fat (21% saturated), 7g protein, 61g carbohydrate, 8.1g fiber, 2mg cholesterol, 627mg sodium

spiced cream of butternut squash soup ▶

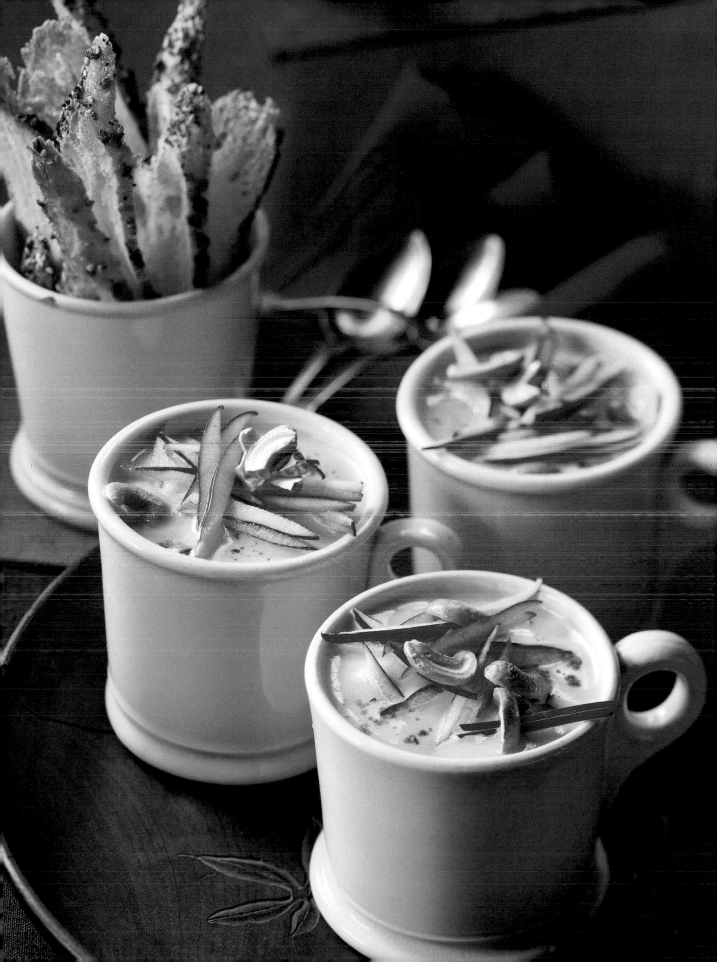

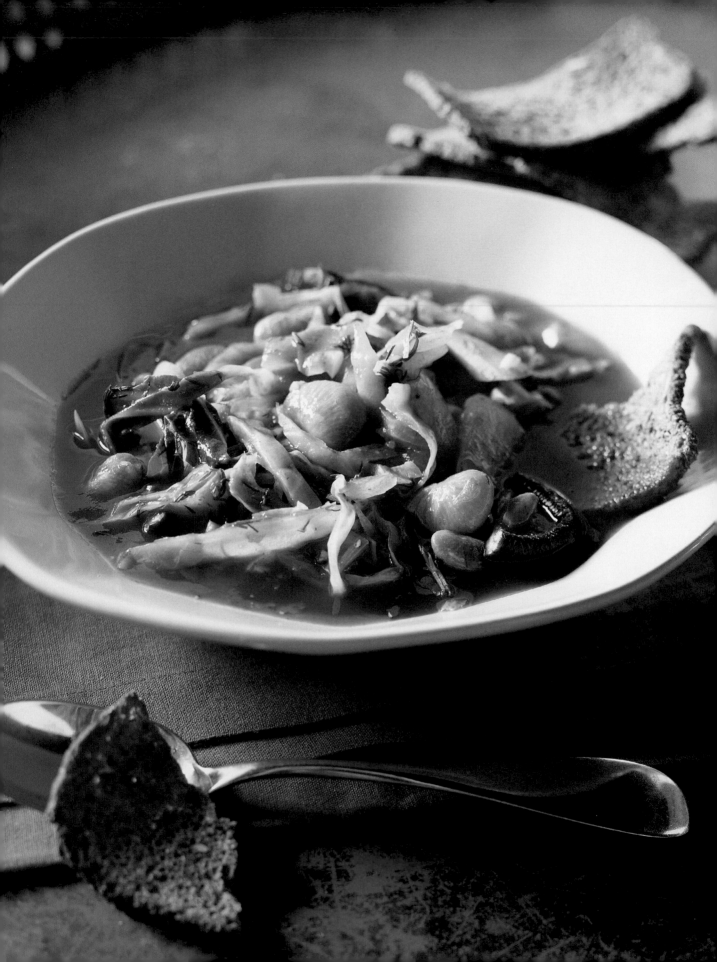

mushroom & winter vegetable soup

Cabbage and mushrooms, two phytochemical-rich foods, team up in this hearty winter soup. Serve with thin dark rye or pumpernickel toast.

½ CUP DRIED SHIITAKE MUSHROOMS

1½ CUPS BOILING WATER

2 TABLESPOONS OLIVE OIL

1 LARGE ONION, FINELY CHOPPED

4 CLOVES GARLIC, MINCED

1 LARGE CARROT, THINLY SLICED

1 LARGE PARSNIP (ABOUT 8 OUNCES), THINLY SLICED

1 SMALL HEAD GREEN CABBAGE (1½ POUNDS), SHREDDED (ABOUT 8 CUPS)

1¼ CUPS FROZEN BABY LIMA BEANS

⅓ CUP CHOPPED FRESH DILL

⅓ CUP TOMATO PASTE

¼ CUP RED WINE VINEGAR

¾ TEASPOON SALT

1 In a small bowl, combine the shiitake mushrooms and boiling water. Let stand for 20 minutes, or until softened. With your fingers, remove the mushrooms from the soaking liquid, reserving the liquid. Trim any stems from the mushrooms and coarsely chop the caps. Strain the reserved liquid through a fine-meshed sieve or coffee filter; set aside.

2 Meanwhile, in a large saucepan or Dutch oven, heat the oil over medium heat. Add the onion and garlic, and cook for 5 minutes, or until the onion is light golden. Add the carrot and parsnip, and cook for 5 minutes, or until the carrot is crisp-tender.

3 Stir in the cabbage. Cover and cook for 5 minutes, or until the cabbage begins to wilt. Stir in the mushrooms and reserved liquid, the lima beans, dill, tomato paste, vinegar, salt, and 3 cups of water; bring to a boil. Reduce to a simmer; cover and cook for 25 minutes, or until the soup is richly flavored.

Makes 4 servings. Per serving: 282 calories, 7.8g total fat (13% saturated), 9g protein, 48g carbohydrate, 13g fiber, 0mg cholesterol, 682mg sodium

spiced moroccan carrot soup

Warm Moroccan spices, tempered by the sweetness of carrots, carrot juice, and tomato paste, add complexity to this thick, creamy soup. The garnish of cilantro, a typical Moroccan seasoning, provides this beta-carotene-packed soup with a fresh, clean finish.

1 TABLESPOON OLIVE OIL

1 MEDIUM ONION, THINLY SLICED

3 CLOVES GARLIC, THINLY SLICED

1 POUND CARROTS, THINLY SLICED

¾ TEASPOON CINNAMON

¾ TEASPOON GROUND GINGER

¾ TEASPOON TURMERIC

½ TEASPOON PAPRIKA

1 CUP CARROT JUICE

2 TABLESPOONS TOMATO PASTE

3 TABLESPOONS RICE

¾ TEASPOON SALT

½ TEASPOON PEPPER

½ CUP CHOPPED CILANTRO

1 In a medium saucepan, heat the oil over medium heat. Add the onion and garlic, and cook, stirring frequently for 5 minutes, or until the onion is golden.

2 Stir in the carrots, cinnamon, ginger, turmeric, and paprika, and cook for 1 minute. Stir in the carrot juice, tomato paste, rice, salt, pepper, and 2 cups of water; bring to a boil. Reduce to a simmer; cover and cook for 20 minutes, or until the carrots and rice are tender.

3 Transfer the mixture to a food processor and puree until smooth. Sprinkle the soup with the cilantro when serving.

Makes 4 servings. Per serving: 167 calories, 4g total fat (13% saturated), 4g protein, 31g carbohydrate, 4.9g fiber, 0mg cholesterol, 562mg sodium

orange beef with broccoli & jicama

Crisp, crunchy, and sweet, fresh jicama stands in where you might expect to find canned water chestnuts in this Asian-inspired dish. In addition to vitamin C (which comes from the bell pepper and broccoli), this beef stir-fry also provides good amounts of vitamin B_{12}, niacin, and potassium.

- 12 OUNCES FLANK STEAK
- 2 TEASPOONS CORNSTARCH
- ¼ CUP DRY SHERRY
- 2 TABLESPOONS REDUCED-SODIUM SOY SAUCE
- ¼ TEASPOON BAKING SODA
- 4 TEASPOONS OLIVE OIL
- 4 TABLESPOONS FINELY SLIVERED ORANGE ZEST
- ¼ TEASPOON CRUSHED RED PEPPER FLAKES
- 5 CUPS BROCCOLI FLORETS AND STEMS
- 1 RED BELL PEPPER, CUT INTO MATCHSTICKS
- 4 SCALLIONS, THINLY SLICED
- 3 CLOVES GARLIC, MINCED
- 1 CUP JICAMA MATCHSTICKS

1 Halve the flank steak lengthwise (with the grain), then cut each piece crosswise (against the grain) into thin slices.

2 In a medium bowl, whisk together the cornstarch, sherry, soy sauce, and baking soda until well combined. Add the flank steak, tossing to coat. Refrigerate for 30 minutes.

3 In a large nonstick skillet, heat 3 teaspoons of the oil over medium heat. Lift the beef from its marinade, reserving the marinade. Add the beef, half of the orange zest, and the red pepper flakes, and cook for 3 minutes, or until the beef is just cooked through. Transfer the beef to a plate.

4 Add the remaining 1 teaspoon oil to the pan along with the broccoli, bell pepper, scallions, and garlic, and cook for 3 minutes, or until the broccoli is beginning to soften. Add ½ cup of water, and cook for 2 to 3 minutes, or until the broccoli is crisp-tender.

5 Stir ⅓ cup of water into the reserved marinade and add to the pan; bring to a boil and cook, stirring constantly for 1 minute, or until the sauce is lightly thick-ened. Return the beef to the pan; add the jicama and cook 1 minute, just until the beef is heated through. Serve garnished with the remaining orange zest.

Makes 4 servings. Per serving: 284 calories, 14g total fat (32% saturated), 21g protein, 16g carbohydrate, 5.3g fiber, 44mg cholesterol, 473mg sodium

lamb & spinach stir-fry

Frozen chopped spinach is a convenient (and equally nutritious) alternative to fresh, and there's no need to clean it. If you can't find boneless loin of lamb, buy chops and have the butcher bone them for you.

- 2 TEASPOONS OLIVE OIL
- 6 SCALLIONS, THINLY SLICED
- 3 CLOVES GARLIC, SLIVERED
- 2 YELLOW BELL PEPPERS, CUT INTO MATCHSTICKS
- 1 POUND BONELESS LOIN OF LAMB, CUT INTO ½ X 2-INCH STRIPS
- 1¼ CUPS CANNED CRUSHED TOMATOES
- ¾ TEASPOON SALT
- ¾ TEASPOON GROUND GINGER
- 2 PACKAGES (10 OUNCES EACH) FROZEN CHOPPED SPINACH, THAWED AND SQUEEZED DRY
- ¾ CUP PLAIN LOW-FAT YOGURT
- 1 TABLESPOON FLOUR

1 In a nonstick Dutch oven or flameproof casserole, heat the oil over medium heat. Add the scallions and garlic, and cook, stirring frequently for 2 minutes, or until the scallions are tender.

2 Increase the heat to medium, add the bell peppers, and cook for 2 minutes, or until crisp-tender. Add the lamb, tomatoes, salt, and ginger, and cook for 3 to 4 minutes, or until the lamb is no longer pink.

3 Stir in the spinach, and cook for 2 minutes, or until tender and heated through.

4 In a small bowl, stir together the yogurt and flour. Stir the yogurt mixture into the pan and cook for 2 minutes, or until well absorbed into the spinach.

Makes 4 servings. Per serving: 287 calories, 10g total fat (31% saturated), 32g protein, 18g carbohydrate, 4.8g fiber, 78mg cholesterol, 775mg sodium

orange beef with broccoli & jicama ▶

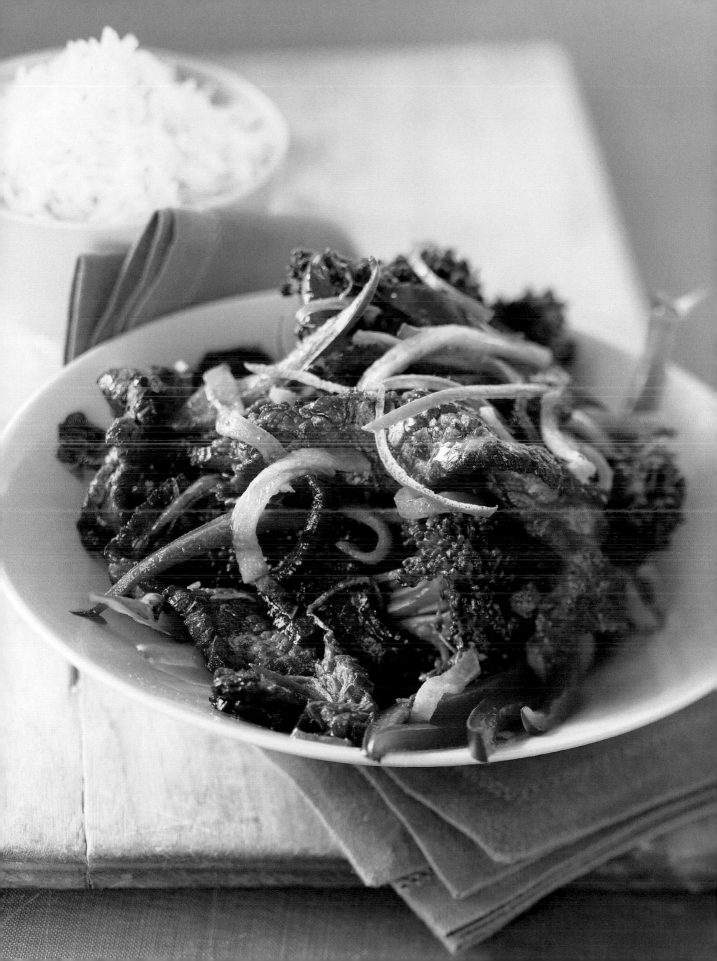

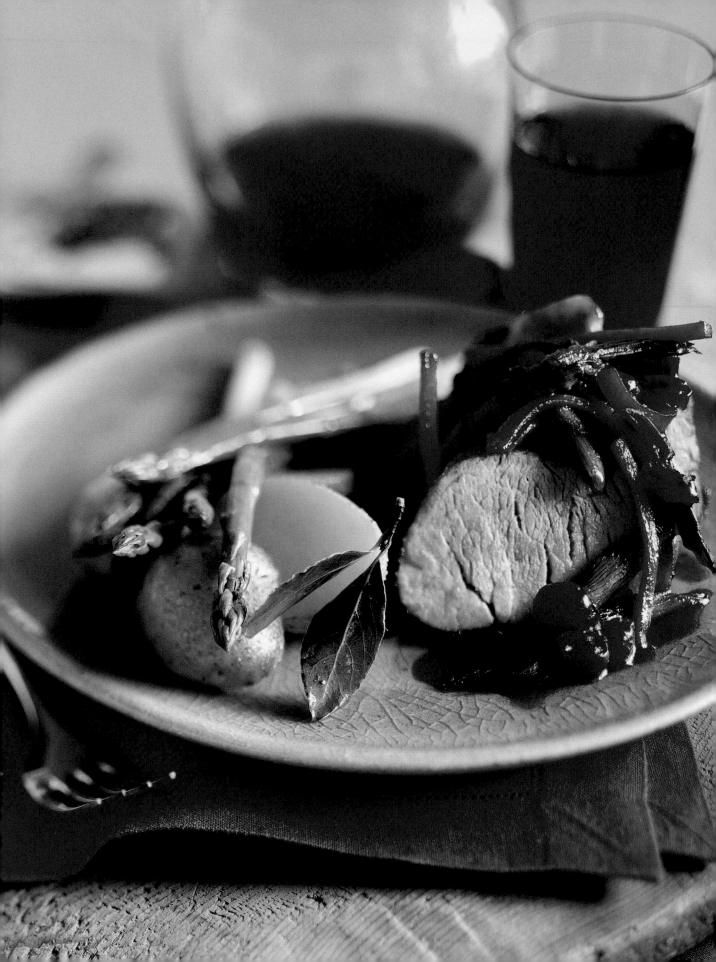

braised pork with cranberries

Cranberries add a tangy undertone to this dish, and provide anthocyanins, ellagic acid, and quercetin.

- ½ CUP SUGAR
- 1 TEASPOON DRIED ROSEMARY, MINCED
- ¾ TEASPOON SALT
- ½ TEASPOON PEPPER
- ½ TEASPOON GROUND GINGER
- 1 POUND WELL-TRIMMED PORK TENDERLOIN, HALVED CROSSWISE
- 1 TABLESPOON OLIVE OIL
- 12 CLOVES GARLIC, PEELED
- 8 SCALLIONS, CUT INTO 2-INCH LENGTHS
- 4 CARROTS, CUT INTO MATCHSTICKS
- 12 OUNCES FRESH OR FROZEN CRANBERRIES
- ⅔ CUP ORANGE JUICE
- 1 BAY LEAF

1 Preheat the oven to 350°F. In a large bowl, stir together ¼ cup of the sugar, the rosemary, salt, pepper, and ginger. Add the pork, and turn to coat with the spice mixture.

2 In a nonstick Dutch oven or flameproof casserole, heat the oil over medium-high heat. Lift the pork from the spice mixture and add to the pan along with the garlic. Cook the pork for 2 minutes per side, or until it is richly browned. Transfer the pork to a plate.

3 Add the scallions and carrots to the pan, and cook for 3 minutes, or until the carrots begin to color. Stir the remaining ¼ cup sugar, the cranberries, orange juice, and bay leaf into the pan; bring to a boil.

4 Return the pork to the pan; reduce to a simmer, cover, and transfer to the oven. Bake for 30 minutes, or until the pork is cooked through but still juicy.

5 Lift the pork from the pan and slice. Remove and discard the bay leaf from the sauce. Serve the pork with vegetables and sauce on top.

Makes 4 servings. Per serving: 380 calories, 7.7g total fat (24% saturated), 26g protein, 53g carbohydrate, 6.6g fiber, 74mg cholesterol, 526mg sodium

roast pork & quinoa salad with arugula

Vitamin C-rich lemon and grapefruit juices enhance the absorption of iron from the quinoa.

- ¼ CUP APRICOT JAM
- 2 TABLESPOONS DIJON MUSTARD
- 1 TEASPOON GRATED LEMON ZEST
- 2 TABLESPOONS FRESH LEMON JUICE
- 1 TEASPOON CHILI POWDER
- 1 POUND WELL-TRIMMED PORK TENDERLOIN
- ¾ TEASPOON SALT
- 1 CUP QUINOA, WELL RINSED
- 1 TABLESPOON OLIVE OIL
- 3 PINK GRAPEFRUITS
- 8 CUPS ARUGULA (ABOUT 2 BUNCHES)

1 Preheat the oven to 400°F. In a large bowl, whisk together the jam, mustard, lemon zest, lemon juice, and ½ teaspoon of the chili powder. Measure out 3 tablespoons of the jam mixture for the pork.

2 Place the pork in a small roasting pan. Rub with ¼ teaspoon of the salt and the remaining ½ teaspoon chili powder. Roast for 15 minutes. Brush the 3 tablespoons jam mixture over the pork and roast for 10 minutes, or until cooked through but still juicy.

3 Meanwhile, in a large saucepan, bring 2 cups of water to a boil. Add the quinoa and remaining ½ teaspoon salt and return to a boil. Reduce to a simmer; cover and cook for 12 minutes, or until tender. Drain.

4 Whisk the oil into the bowl with the remaining jam mixture. Add the quinoa, tossing to combine.

5 With a paring knife, cut off the skin from the grapefruits. Working over a bowl to catch the juice, cut between the membranes to release the sections. Add the grapefruit sections and ¼ cup of the juice to the bowl with the quinoa.

6 Place the quinoa salad on a bed of arugula. Thinly slice the pork and arrange on top.

Makes 4 servings. Per serving: 450 calories, 10g total fat (20% saturated), 31g protein, 59g carbohydrate, 4.8g fiber, 65mg cholesterol, 697mg sodium

◀ **braised pork with cranberries**

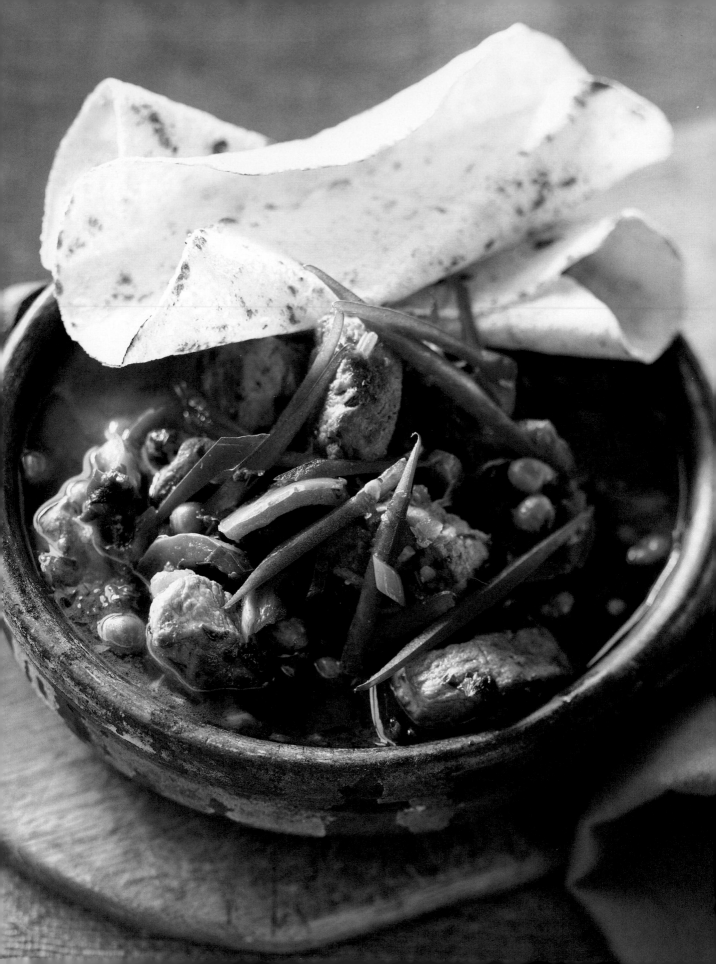

green pork chili

Although 1½ cups may seem like a lot, the cilantro lends a distinctive southwestern flavor (and color) to the chili. Stirring in half of this pungent herb at the end gives the chili a final, fresh burst of cilantro.

- 2 TABLESPOONS OLIVE OIL
- 1 POUND PORK TENDERLOIN, CUT INTO 1-INCH CHUNKS
- 2 TABLESPOONS FLOUR
- 6 SCALLIONS, THINLY SLICED
- 3 CLOVES GARLIC, MINCED
- 1 LARGE GREEN BELL PEPPER, CUT INTO ½-INCH CHUNKS
- 1 PICKLED JALAPEÑO PEPPER, FINELY CHOPPED
- 1 CAN (4½ OUNCES) CHOPPED MILD GREEN CHILIES
- 1½ CUPS PACKED CILANTRO SPRIGS, CHOPPED
- ¾ TEASPOON SALT
- ½ TEASPOON GROUND CORIANDER
- 1½ CUPS FROZEN PEAS, THAWED
- 2 TABLESPOONS FRESH LIME JUICE
- 1 RED BELL PEPPER, SLIVERED

1 Preheat the oven to 350°F. In a nonstick Dutch oven or flameproof casserole, heat the oil over medium heat. Dredge the pork in the flour, shaking off the excess. Add the pork, and sauté for 4 minutes, or until golden brown. With a slotted spoon, transfer the pork to a plate.

2 Add the scallions and garlic to the pan, and cook for 1 minute, or until the scallions are tender. Add the green bell pepper and jalapeño, and cook for 4 minutes, or until the bell pepper is crisp-tender. Stir in the mild green chilies, half the cilantro, the salt, ground coriander, and 1¼ cups of water; bring to a boil.

3 Return the pork to the pan. Cover, place in the oven, and bake for 25 minutes, or until the pork is tender.

4 Stir in the peas, lime juice, and the remaining cilantro. Re-cover and let stand for 3 minutes. Serve topped with the red bell pepper.

Makes 4 servings. Per serving: 306 calories, 13g total fat (23% saturated), 28g protein, 19g carbohydrate, 4.3g fiber, 75mg cholesterol, 810mg sodium

spicy mexican-style stuffed beef burgers

Flaxseeds, rich in antioxidants called lignans, are also a good source of fiber and omega-3 fatty acids. Flaxseeds add a slightly nutty flavor and some good-for-you fat to these burgers.

- 1 POUND WELL-TRIMMED BEEF TOP ROUND, CUT INTO CHUNKS
- ¼ CUP FLAXSEEDS
- 2 PICKLED JALAPEÑO PEPPERS, MINCED
- 1 TEASPOON GROUND CUMIN
- ½ TEASPOON SALT
- ½ CUP CORN KERNELS
- ⅓ CUP CHOPPED CILANTRO
- ¼ CUP OIL-PACKED SUN-DRIED TOMATOES, DRAINED AND COARSELY CHOPPED
- ¼ CUP DIJON MUSTARD
- 2 TABLESPOONS FRESH LIME JUICE
- 1 TABLESPOON RED WINE VINEGAR
- 2 TEASPOONS HONEY
- 1 RED BELL PEPPER, DICED

1 In a food processor, process the beef until finely chopped. In a mini food processor, spice grinder, or coffee grinder, grind the flaxseeds until finely ground.

2 In a medium bowl, combine the beef, ground flaxseeds, jalapeño peppers, cumin, and salt until well mixed. In a small bowl, combine the corn, cilantro, and sun-dried tomatoes.

3 Shape the beef mixture into 4 patties. Make a well in the center of each patty and stuff with the corn mixture. Shape the meat around the filling.

4 Preheat the broiler. Broil the burgers 6 inches from the heat for 4 minutes per side for medium.

5 Meanwhile, in a small bowl, stir together the mustard, lime juice, vinegar, and honey. Stir in the red bell pepper. Serve the burgers topped with the red pepper relish.

Makes 4 servings. Per serving: 290 calories, 9.9g total fat (18% saturated), 31g protein, 17g carbohydrate, 4.7g fiber, 72mg cholesterol, 879mg sodium

pork & root vegetable stew

Gingersnap cookies work as both a thickener and a flavor enhancer in this winter stew. Rutabaga, a type of turnip, has a sweet and peppery taste. If only huge rutabagas are available, save the leftover for other uses, such as mashed rutabaga.

- 1 TABLESPOON OLIVE OIL
- 3 LEEKS, HALVED LENGTHWISE, THINLY SLICED CROSSWISE, AND WELL WASHED
- 3 CLOVES GARLIC, THINLY SLICED
- 2 CARROTS, HALVED LENGTHWISE AND THINLY SLICED CROSSWISE
- 2 MEDIUM PARSNIPS, HALVED LENGTHWISE AND THINLY SLICED CROSSWISE
- 1 SMALL RUTABAGA (ABOUT 10 OUNCES), PEELED AND CUT INTO ½-INCH CHUNKS (ABOUT 2 CUPS)
- 1¼ CUPS CANNED CRUSHED TOMATOES
- 6 GINGERSNAP COOKIES (1½ OUNCES), CRUMBLED
- 3 TABLESPOONS CIDER VINEGAR
- 2 TEASPOONS LIGHT BROWN SUGAR
- ¾ TEASPOON SALT
- 1 POUND WELL-TRIMMED PORK TENDERLOIN, CUT INTO 1-INCH CHUNKS

1 In a nonstick Dutch oven or flameproof casserole, heat the oil over medium heat. Add the leeks and garlic, and cook, stirring occasionally for 5 minutes, or until tender.

2 Stir in the carrots, parsnips, and rutabaga, and cook for 7 minutes, or until the vegetables are crisp-tender.

3 Add the tomatoes, gingersnaps, vinegar, brown sugar, salt, and 1 cup of water; bring to a boil. Add the pork and reduce to a simmer; cover and cook for 30 minutes, or until the pork and vegetables are tender.

Makes 4 servings. Per serving: 373 calories, 9.1g total fat (23% saturated), 28g protein, 46g carbohydrate, 7.3g fiber, 74mg cholesterol, 733mg sodium

thai-style beef sandwich

There's enough of this spicy, refreshing slaw to serve on the side as well as on the sandwich.

- 2 TABLESPOONS TOMATO PASTE
- ½ CUP FRESH LIME JUICE (ABOUT 3 LIMES)
- 1½ TEASPOONS GROUND CORIANDER
- 1 POUND WELL-TRIMMED FLANK STEAK
- 1 TEASPOON SUGAR
- ¾ TEASPOON SALT
- ¾ TEASPOON RED PEPPER FLAKES
- 3 CUPS PACKED SHREDDED GREEN CABBAGE (ABOUT 12 OUNCES)
- 2 CARROTS, SHREDDED
- 1 LARGE RED BELL PEPPER, CUT INTO MATCHSTICKS
- ½ CUP CHOPPED CILANTRO
- ⅓ CUP CHOPPED FRESH MINT
- 4 HARD ROLLS, HALVED CROSSWISE

1 In a shallow nonaluminum pan, stir together the tomato paste, ¼ cup of the lime juice, and the ground coriander. Add the flank steak, turning it to coat. Refrigerate for 30 minutes.

2 In a large bowl, whisk together the remaining ¼ cup lime juice, the sugar, salt, and red pepper flakes. Add the cabbage, carrots, bell pepper, cilantro, and mint; toss well to combine. Refrigerate the slaw until serving time.

3 Preheat the broiler. Remove the steak from its marinade. Broil 6 inches from the heat for 4 minutes per side for medium-rare, brushing any remaining marinade over the steak. Let stand for 10 minutes before thinly slicing across the grain on the diagonal.

4 To serve, place the cabbage slaw on the bottom half of each cut roll. Top with ribbons of sliced steak.

Makes 4 servings. Per serving: 410 calories, 12g total fat (36% saturated), 31g protein, 46g carbohydrate, 5.7g fiber, 57mg cholesterol, 913mg sodium

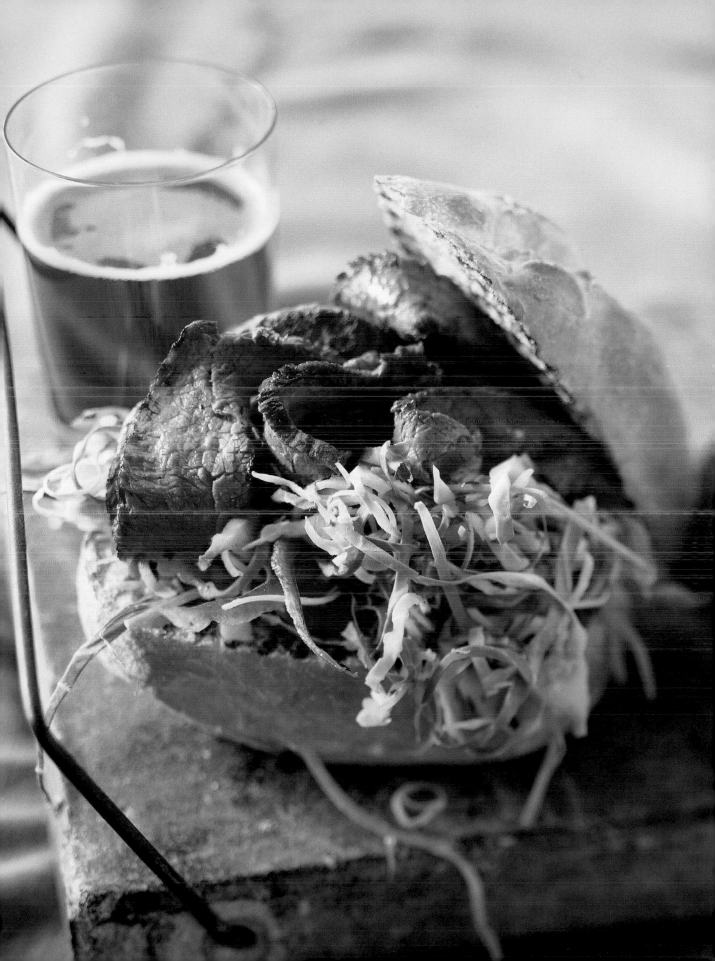

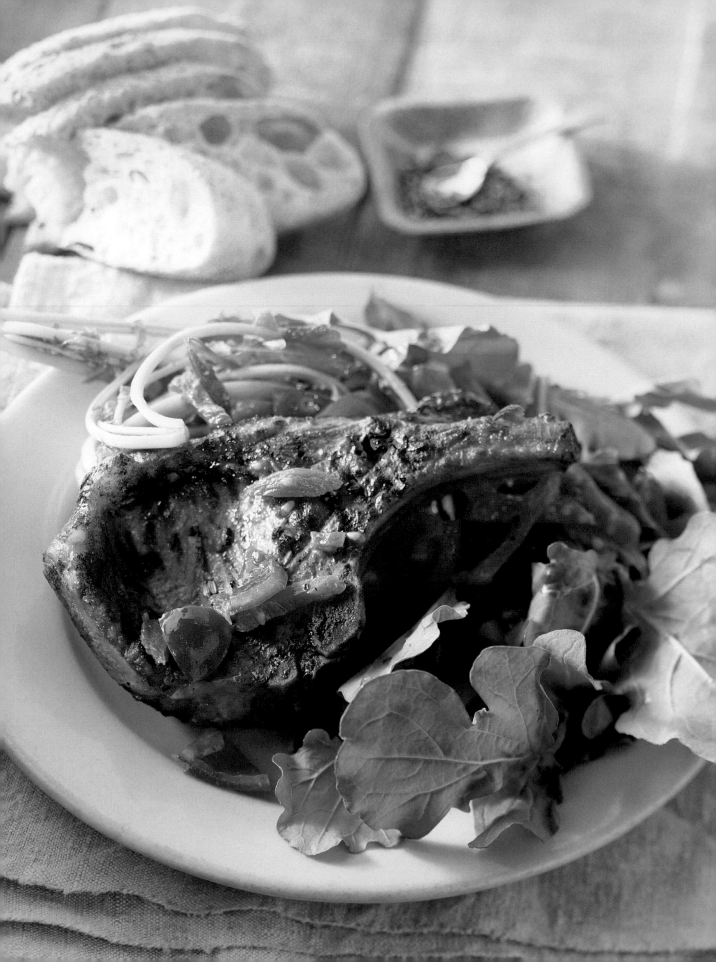

pan-grilled pork chops with arugula

Hot grilled chops served on a bed of greens tossed in a lemony vinaigrette is a symphony of flavors and textures. Fennel and coriander seeds provide earthy undertones along with the phytochemical limonene.

1¼ TEASPOONS FENNEL SEEDS

¾ TEASPOON GROUND CUMIN

¾ TEASPOON GROUND CORIANDER

¾ TEASPOON SALT

4 CENTER-CUT PORK CHOPS (¾ INCH THICK, ABOUT 6 OUNCES EACH)

4 TEASPOONS OLIVE OIL

3 TABLESPOONS FRESH LEMON JUICE

1 TEASPOON DIJON MUSTARD

2 BUNCHES ARUGULA, TOUGH STEMS REMOVED (ABOUT 8 CUPS)

4 PLUM TOMATOES, DICED

¼ CUP DRIED APRICOTS, DICED

1 In a small bowl, stir together 1 teaspoon of the fennel seeds, the cumin, coriander, and ½ teaspoon of the salt. Rub the spice mixture into both sides of the pork chops.

2 Brush a grill pan with 1 teaspoon of the oil. Heat the pan over medium heat. Add the chops and cook for 4 minutes per side, or until cooked through but still juicy.

3 Meanwhile, in a large bowl, whisk together the remaining ¼ teaspoon fennel seeds, ¼ teaspoon salt, 3 teaspoons olive oil, the lemon juice, and mustard. Add the arugula, tomatoes, and apricots; toss to combine.

4 To serve, divide the salad among 4 plates and top each with a pork chop.

Makes 4 servings. Per serving: 306 calories, 17g total fat (30% saturated), 28g protein, 10g carbohydrate, 2.1g fiber, 75mg cholesterol, 536mg sodium

greek-style meatloaf

The typical Greek seasonings of dill, mint, and lemon zest add a handful of phytochemicals to the more standard nutrients—zinc, vitamin B$_{12}$, niacin, and thiamin—provided by this delicious meatloaf. For even more of a Greek taste, replace the pork with an equal amount of lean ground lamb.

2 TEASPOONS OLIVE OIL

4 SCALLIONS, THINLY SLICED

3 CLOVES GARLIC, MINCED

8 OUNCES WELL-TRIMMED PORK TENDERLOIN

8 OUNCES WELL-TRIMMED BEEF TOP ROUND

½ CUP COOKED RICE

2 TABLESPOONS TOMATO PASTE

⅓ CUP CHOPPED FRESH DILL

¼ CUP CHOPPED FRESH MINT

2 TEASPOONS GRATED LEMON ZEST

½ TEASPOON DRIED OREGANO

½ TEASPOON SALT

4 OUNCES CRUMBLED FETA CHEESE

1 In a small skillet, heat the oil over low heat. Add the scallions and garlic, and cook for 3 minutes, or until the scallions are tender. Transfer the mixture to a large bowl.

2 Preheat the oven to 350°F. In a food processor, combine the pork and beef and process until finely ground. Transfer to the bowl with the scallion mixture. Add the rice, tomato paste, dill, mint, lemon zest, oregano, salt, and 2 tablespoons of water. Mix until well combined.

3 Spoon half the meat mixture into an 8½ x 4½-inch metal loaf pan. Sprinkle with the feta cheese and top with the remaining meat mixture. Tap the pan on the work surface several times to pack the mixture.

4 Bake for 25 minutes, or until the juices run clear when the loaf is poked with a toothpick. Serve hot, warm, or chilled.

Makes 4 servings. Per serving: 279 calories, 12g total fat (48% saturated), 30g protein, 11g carbohydrate, 1.3g fiber, 94mg cholesterol, 734mg sodium

caraway-coated pepper steak with cherry sauce

Juicy sirloin steaks, coated with caraway seeds and peppercorns, then topped with a tangy cherry sauce, are mouthwatering and good for you. The caraway seeds and cherries are a good source of the phytochemical perillyl alcohol, and the beef provides good amounts of zinc, iron, and vitamins B_6 and B_{12}.

- 1 TABLESPOON COARSELY CRACKED BLACK PEPPERCORNS
- 2 TEASPOONS CARAWAY SEEDS
- 4 LEAN SIRLOIN STEAKS (ABOUT 4 OUNCES EACH)
- 1 TABLESPOON OLIVE OIL
- 1 MEDIUM RED ONION, FINELY CHOPPED
- 1 CUP DRY RED WINE
- 1 BAG (20 OUNCES) FROZEN PITTED SWEET CHERRIES, THAWED, DRAINED, AND COARSELY CHOPPED
- 2 TEASPOONS DIJON MUSTARD
- 1 TABLESPOON RED WINE VINEGAR
- ½ TEASPOON SALT
- ¼ TEASPOON GROUND GINGER
- ¼ CUP CHOPPED PARSLEY

1 In a shallow bowl, combine the peppercorns and caraway seeds. Dip the steaks in the spice mixture, pressing it into both sides.

2 In a large nonstick skillet, heat the oil over medium heat. Add the steaks, and cook for 3 minutes per side for medium-rare. Transfer the steaks to a platter and keep warm.

3 Add the onion to the skillet and sauté for 4 minutes, or until tender. Add the wine, increase the heat to high, and cook for 2 minutes. Stir in the cherries, mustard, vinegar, salt, and ginger; cook for 5 minutes, or until the cherries are very tender.

4 Return the steaks to the pan and cook for 1 minute per side to heat through. Transfer the steaks to 4 plates. Stir the parsley into the sauce and spoon the sauce over the steaks.

Makes 4 servings. Per serving: 351 calories, 10g total fat (25% saturated), 27g protein, 30g carbohydrate, 3.9g fiber, 69mg cholesterol, 425mg sodium

savory lamb stew with sweet potatoes

Okra and peanut butter contribute to the thickness and heartiness of this West African-inspired stew (these ingredients are common to West African cooking). In addition to huge amounts of beta-carotene supplied by the sweet potatoes, this dish is rich in zinc and B vitamins from the lamb.

- 3 TEASPOONS OLIVE OIL
- 1 POUND WELL-TRIMMED LEAN LEG OF LAMB, CUT INTO 1-INCH CHUNKS
- 1 MEDIUM ONION, FINELY CHOPPED
- 4 CLOVES GARLIC, MINCED
- 1 CUP CANNED CRUSHED TOMATOES
- 1 POUND SWEET POTATOES, PEELED AND CUT INTO ½-INCH CHUNKS
- 2 TABLESPOONS CREAMY PEANUT BUTTER
- 1 TEASPOON SALT
- ½ TEASPOON CAYENNE PEPPER
- 1 PACKAGE (10 OUNCES) FROZEN CUT OR WHOLE OKRA, THAWED

1 Preheat the oven to 350°F. In a large nonstick Dutch oven or flameproof casserole, heat 2 teaspoons of the oil over medium-high heat. Add the lamb and sauté for 5 minutes, or until browned. With a slotted spoon, transfer the lamb to a plate.

2 Reduce the heat to medium and add the remaining 1 teaspoon oil, the onion, and garlic; cook for 2 minutes. Stir in ⅓ cup of water, and cook until the onion is golden brown and tender.

3 Stir in the tomatoes, sweet potatoes, peanut butter, salt, cayenne, and 1½ cups of water; bring to a boil. Return the lamb to the pan. Cover, transfer to the oven, and bake for 25 minutes.

4 Stir in the okra, return the pan to the oven, and bake for 15 minutes, or until the lamb and okra are tender.

Makes 4 servings. Per serving: 363 calories, 13g total fat (23% saturated), 29g protein, 33g carbohydrate, 6.5g fiber, 73mg cholesterol, 803mg sodium

savory lamb stew with sweet potatoes ▶

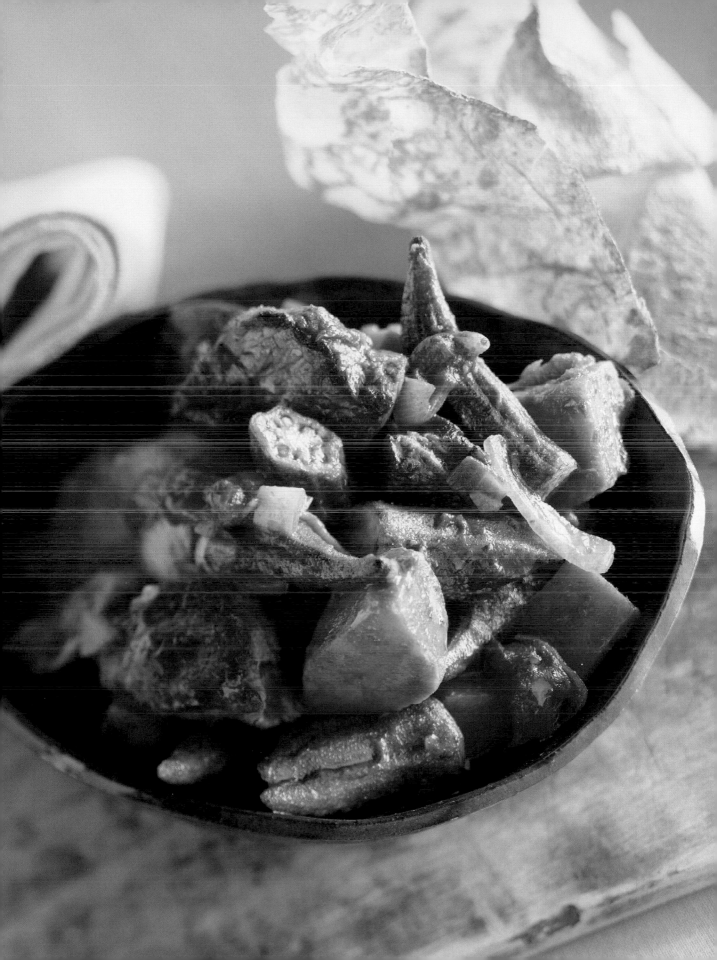

black bean & turkey soup with winter squash

The black beans add a rich, almost smoky flavor, and a dark purplish hue. Corn and butternut squash provide a sweet counterpoint to the earthy turkey and beans, as well as good amounts of beta-carotene and lutein.

1½ CUPS DRIED BLACK BEANS, PICKED OVER AND RINSED (**10** OUNCES)

3½ POUNDS TURKEY DRUMSTICKS, SKINNED

1 GREEN BELL PEPPER, CUT INTO ½-INCH SQUARES

1 CUP CHOPPED CILANTRO

4 SCALLIONS, THINLY SLICED

1 TABLESPOON GRATED LEMON ZEST

1 TABLESPOON CHILI POWDER

2½ TEASPOONS GROUND CUMIN

2½ TEASPOONS GROUND CORIANDER

1 TEASPOON GROUND GINGER

5 CUPS DICED (½-INCH) BUTTERNUT SQUASH

1 PACKAGE (**10** OUNCES) FROZEN CORN KERNELS

2¼ TEASPOONS SALT

¼ CUP FRESH LEMON JUICE

1 In a large saucepan or stockpot, combine the beans with water to cover by 3 inches; bring to a boil.

2 Add the turkey drumsticks, bell pepper, ½ cup of the cilantro, the scallions, lemon zest, chili powder, cumin, coriander, and ginger; return the mixture to a boil. Reduce to a simmer; partially cover and cook for 1 hour, 15 minutes.

3 Add the squash, corn, and salt, and cook, uncovered, for 15 minutes, or until the beans and turkey are tender.

4 Remove from the heat. Remove the turkey legs from the soup, and when cool enough to handle, cut the meat from the bones. Discard any ligaments and cartilage, and cut the turkey into bite-size pieces.

5 Return the turkey meat to the pan. Add the lemon juice and the remaining ½ cup cilantro, and cook for 3 minutes to heat through.

Makes 8 servings. Per serving: 339 calories, 5.6g total fat (30% saturated), 32g protein, 43g carbohydrate, 8g fiber, 80 mg cholesterol, 832mg sodium

chicken-kale soup with roasted pepper puree

Nutty-flavored flaxseed oil, high in omega-3 fatty acids, is available in the refrigerated section of many health-food stores. If you can't find it, substitute dark sesame oil.

1¼ POUNDS SKINLESS, BONELESS CHICKEN THIGHS, CUT INTO **1**-INCH CHUNKS

4 CARROTS, THINLY SLICED

3 LARGE RED ONIONS, CUT INTO ½-INCH CHUNKS

5 CLOVES GARLIC, MINCED, PLUS **1** WHOLE CLOVE GARLIC

2 TABLESPOONS FINELY CHOPPED FRESH GINGER

1 TEASPOON CAYENNE PEPPER

¾ TEASPOON SALT

2 RED BELL PEPPERS, CUT LENGTHWISE INTO FLAT PANELS

1 TABLESPOON HULLED ROASTED PUMPKIN SEEDS

1 TABLESPOON FLAXSEED OIL

¼ CUP ORZO PASTA (1½ OUNCES)

8 CUPS SHREDDED KALE

1 In a large saucepan or stockpot, combine 4 cups of water, the chicken, carrots, onions, minced garlic, ginger, cayenne, and salt; bring to a boil over high heat. Reduce to a simmer; partially cover and cook for 25 minutes.

2 Meanwhile, preheat the broiler. Place the pepper pieces, skin-side up, on a broiler pan and broil 6 inches from the heat for 10 minutes, or until the skin is well charred. When cool enough to handle, peel the peppers and transfer them to a food processor along with the pumpkin seeds, flaxseed oil, and whole garlic clove; process until pureed.

3 Add the orzo to the soup, and cook, uncovered, for 5 minutes. Stir in the kale, and cook for 5 minutes, or until the kale and orzo are tender.

4 Serve the soup with the roasted pepper puree.

Makes 4 servings. Per serving: 433 calories, 12g total fat (18% saturated), 38g protein, 48g carbohydrate, 9.1g fiber, 118mg cholesterol, 649mg sodium

chicken-kale soup with roasted pepper puree ▶

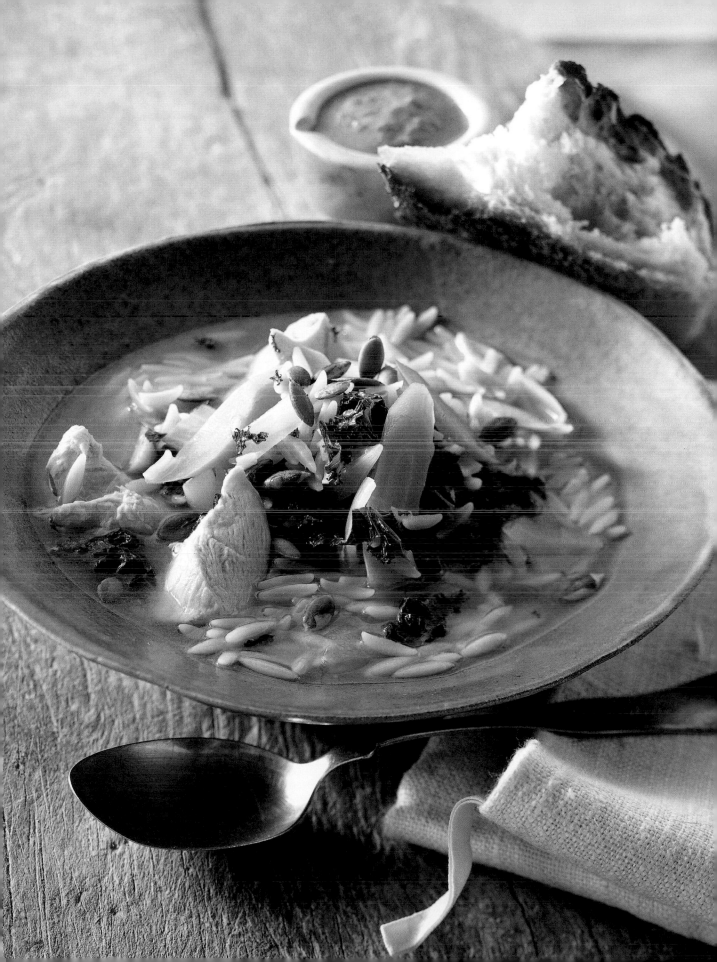

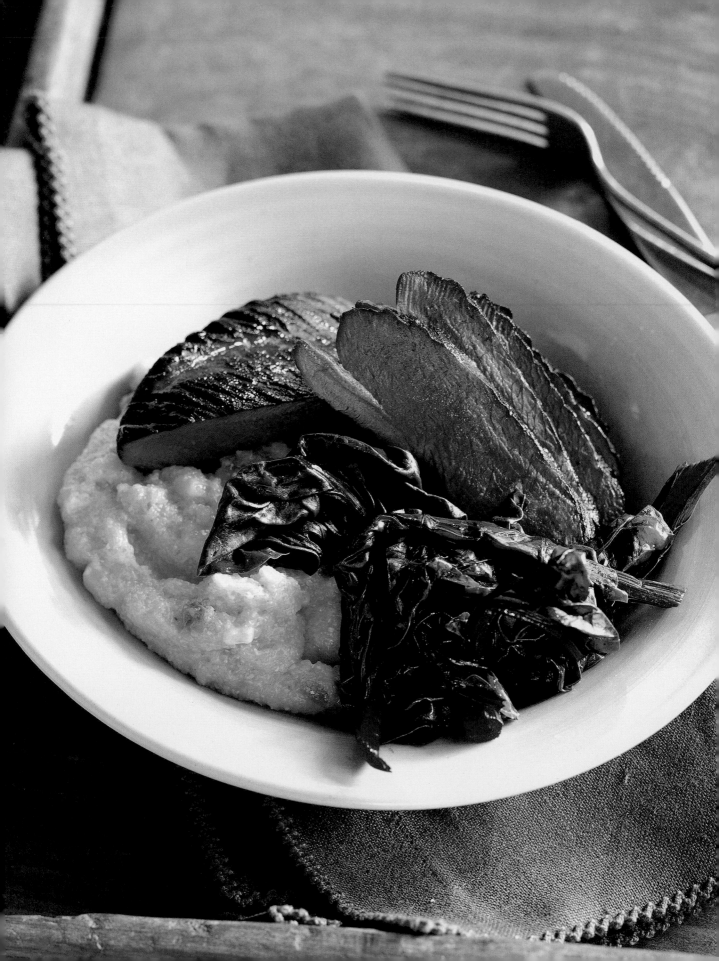

grilled duck breast with polenta

Despite its reputation as a high-fat food, duck breast is actually a very lean cut (a 3-ounce serving of skinless cooked duck breast has 30% less fat than skinless chicken breast). Here the duck is rubbed with an Indian-inspired spice mixture and served with a soft polenta that is studded with corn and peas and seasoned with mango chutney.

- 2 TEASPOONS TURMERIC
- 1 TEASPOON SALT
- ¾ TEASPOON SUGAR
- ½ TEASPOON GROUND GINGER
- 4 SKINLESS, BONELESS DUCK BREAST HALVES (ABOUT 5 OUNCES EACH)
- 1 TABLESPOON OLIVE OIL
- ¾ CUP YELLOW CORNMEAL
- 1½ CUPS FROZEN PEAS
- 1½ CUPS FROZEN CORN KERNELS
- 3 TABLESPOONS MANGO CHUTNEY, FINELY CHOPPED

1 In a small bowl, stir together the turmeric, ¼ teaspoon of the salt, the sugar, and ginger. Rub the mixture into both sides of the duck breasts.

2 Brush a grill pan or skillet with the oil. Add the duck breasts, and cook for 3 minutes per side for medium-rare.

3 Meanwhile, in a small bowl, combine the cornmeal and 1 cup of cold water, stirring until smooth. In a medium saucepan, bring 1¼ cups of water to a boil over high heat. Stir in the cornmeal mixture and the remaining ¾ teaspoon salt, and reduce the heat to low; cook, stirring frequently for 7 minutes, or until the polenta is thickened and tender.

4 Stir the peas, corn, and chutney into the polenta, and cook for 2 minutes, or until the vegetables are heated through. Slice the duck across the grain on the diagonal and serve alongside the polenta.

Makes 4 servings. Per serving: *415 calories, 5.3g total fat (11% saturated), 35g protein, 57g carbohydrate, 4.7g fiber, 149mg cholesterol, 920mg sodium*

chicken arrabbiata with shiitakes & artichokes

A large quantity of dried shiitake mushrooms adds deep flavor to this dish and also provides a boost to the immune system.

- 1 CUP DRIED SHIITAKE MUSHROOMS
- 1½ CUPS BOILING WATER
- 3 TEASPOONS OLIVE OIL
- 2¼ POUNDS SKINLESS CHICKEN DRUMSTICKS AND THIGHS
- 2 TABLESPOONS FLOUR
- 1 MEDIUM ONION, FINELY CHOPPED
- 6 CLOVES GARLIC, SLICED
- 1 TABLESPOON DRIED ROSEMARY, MINCED
- ¾ TEASPOON CRUSHED RED PEPPER FLAKES
- 1½ CUPS CANNED CRUSHED TOMATOES
- 1 PACKAGE (9 OUNCES) FROZEN ARTICHOKE HEARTS
- ½ TEASPOON SALT

1 In a small bowl, combine the shiitake mushrooms and boiling water. Let stand for 20 minutes, or until softened. With your fingers, remove the mushrooms from the soaking liquid, reserving the liquid. Trim any stems from the mushrooms and thinly slice the caps. Strain the reserved liquid through a fine-meshed sieve or coffee filter; set aside.

2 In a large nonstick skillet, heat 2 teaspoons of the oil over medium heat. Dredge the chicken in the flour, shaking off the excess. Add the chicken to the pan, and sauté for 3 minutes per side, or until golden brown. Transfer the chicken to a plate.

3 Add the remaining 1 teaspoon oil, the onion, and garlic to the pan, and cook for 3 minutes. Add the mushrooms, rosemary, and red pepper flakes, and cook for 1 minute. Add the reserved liquid and bring to a boil. Boil for 2 minutes, or until slightly reduced.

4 Stir in the tomatoes, artichokes, and salt; return to a boil. Return the chicken to the pan and reduce to a simmer; cover and cook for 30 minutes, or until the chicken is cooked through.

Makes 4 servings. Per serving: *345 calories, 11g total fat (22% saturated), 40g protein, 24g carbohydrate, 7.3g fiber, 139mg cholesterol, 619mg sodium*

chicken piccata

The small amount of cold butter added to the sage, rosemary, and lemon sauce at the end softens it and lends a creamy texture to it. Elegant, yet quick and easy to make, this chicken dish is high in niacin and selenium.

- 2 TABLESPOONS FLOUR
- ½ TEASPOON RUBBED SAGE
- ½ TEASPOON DRIED ROSEMARY, MINCED
- ½ TEASPOON SALT
- 8 CHICKEN CUTLETS (ABOUT 1¼ POUNDS TOTAL)
- 4 TEASPOONS OLIVE OIL
- 4 CLOVES GARLIC, MINCED
- 1 TEASPOON GRATED LEMON ZEST
- ⅓ CUP FRESH LEMON JUICE
- 2 TEASPOONS SMALL CAPERS, DRAINED
- 3 TABLESPOONS CHOPPED PARSLEY
- 2 TEASPOONS COLD UNSALTED BUTTER, CUT UP

1 On a sheet of wax paper, combine the flour, sage, rosemary, and salt. Dredge the chicken in the seasoned flour mixture until well coated.

2 In a large nonstick skillet, heat 3 teaspoons of the oil over medium heat. Add the chicken, and cook for 2 minutes per side, or until golden brown and cooked through. Transfer to a platter.

3 Add the remaining 1 teaspoon oil and the garlic to the pan, and cook for 10 seconds. Add the lemon zest, lemon juice, and capers, and cook for 1 minute, scraping up any browned bits clinging to the pan.

4 Remove the pan from the heat, add the parsley, and swirl in the butter until the sauce is slightly thickened. Serve the sauce over the chicken.

Makes 4 servings. Per serving: *239 calories, 8.2g total fat (27% saturated), 33g protein, 6g carbohydrate, 0.5g fiber, 87mg cholesterol, 447mg sodium*

rich curried chicken & vegetables

The homemade curry powder for this chicken dish has an especially high proportion of phytochemical-rich turmeric and ginger.

- 1 TABLESPOON TURMERIC
- 1½ TEASPOONS GROUND GINGER
- 1 TEASPOON SALT
- ½ TEASPOON CINNAMON
- ½ TEASPOON SUGAR
- ½ TEASPOON PEPPER
- 1¼ POUNDS SKINLESS, BONELESS CHICKEN THIGHS, CUT INTO 1-INCH CHUNKS
- 2 TEASPOONS OLIVE OIL
- 1 MEDIUM ONION, HALVED AND THICKLY SLICED
- 4 CLOVES GARLIC, MINCED
- 3 CARROTS, THICKLY SLICED
- 1 POUND SMALL RED-SKINNED POTATOES, QUARTERED
- 2 TEASPOONS CREAMY PEANUT BUTTER
- 4 CUPS BROCCOLI FLORETS

1 In a medium bowl, stir together the turmeric, ginger, ½ teaspoon of the salt, the cinnamon, sugar, and pepper. Add the chicken, tossing to coat.

2 In a nonstick Dutch oven, heat the oil over medium heat. Add the onion and garlic, and cook, stirring frequently for 7 minutes, or until the onion is tender.

3 Add ½ cup of water, the carrots, potatoes, peanut butter, and the remaining ½ teaspoon salt; bring to a boil. Cook for 5 minutes, or until the carrots begin to soften.

4 Add the chicken, and cook for 2 minutes, or until no longer pink. Stir in 2 cups of water and bring to a boil. Reduce to a simmer; cover and cook for 15 minutes, or until the chicken is cooked through and the potatoes are tender.

5 Add the broccoli; cover and cook for 5 minutes, or until the broccoli is tender.

Makes 4 servings. Per serving: *394 calories, 9.7g total fat (20% saturated), 37g protein, 38g carbohydrate, 7.9g fiber, 118mg cholesterol, 789mg sodium*

rich curried chicken & vegetables ▶

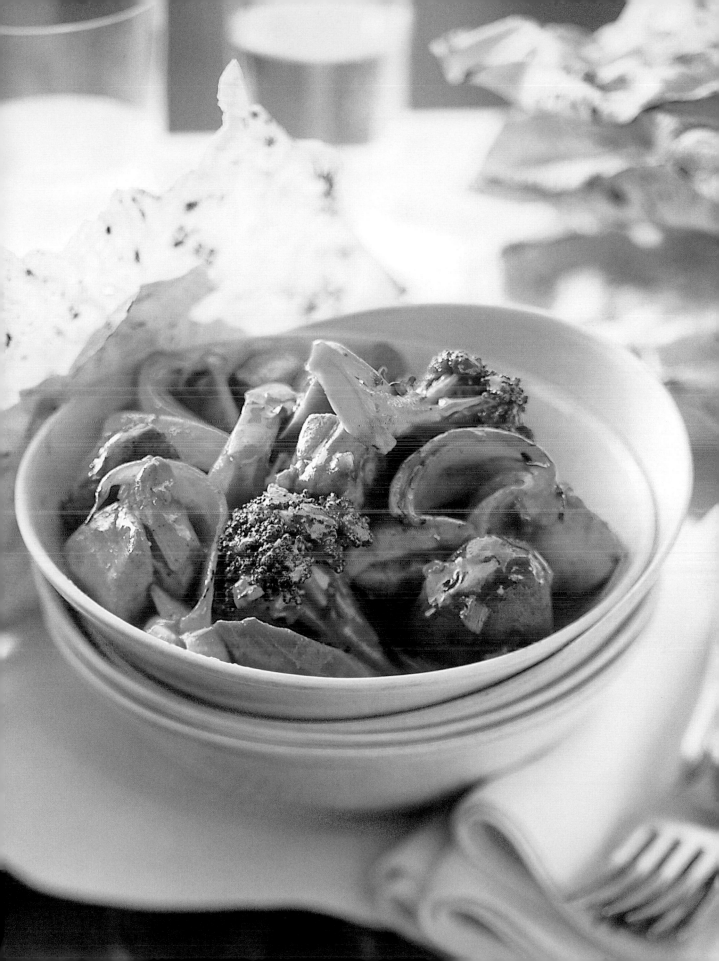

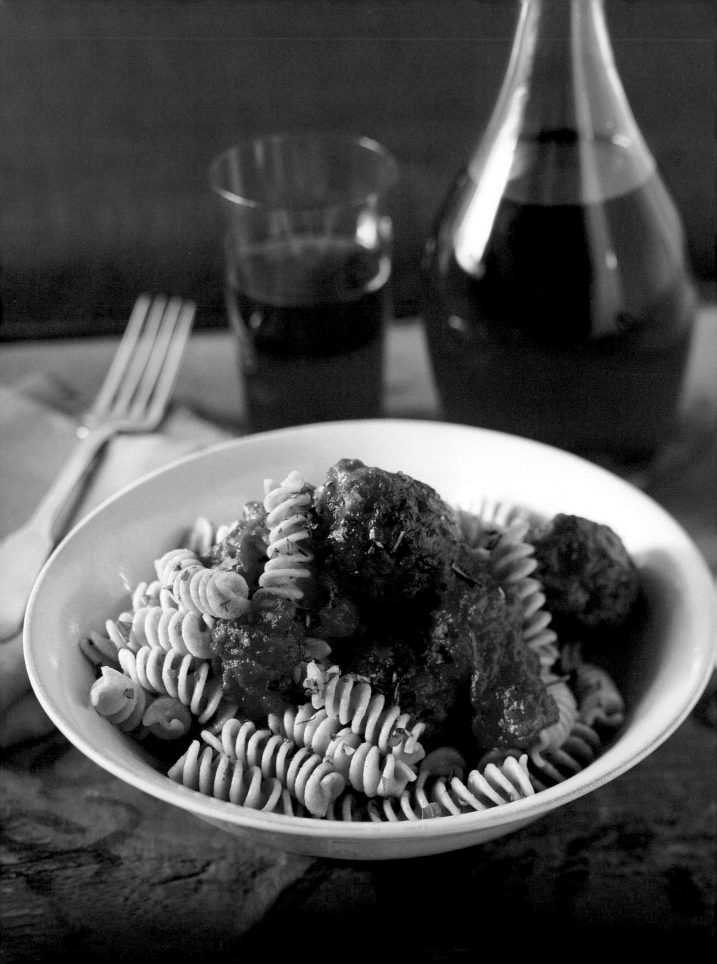

herbed turkey meatballs & fusilli

Turkey, herbs, cheese, and currants combine to make tender, flavorful meatballs packed with zinc, selenium, calcium, magnesium, and B vitamins.

- 2 TABLESPOONS OLIVE OIL
- 1 MEDIUM ONION, FINELY CHOPPED
- 3 CLOVES GARLIC, MINCED
- 2 SLICES FIRM WHITE SANDWICH BREAD, CRUMBLED
- ¼ CUP LOW-FAT (1%) MILK
- 1 POUND LEAN GROUND TURKEY BREAST
- ½ CUP CHOPPED PARSLEY
- 1 LARGE EGG
- ⅓ CUP GRATED PARMESAN CHEESE
- ¼ CUP DRIED CURRANTS
- ¾ TEASPOON RUBBED SAGE
- ½ TEASPOON SALT
- 2 TABLESPOONS FLOUR
- 1 CAN (28 OUNCES) CRUSHED TOMATOES
- 3 STRIPS (3 x ½-INCH EACH) ORANGE ZEST
- 8 OUNCES WHOLE WHEAT FUSILLI

1 In a large skillet, heat 1 tablespoon of the oil over medium heat. Add the onion and garlic, and cook for 7 minutes, or until golden. Transfer to a large bowl. Add the crumbled bread and milk to the bowl; let stand for 1 minute to soften the bread.

2 Add the turkey, parsley, egg, Parmesan, currants, sage, and salt; mix well. Shape the mixture into 24 walnut-size meatballs. Dredge the meatballs in the flour, shaking off the excess.

3 In the same skillet, heat the remaining 1 tablespoon oil over medium heat. Add the meatballs, and sauté for 3 minutes, or until golden brown. Add the tomatoes and orange zest, and bring to a boil. Reduce to a simmer; cover and cook for 12 minutes, or until the meatballs are cooked through.

4 Meanwhile, in a large pot of boiling water, cook the fusilli according to package directions. Drain and toss in a large bowl with the meatballs and sauce.

Makes 4 servings. Per serving: 579 calories, 13g total fat (25% saturated), 46g protein, 74g carbohydrate, 10g fiber, 130mg cholesterol, 901mg sodium

braised chicken thighs with winter vegetables

Shiitake mushrooms, brussels sprouts, and potatoes are all earthy vegetables that marry well with rich, dark-meat chicken.

- ½ CUP DRIED SHIITAKE MUSHROOMS
- 1 CUP BOILING WATER
- 8 SKINLESS BONE-IN CHICKEN THIGHS (ABOUT 5 OUNCES EACH)
- 2 TABLESPOONS FLOUR
- 3 TEASPOONS OLIVE OIL
- 2 LEEKS, HALVED LENGTHWISE, CUT CROSSWISE INTO 1-INCH LENGTHS, AND WELL WASHED
- 1½ POUNDS SMALL RED-SKINNED POTATOES, CUT INTO ½-INCH CHUNKS
- 1 PACKAGE (10 OUNCES) FROZEN BRUSSELS SPROUTS
- 1 TEASPOON SALT
- ½ TEASPOON DRIED THYME

1 In a small bowl, combine the shiitake mushrooms and boiling water. Let stand for 20 minutes, or until softened. With your fingers, remove the mushrooms from the soaking liquid, reserving the liquid. Trim any stems from the mushrooms and thinly slice the caps. Strain the reserved liquid through a fine-meshed sieve or coffee filter; set aside.

2 Dredge the chicken in the flour, shaking off the excess. In a nonstick Dutch oven, heat 2 teaspoons of the oil over medium heat. Add the chicken, and cook for 3 minutes per side, or until golden brown. Transfer the chicken to a plate.

3 Add the remaining 1 teaspoon oil, the leeks, and mushrooms to the pan; cook, stirring frequently for 2 minutes, or until the leeks are golden.

4 Add the reserved liquid, the potatoes, brussels sprouts, salt, thyme, and 1 cup of water; bring to a boil. Return the chicken to the pan and reduce to a simmer; cover and cook, stirring occasionally for 25 minutes, or until the chicken is cooked through and the brussels sprouts and potatoes are tender.

Makes 4 servings. Per serving: 501 calories, 12.3g total fat (21% saturated), 48g protein, 50g carbohydrate, 5.9g fiber, 172mg cholesterol, 792mg sodium

◀ **herbed turkey meatballs & fusilli**

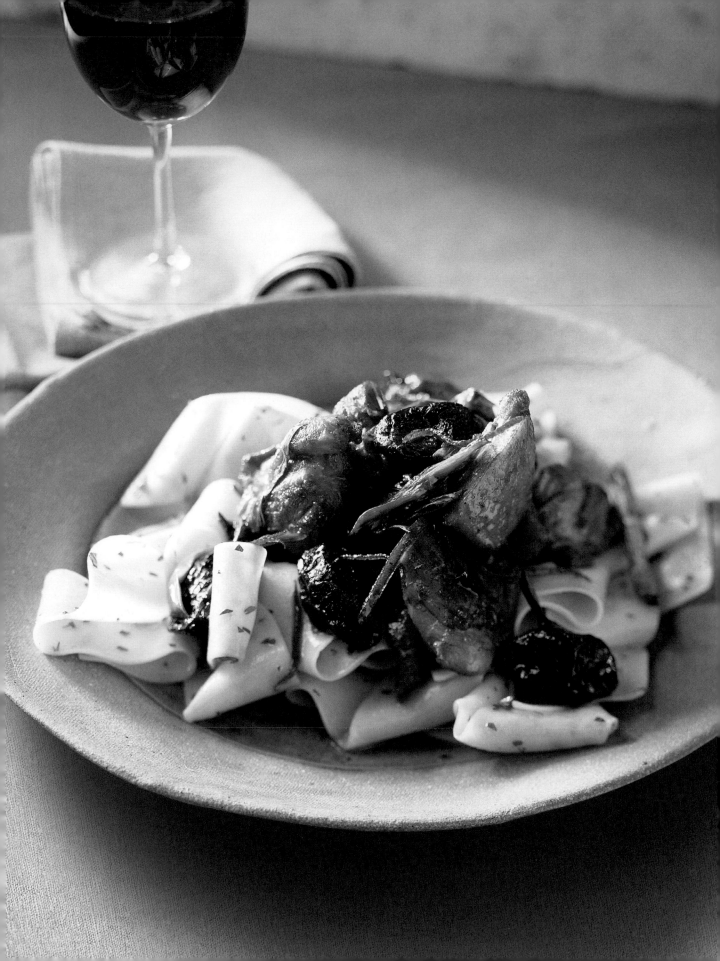

roast turkey breast with preserved lemons & rosemary

Preserved lemons, a Moroccan staple, generally take a month to prepare. However, this recipe calls for a quick version (made in 20 minutes). The lemon adds wonderful flavor as well as a number of phytochemicals found only in the peel.

- 1 LEMON
- ¼ CUP FRESH LEMON JUICE
- ¼ CUP SALT
- 1 STICK CINNAMON
- ½ TEASPOON CORIANDER SEEDS
- ⅓ CUP CHOPPED PARSLEY
- 1 TABLESPOON FRESH ROSEMARY, MINCED
- 6 CLOVES GARLIC, MINCED
- 1 SMALL WHOLE TURKEY BREAST (ABOUT 4½ POUNDS)
- 1 TABLESPOON OLIVE OIL
- 1 MEDIUM ONION, THICKLY SLICED
- 1 CARROT, THINLY SLICED

1 Halve the lemon lengthwise. Then cut each half lengthwise into ½-inch-wide strips.

2 In a small saucepan, combine the lemon strips, lemon juice, 1 cup of water, the salt, cinnamon stick, and coriander; bring to a boil, stirring until the salt dissolves. Cook for 20 minutes, or until very soft.

3 Preheat the oven to 350°F. Lift half of the lemon strips from the cooking liquid and mince. Set aside the remaining lemon strips in the cooking liquid.

4 Transfer the minced lemon to a small bowl and combine with the parsley, rosemary, and garlic. Carefully lift the skin of the turkey breast, without removing it. With a small knife, make incisions all over the turkey breast and push the lemon mixture into the incisions. Rub any remaining mixture and the oil over the turkey flesh and replace the skin.

5 Remove the remaining lemon strips from the cooking liquid (discard the liquid and spices). Place the lemon strips, onion, and carrot inside the turkey cavity. Place breast-side down on a rack in a roasting pan, and roast for 1 hour, 15 minutes.

6 Turn the turkey breast-side up and roast for 30 minutes, or until a meat thermometer registers 165°F (the temperature will rise to 170°F as the turkey stands). Let stand for 10 minutes before carving.

Makes 8 servings. Per serving: 248 calories, 3g total fat (20% saturated), 48g protein, 5g carbohydrate, 1.4g fiber, 132mg cholesterol, 671mg sodium

chicken with red wine, port & prunes

Red wine, with its phytochemical resveratrol, gives this dish depth as well as health benefits.

- 1 CUP PITTED PRUNES
- ⅔ CUP DRY RED WINE
- ⅓ CUP PORT
- 2 TEASPOONS OLIVE OIL
- 1 POUND SKINLESS, BONELESS CHICKEN THIGHS, CUT INTO 2-INCH CHUNKS
- 2 TABLESPOONS FLOUR
- 8 SCALLIONS, CUT INTO 2-INCH LENGTHS
- 2 TEASPOONS SLIVERED ORANGE ZEST
- ¼ CUP ORANGE JUICE
- 2 TEASPOONS BALSAMIC VINEGAR
- ½ TEASPOON SALT
- ½ TEASPOON PEPPER
- 3 TABLESPOONS CHOPPED PARSLEY

1 In a medium bowl, combine the prunes, wine, and port; let stand for 30 minutes at room temperature.

2 In a large nonstick skillet, heat the oil over medium heat. Dredge the chicken in the flour, shaking off the excess. Add the chicken to the pan, and sauté for 3 minutes, or until golden brown. Add the scallions, and cook for 1 minute, or until wilted.

3 Stir in the prunes and their soaking liquid, the orange zest, orange juice, vinegar, salt, and pepper; bring to a boil. Reduce to a simmer; cover and cook for 20 minutes, or until the chicken and prunes are tender. Stir in the parsley.

Makes 4 servings. Per serving: 298 calories, 7g total fat (21% saturated), 25g protein, 36g carbohydrate, 3.9g fiber, 94mg cholesterol, 399mg sodium

chicken waldorf salad with toasted walnuts

Horseradish and black pepper add a nice kick to this classic American salad.

- ⅓ CUP WALNUTS
- 1 POUND SKINLESS, BONELESS CHICKEN BREASTS
- ½ TEASPOON SALT
- ½ TEASPOON PEPPER
- ¾ CUP PLAIN LOW-FAT YOGURT
- 3 TABLESPOONS HORSERADISH
- 2 TABLESPOONS LIGHT MAYONNAISE
- 2 TABLESPOONS FRESH LEMON JUICE
- 2 CUPS SEEDLESS RED GRAPES, HALVED
- 1½ CUPS THINLY SLICED CELERY (ABOUT 3 STALKS)
- 2 RED APPLES (UNPEELED), CUT INTO ½-INCH CUBES
- 4 CUPS SHREDDED ROMAINE LETTUCE

1 Preheat the oven to 350°F. Place the walnuts on a baking sheet, and bake for 7 minutes, or until slightly crisped and fragrant. When cool enough to handle, coarsely chop.

2 Preheat the broiler. Sprinkle the chicken with ¼ teaspoon of the salt and ¼ teaspoon of the pepper. Broil 6 inches from the heat for 4 to 5 minutes per side, or until cooked through. Cool to room temperature, then cut into 1-inch chunks.

3 In a large bowl, whisk together the yogurt, horseradish, mayonnaise, lemon juice, and the remaining ¼ teaspoon salt and ¼ teaspoon pepper.

4 Add the walnuts, chicken, grapes, celery, and apples; toss to coat. Add the romaine and toss again.

Makes 4 servings. Per serving: 351 calories, 11g total fat (19% saturated), 32g protein, 35g carbohydrate, 5g fiber, 71mg cholesterol, 508mg sodium

moroccan braised chicken

In this braise, chicken breasts are cooked with a hearty mixture of typical North African ingredients: chickpeas, lemon, cilantro, and apricots.

- ½ CUP DRIED APRICOTS
- 1 CUP BOILING WATER
- 1 TABLESPOON OLIVE OIL
- 4 SKINLESS, BONELESS CHICKEN BREAST HALVES (ABOUT 6 OUNCES EACH)
- 1 LARGE ONION, FINELY CHOPPED
- 6 CLOVES GARLIC, MINCED
- 2 CELERY STALKS, THINLY SLICED
- 1 CUP CANNED CHICKPEAS, DRAINED AND RINSED
- 1 CAN (14½ OUNCES) NO-SALT-ADDED STEWED TOMATOES
- 2 TEASPOONS GRATED LEMON ZEST
- 2 TABLESPOONS FRESH LEMON JUICE
- 1½ TEASPOONS GROUND CORIANDER
- ½ TEASPOON PEPPER
- ½ CUP CHOPPED CILANTRO

1 In a small bowl, combine the apricots and boiling water, and let stand for 10 minutes at room temperature. Strain the apricots, reserving the soaking liquid, then dice the apricots.

2 Meanwhile, in a large skillet, heat the oil over medium heat. Add the chicken, and sauté for 3 minutes per side, or until golden brown. Transfer the chicken to a plate.

3 Add the onion and garlic to the skillet, and cook, stirring frequently for 7 minutes, or until the onion is tender. Add the celery and cook for 3 minutes.

4 Stir in the apricots, the reserved liquid, the chickpeas, tomatoes, lemon zest, lemon juice, coriander, and pepper.

5 Bring to a boil and return the chicken to the pan. Reduce to a simmer; cover and cook for 15 minutes, or until the chicken is cooked through. Stir in the cilantro and serve.

Makes 4 servings. Per serving: 367 calories, 7g total fat (16% saturated), 45g protein, 32g carbohydrate, 7.2g fiber, 99mg cholesterol, 232mg sodium

moroccan braised chicken ▶

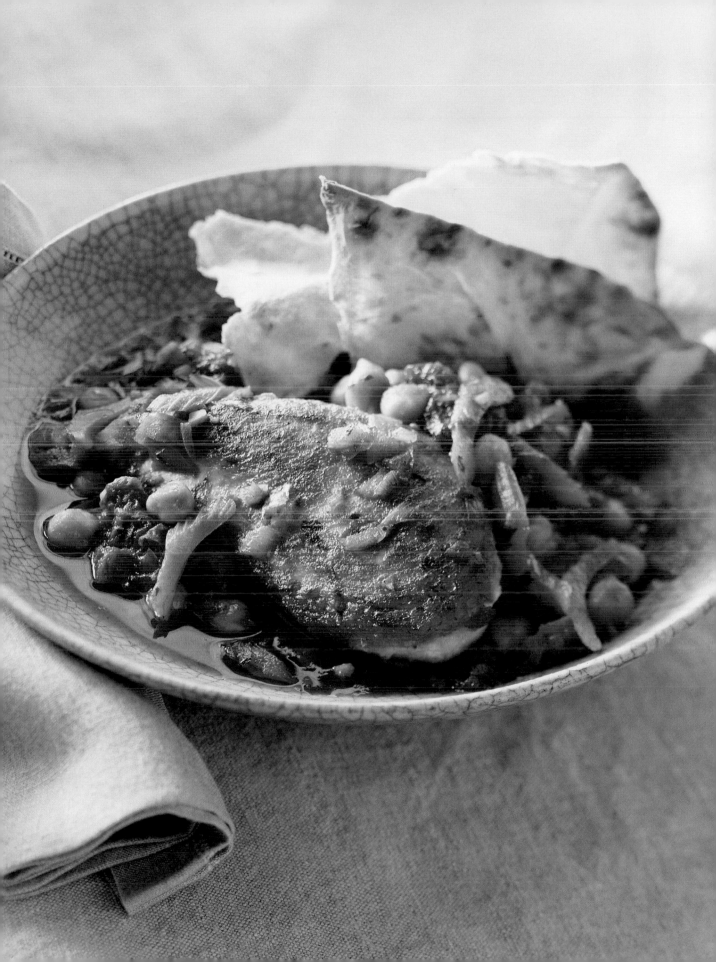

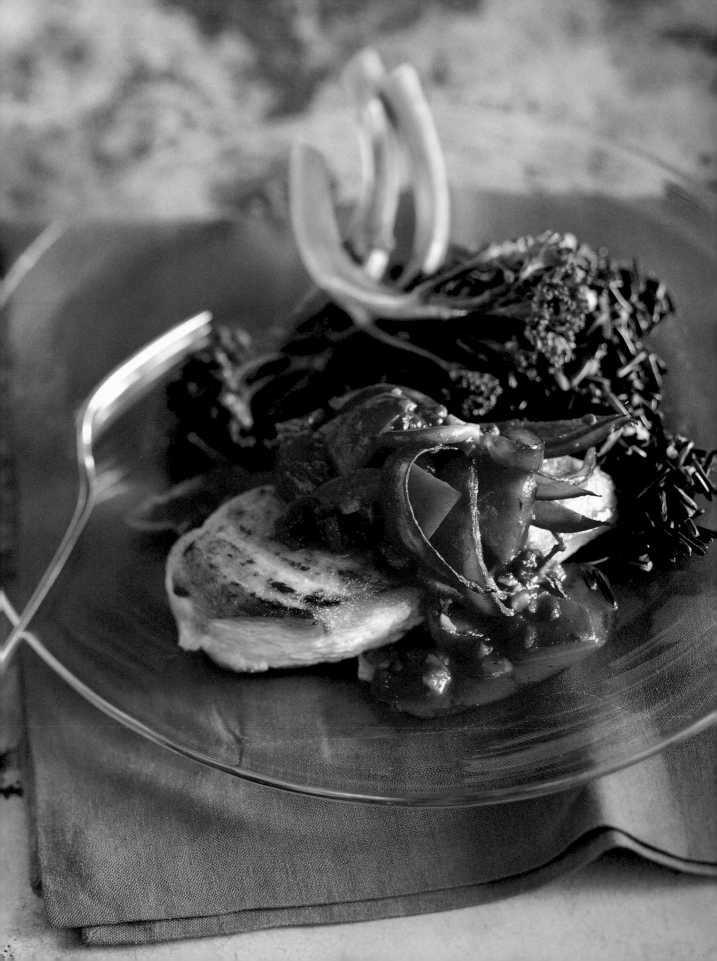

pineapple-chipotle chicken

Pineapple juice, tomato paste, fresh ginger, and smoky-hot chipotle peppers in adobo sauce (a spicy, chili- and vinegar-based sauce) give the sauce for this chicken a pleasing balance of spicy, sweet, and savory flavors. If you can't find chipotle peppers, substitute 1 to 1½ teaspoons of medium-hot chili powder.

- 1 TABLESPOON PLUS 2 TEASPOONS OLIVE OIL
- 4 SKINLESS, BONELESS CHICKEN BREAST HALVES (ABOUT 5 OUNCES EACH)
- 2 TABLESPOONS FLOUR
- 1 MEDIUM RED ONION, HALVED AND SLICED ½ INCH THICK
- 3 CLOVES GARLIC, MINCED
- 1 RED BELL PEPPER, CUT INTO ½-INCH CHUNKS
- ¼ CUP MINCED FRESH GINGER
- 2½ CUPS PINEAPPLE JUICE
- ¼ CUP TOMATO PASTE
- 2 CHIPOTLE PEPPERS IN ADOBO, MINCED (4 TEASPOONS)
- ¾ TEASPOON SALT

1 In a large nonstick skillet, heat 1 tablespoon of the oil over medium heat. Dredge the chicken in the flour, shaking off the excess. Add the chicken to the skillet, and cook for 2 minutes per side, or until golden brown. Transfer the chicken to a plate.

2 Add the remaining 2 teaspoons oil to the pan along with the onion and garlic, and cook, stirring frequently for 5 minutes, or until the onion is tender.

3 Add the bell pepper and ginger, and cook for 3 minutes. Stir in the pineapple juice, tomato paste, chipotle pepper, and salt; bring to a boil. Boil for 5 minutes.

4 Return the chicken to the pan. Reduce to a simmer and cook for 10 minutes, or until the chicken is cooked through.

Makes 4 servings. Per serving: 350 calories, 7.9g total fat (16% saturated), 36g protein, 34g carbohydrate, 2.1g fiber, 82mg cholesterol, 709mg sodium

indian-style turkey burgers

If you like spicy food, look for a container of hot Madras curry and use it in place of the regular curry powder. Grinding your own turkey guarantees that it will be lean (store-bought turkey often has skin ground in with the breast meat).

- 1 TABLESPOON OLIVE OIL
- 1 LARGE RED ONION, FINELY CHOPPED,
- 3 CLOVES GARLIC, MINCED
- 2 TABLESPOONS MINCED FRESH GINGER
- 1 RED BELL PEPPER, DICED
- 1½ TEASPOONS CURRY POWDER
- ½ CUP TOMATO JUICE
- 4 TABLESPOONS CHOPPED MANGO CHUTNEY
- 1 POUND LEAN GROUND TURKEY BREAST
- ⅓ CUP PLAIN LOW FAT YOGURT
- ¼ CUP CHOPPED CILANTRO
- 1 SLICE FIRM WHITE SANDWICH BREAD, CRUMBLED
- ½ TEASPOON SALT

1 In a small skillet, heat the oil over medium heat. Add the onion, garlic, and ginger, and cook, stirring frequently for 5 minutes, or until the onion is lightly browned. Measure out ½ cup of the onion-ginger mixture and transfer it to a large bowl.

2 To the mixture remaining in the skillet, add the bell pepper, and cook for 4 minutes, or until crisp-tender. Stir in 1 teaspoon of the curry powder, and cook for 1 minute. Stir in the tomato juice and 2 tablespoons of the chutney; bring to a boil. Boil for 1 minute.

3 To the reserved onion-ginger mixture, add the remaining ½ teaspoon curry powder, 2 tablespoons chutney, the turkey, yogurt, cilantro, crumbled bread, and salt. Gently shape the mixture into 4 patties.

4 Preheat the broiler. Broil the patties 6 inches from the heat for 3½ minutes per side, or until cooked through. Serve the burgers with the sautéed pepper mixture on top.

Makes 4 servings. Per serving: 288 calories, 4.9g total fat (19% saturated), 31g protein, 28g carbohydrate, 2g fiber, 72mg cholesterol, 685mg sodium

chicken-melon salad

Broiled chicken tossed in a lime-mustard dressing with cantaloupe, cherry tomatoes, and peppery watercress adds up to a nutrient-packed salad rich in lycopene, beta-carotene, and vitamin C.

- 1 TABLESPOON CHILI POWDER
- 1 TEASPOON DRIED OREGANO
- 1 POUND SKINLESS, BONELESS CHICKEN BREASTS
- 1 TABLESPOON OLIVE OIL
- 5 TABLESPOONS FRESH LIME JUICE
- ½ TEASPOON SALT
- 2 CORN TORTILLAS (6-INCH DIAMETER), CUT INTO 8 WEDGES EACH
- 2 TABLESPOONS LIGHT MAYONNAISE
- 2 TEASPOONS DIJON MUSTARD
- 2 BUNCHES WATERCRESS, TOUGH STEMS TRIMMED (ABOUT 6 CUPS)
- 3 CUPS CANTALOUPE CHUNKS (½-INCH)
- 2 CUPS CHERRY TOMATOES, HALVED
- 2 SCALLIONS, THINLY SLICED

1 Preheat the oven to 450°F. In a small bowl, stir together the chili powder and oregano. Measure out 1 teaspoon of the mixture and set aside. Rub the remaining mixture into the chicken.

2 In a small bowl, whisk together the reserved 1 teaspoon spice mixture, the olive oil, 1 tablespoon of the lime juice, and ¼ teaspoon of the salt. Dip the tortilla wedges into the chili mixture. Transfer the wedges to a baking sheet and bake for 5 minutes, or until crisp. Remove the tortilla wedges from the oven and preheat the broiler.

3 Broil the chicken 6 inches from the heat for 4 minutes per side, or until cooked through. When cool enough to handle, slice into bite-size pieces.

4 Meanwhile, in a large bowl, whisk together the remaining 4 tablespoons lime juice, ¼ teaspoon salt, the mayonnaise, and mustard. Add the chicken, watercress, cantaloupe, tomatoes, and scallions. Serve topped with the tortilla wedges.

Makes 4 servings. Per serving: 283 calories, 8.5g total fat (16% saturated), 30g protein, 23g carbohydrate, 4.3g fiber, 68mg cholesterol, 558mg sodium

balsamic-glazed turkey cutlets

Butternut squash, sage, and turkey lend an autumnal feel to this dish. One serving provides nearly half of the recommended daily intake for beta-carotene, selenium, niacin, and vitamin B_6.

- 1 POUND TURKEY CUTLETS
- 2 TABLESPOONS FLOUR
- 2 TABLESPOONS OLIVE OIL
- 2 CUPS CUBED (½-INCH) BUTTERNUT SQUASH (ABOUT 12 OUNCES)
- 2 TEASPOONS SUGAR
- ¼ CUP BALSAMIC VINEGAR
- ½ TEASPOON SALT
- ½ TEASPOON LEAF SAGE
- 2 RED APPLES (UNPEELED), THINLY SLICED
- 1 TEASPOON CORNSTARCH BLENDED WITH 1 TABLESPOON WATER

1 Dredge the turkey in the flour, shaking off the excess. In a large nonstick skillet, heat 1 tablespoon of the oil over medium heat. Add half the turkey, and cook for 1 minute per side, or until golden brown and just cooked through. Transfer the turkey to a plate. Repeat with the remaining 1 tablespoon oil and remaining turkey.

2 Add the squash to the pan, sprinkle with the sugar, and cook for 3 minutes, or until lightly browned. Add the vinegar, and cook for 1 minute.

3 Stir in 1¼ cups of water, the salt, and sage; bring to a boil. Reduce to a simmer and stir in the apples; cover and cook for 2 minutes, or until the squash and apples are tender.

4 Stir in the cornstarch mixture, and cook for 1 minute, or until lightly thickened. Return the turkey to the pan, and simmer gently for 1 minute, or until heated through.

Makes 4 servings. Per serving: 283 calories, 7.8g total fat (15% saturated), 29g protein, 25g carbohydrate, 2.8g fiber, 70mg cholesterol, 350mg sodium

balsamic-glazed turkey cutlets ▶

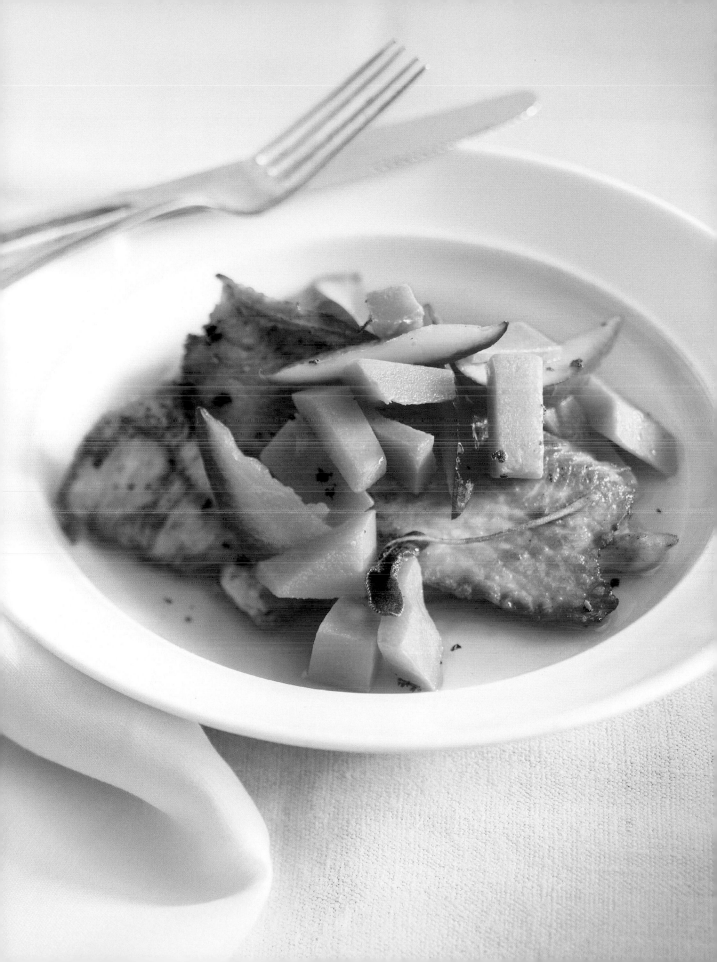

turkey braciole stuffed with provolone & spinach

More commonly made from thin slices of beef, braciole are simply meat rolled around a filling. Turkey cutlets lend themselves to this preparation, and when filled with spinach and provolone are a good source of folate, calcium, beta-carotene, selenium, and niacin.

- 8   TURKEY CUTLETS (1 POUND TOTAL)
- 1   TEASPOON RUBBED SAGE
- ¼   TEASPOON SALT
- 4   SLICES (4 OUNCES) THINLY SLICED PROVOLONE CHEESE, HALVED
- 1   PACKAGE (10 OUNCES) FROZEN CHOPPED SPINACH, THAWED AND SQUEEZED DRY
- 3   TABLESPOONS FLOUR
- 1   TABLESPOON OLIVE OIL
- 1¼ CUPS CANNED CRUSHED TOMATOES
- 1   TEASPOON GRATED ORANGE ZEST
- ¼   CUP FRESH ORANGE JUICE
- 2   TABLESPOONS DRIED CURRANTS OR CHOPPED RAISINS

1 Sprinkle one side of each cutlet with the sage and the salt. Lay 1 half-slice of provolone on top of the sage and top with the spinach. Roll up the cutlets and secure with a toothpick.

2 Dredge the turkey rolls in the flour, shaking off the excess. In a large nonstick skillet, heat the oil over medium heat. Add the rolls, and sauté for 2 minutes per side, or until golden brown.

3 Add the tomatoes, orange zest, orange juice, and currants; bring to a boil. Reduce to a simmer; cover and cook for 10 minutes, or until the turkey is cooked through.

4 To serve, remove the toothpicks and spoon the sauce over the turkey rolls.

Makes 4 servings. Per serving: 329 calories, 12g total fat (46% saturated), 39g protein, 16g carbohydrate, 2.6g fiber, 90mg cholesterol, 622mg sodium

jamaican jerked chicken salad

Assemble this salad at serving time, because an enzyme in kiwifruit, actinidin, quickly starts to break down any protein it happens to be in contact with. If the chicken and kiwi sit too long, the chicken begins to get mushy, so eat this spicy and refreshing salad while the chicken is still warm.

- 4   SCALLIONS, THINLY SLICED
- 3   CLOVES GARLIC, MINCED
- 1¼ TEASPOONS DRIED THYME
- 1   TEASPOON BLACK PEPPER
- ¾   TEASPOON GROUND ALLSPICE
- ¾   TEASPOON SALT
- 4   TABLESPOONS RED WINE VINEGAR
- 2   TABLESPOONS DIJON MUSTARD
- 2   TEASPOONS DARK BROWN SUGAR
- 1   POUND SKINLESS, BONELESS CHICKEN BREASTS
- 1   TABLESPOON OLIVE OIL
- 2   CUPS PINEAPPLE CHUNKS
- 4   KIWIFRUIT, PEELED AND CUT INTO WEDGES
- 1   LARGE RED BELL PEPPER, CUT INTO MATCHSTICKS
- 1   CUP JICAMA MATCHSTICKS

1 In a large bowl, stir together half the scallions, the garlic, thyme, black pepper, allspice, and ½ teaspoon of the salt. Stir in 2 tablespoons of the vinegar, 1 tablespoon of the mustard, and the brown sugar; mix well. Add the chicken, rubbing the mixture into the chicken. Cover and set aside.

2 In a separate bowl, whisk together the remaining 2 tablespoons vinegar, 1 tablespoon mustard, ¼ teaspoon salt, and the oil. Add the remaining scallions, the pineapple, kiwifruit, bell pepper, and jicama; toss to combine.

3 Preheat the broiler. Broil the chicken 6 inches from the heat for 4 minutes per side, or until cooked through. When cool enough to handle, slice the chicken on the diagonal. Add to the bowl and toss.

Makes 4 servings. Per serving: 287 calories, 5.6g total fat (15% saturated), 28g protein, 31g carbohydrate, 5.9g fiber, 66mg cholesterol, 701mg sodium

jamaican jerked chicken salad ▶

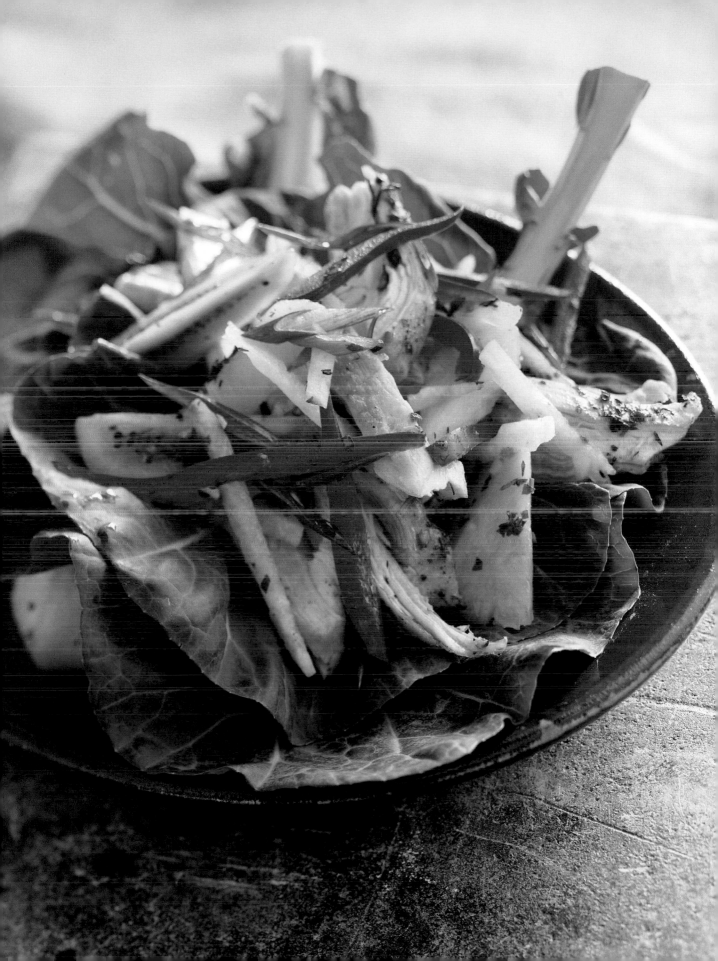

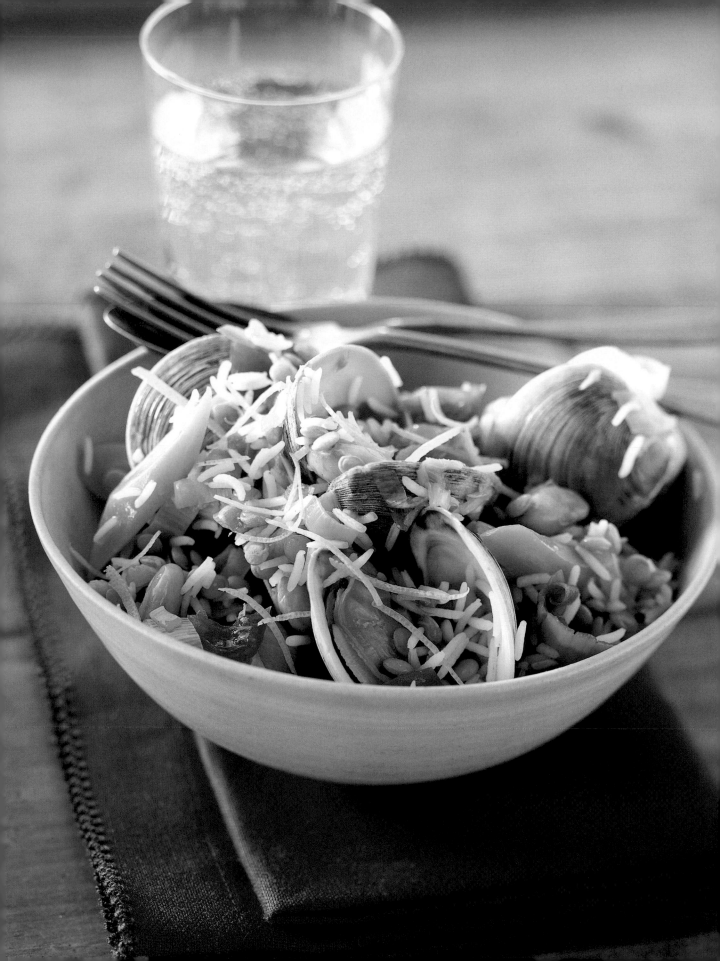

lentil & rice paella with clams

An excellent source of vitamin B₁₂, clams also provide a tremendous amount of iron. Between the clams, lentils, and lima beans in this dish you'll get almost all the iron you need for the day.

1	TABLESPOON OLIVE OIL
2	LARGE LEEKS, QUARTERED LENGTHWISE, THINLY SLICED CROSSWISE, AND WELL WASHED
5	CLOVES GARLIC, MINCED
3	LARGE CARROTS, CUT CROSSWISE INTO ½-INCH SLICES
1	PICKLED JALAPEÑO PEPPER, MINCED
⅔	CUP LENTILS, PICKED OVER AND RINSED
½	TEASPOON SALT
⅔	CUP RICE
1⅓	CUPS FROZEN LIMA BEANS
1	LARGE TOMATO, COARSELY CHOPPED
2	TEASPOONS FINELY SLIVERED LEMON ZEST
1½	DOZEN LITTLENECK CLAMS, WELL SCRUBBED

1 In a nonstick Dutch oven or flameproof casserole, heat the oil over medium heat. Add the leeks and garlic, and cook, stirring frequently for 7 minutes, or until the leeks are tender.

2 Add the carrots and jalapeño, and cook for 5 minutes, or until the carrots are crisp-tender.

3 Add the lentils, stirring to coat. Add 3 cups of water and the salt, and bring to a boil over high heat. Reduce to a simmer; cover and cook for 10 minutes.

4 Add the rice; cover and simmer for 10 minutes. Stir in the lima beans, tomato, and lemon zest; cook for 2 minutes. Place the clams on top of the lentil-rice mixture; cover and cook for 5 to 7 minutes, or until the clams open (check after 3 minutes as some will open before others; discard any that do not open).

Makes 4 servings. *Per serving: 457 calories, 5.3g total fat (13% saturated), 25g protein, 79g carbohydrate, 11g fiber, 21mg cholesterol, 464mg sodium*

broiled shrimp with tomato cocktail sauce

The cocktail sauce for these broiled shrimp is spiced with both a jalapeño pepper and chili powder (good sources of capsaicin) in addition to the traditional heat-generating horseradish. The dish is also rich in selenium (from the shrimp) and lycopene (from the tomatoes in the cocktail sauce).

3½	TEASPOONS CHILI POWDER
1¾	TEASPOONS GROUND CORIANDER
¾	TEASPOON GROUND GINGER
½	TEASPOON SALT
1	CUP CANNED CRUSHED TOMATOES
2	TABLESPOONS TOMATO PASTE
2	TEASPOONS HORSERADISH
2	TEASPOONS BALSAMIC VINEGAR
2	TEASPOONS HONEY
2	TEASPOONS MINCED PICKLED JALAPEÑO PEPPER (1 MEDIUM)
1½	POUNDS LARGE SHRIMP (ABOUT 28), SHELLED AND DEVEINED
1	TABLESPOON OLIVE OIL

1 In a medium bowl, stir together 1½ teaspoons of the chili powder, ¾ teaspoon of the coriander, ¼ teaspoon of the ginger, and ¼ teaspoon of the salt. Add the crushed tomatoes, tomato paste, horseradish, vinegar, honey, and jalapeño. Refrigerate until ready to use.

2 In a large bowl, combine the remaining 2 teaspoons chili powder, 1 teaspoon coriander, ½ teaspoon ginger, and ¼ teaspoon salt. Add the shrimp, and toss well to coat. Add the olive oil, and toss again.

3 Preheat the broiler. Broil the shrimp 6 inches from the heat for 2 minutes per side, or until cooked through. To serve, place a mound of sauce in the center of each of 4 plates and arrange the shrimp around it.

Makes 4 servings. *Per serving: 218 calories, 6.4g total fat (14% saturated), 29g protein, 11g carbohydrate, 1.6g fiber, 211mg cholesterol, 704mg sodium*

◀ **lentil & rice paella with clams**

sicilian pasta salad

This is a take-off on a Sicilian pasta and sardine dish traditionally made for St. Joseph's Day. High in calcium and vitamin B$_{12}$, sardines are also a good source of omega-3 fatty acids.

- 8   OUNCES MEDIUM PASTA SHELLS
- ½   CUP FRESH LEMON JUICE
- 3   TABLESPOONS TOMATO PASTE
- 1   TEASPOON FENNEL SEEDS
- ½   TEASPOON SALT
- 1   BULB FENNEL, STALKS REMOVED (FRONDS RESERVED), BULB CUT INTO ½-INCH CHUNKS
- ⅓   CUP RAISINS
- 3   CANS (4⅜ OUNCES EACH) SARDINES PACKED IN OIL, DRAINED

1 In a large pot of boiling water, cook the pasta according to package directions. Drain, reserving ½ cup of the pasta cooking liquid.

2 Meanwhile, in a large bowl, whisk together the lemon juice, tomato paste, fennel seeds, and salt. Whisk in the reserved liquid.

3 Add the drained pasta, fresh fennel, and raisins to the dressing; toss well.

4 Mince enough of the reserved fennel fronds to get ½ cup. Add the minced fronds and the sardines to the bowl, and toss gently to combine. Serve at room temperature or chilled.

Makes 4 servings. Per serving: 452 calories, 10g total fat (13% saturated), 29g protein, 61g carbohydrate, 4.6g fiber, 114mg cholesterol, 830mg sodium

shrimp & barley gumbo

The combination of collard greens, butternut squash, red and green peppers, and tomatoes makes this Louisiana-influenced stew rich in vitamin C, beta-carotene, and calcium. For a more attractive presentation, leave the shells on the shrimp tails.

- 1   TABLESPOON OLIVE OIL
- 1   LARGE ONION, FINELY CHOPPED
- 3   CLOVES GARLIC, MINCED
- 1   GREEN BELL PEPPER, DICED
- 1   RED BELL PEPPER, DICED
- 1   SMALL BUTTERNUT SQUASH (ABOUT 1½ POUNDS), PEELED AND CUT INTO ½-INCH CHUNKS
- 1   CUP QUICK-COOKING BARLEY
- 1¼ TEASPOONS LOUISIANA-STYLE RED PEPPER SAUCE
- 1   TEASPOON SALT
- ½   TEASPOON DRIED THYME
- 2   PACKAGES (9 OUNCES EACH) FROZEN CHOPPED COLLARD GREENS
- 1   CUP CANNED CRUSHED TOMATOES
- 1   POUND MEDIUM SHRIMP, SHELLED AND DEVEINED

1 In a Dutch oven, heat the oil over medium-low heat. Add the onion and garlic, and cook, stirring frequently for 7 minutes, or until the onion is tender. Add the bell peppers and squash; cook, stirring frequently for 5 minutes, or until the peppers are crisp-tender.

2 Add the barley, red pepper sauce, salt, thyme, and 3½ cups of water; bring to a boil. Stir in the collards and tomatoes, and return to a boil. Reduce to a simmer; cover and cook for 10 minutes, or until the barley is tender.

3 Place the shrimp on top of the stew; cover and cook for 4 to 5 minutes, or until the shrimp are cooked through.

Makes 4 servings. Per serving: 409 calories, 6.6g total fat (12% saturated), 29g protein, 64g carbohydrate, 11g fiber, 140mg cholesterol, 927mg sodium

shrimp & barley gumbo ▶

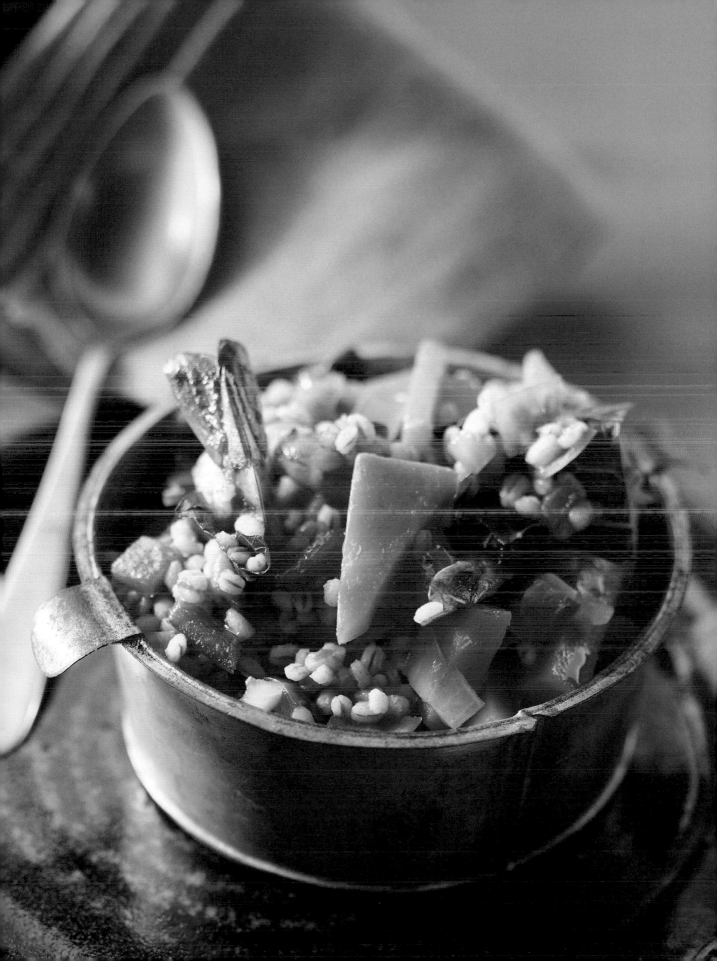

roasted beet & salmon salad

Roasted beets are wonderfully sweet, and while they may take a long time to cook, they do so unattended. Or, to speed up the process, microwave the beets, whole and unpeeled, in a loosely covered microwave-safe container (and, of course, not wrapped in foil). Wear kitchen gloves or use paper towels when peeling the beets to prevent your hands from getting stained.

2 POUNDS BEETS (ABOUT 8), WELL SCRUBBED

⅓ CUP NATURAL (UNBLANCHED) ALMONDS, COARSELY CHOPPED

8 OUNCES WHOLE WHEAT PENNE OR ZITI

1 CUP PLAIN NONFAT YOGURT

¼ CUP FRESH LEMON JUICE

3 TABLESPOONS BALSAMIC VINEGAR

1 TABLESPOON LIGHT MAYONNAISE

¼ TEASPOON SALT

1 CAN (15 OUNCES) SOCKEYE SALMON, DRAINED

3 SCALLIONS, THINLY SLICED

1 Preheat the oven to 400°F. Wrap the beets in foil, place on a baking sheet, and bake for 1 hour, or until tender. While the oven is on, place the almonds on another baking sheet, and toast for 5 to 7 minutes, or until golden brown.

2 Meanwhile, in a large pot of boiling water, cook the pasta according to package directions. Drain.

3 Unwrap the beets. When they're cool enough to handle, peel them and cut into ½-inch chunks.

4 In a large bowl, stir together the yogurt, lemon juice, vinegar, mayonnaise, and salt. Add the toasted almonds, pasta, beets, salmon, and scallions; toss to combine.

Makes 4 servings. **Per serving:** *516 calories, 14g total fat (17% saturated), 34g protein, 68g carbohydrate, 9.8g fiber, 40mg cholesterol, 802mg sodium*

broiled salmon with avocado-mango salsa

If you like, make a small amount of lemon vinaigrette and toss with the lettuce before placing the salmon and salsa on top.

2½ TEASPOONS PAPRIKA

2 TEASPOONS GROUND CORIANDER

¾ TEASPOON SALT

4 SKINLESS, BONELESS SALMON FILLETS (ABOUT 6 OUNCES EACH)

1 LARGE MANGO, PEELED AND CUT INTO ½-INCH CHUNKS (ABOUT 1½ CUPS)

1 HASS AVOCADO, PEELED AND CUT INTO ½-INCH CHUNKS

1 CUP CANNED CHICKPEAS, DRAINED AND RINSED

⅓ CUP CHOPPED CILANTRO

1 TEASPOON GRATED LEMON ZEST

2 TABLESPOONS FRESH LEMON JUICE

2 TEASPOONS OLIVE OIL

6 CUPS MESCLUN OR FRISÉE LETTUCE, TORN INTO BITE-SIZE PIECES

1 In a large bowl, stir together the paprika, coriander, and salt. Measure out 2 teaspoons of the spice mixture and sprinkle over the salmon, rubbing it into the fish. Place the salmon, skinned-side down, on a broiler pan.

2 To the spice mixture remaining in the bowl, add the mango, avocado, chickpeas, cilantro, lemon zest, lemon juice, and oil; toss to combine.

3 Broil the salmon 6 inches from heat for 5 minutes for medium. Serve the salmon and salsa on a bed of frisée lettuce.

Makes 4 servings. **Per serving:** *551 calories, 29g total fat (18% saturated), 42g protein, 35g carbohydrate, 7.8g fiber, 100mg cholesterol, 745mg sodium*

broiled salmon with avocado-mango salsa ▶

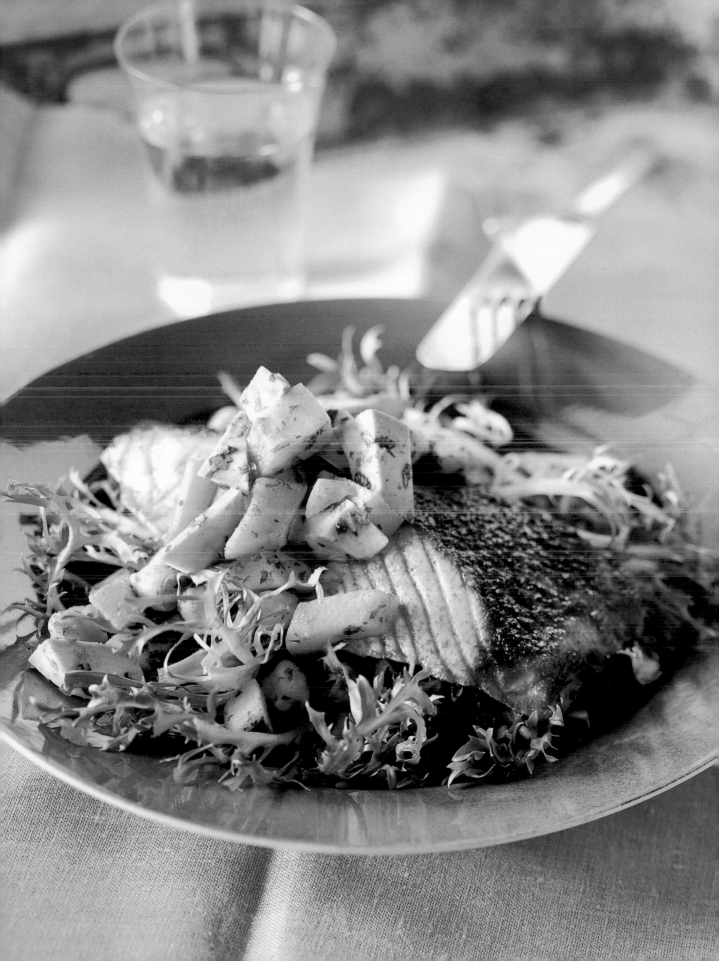

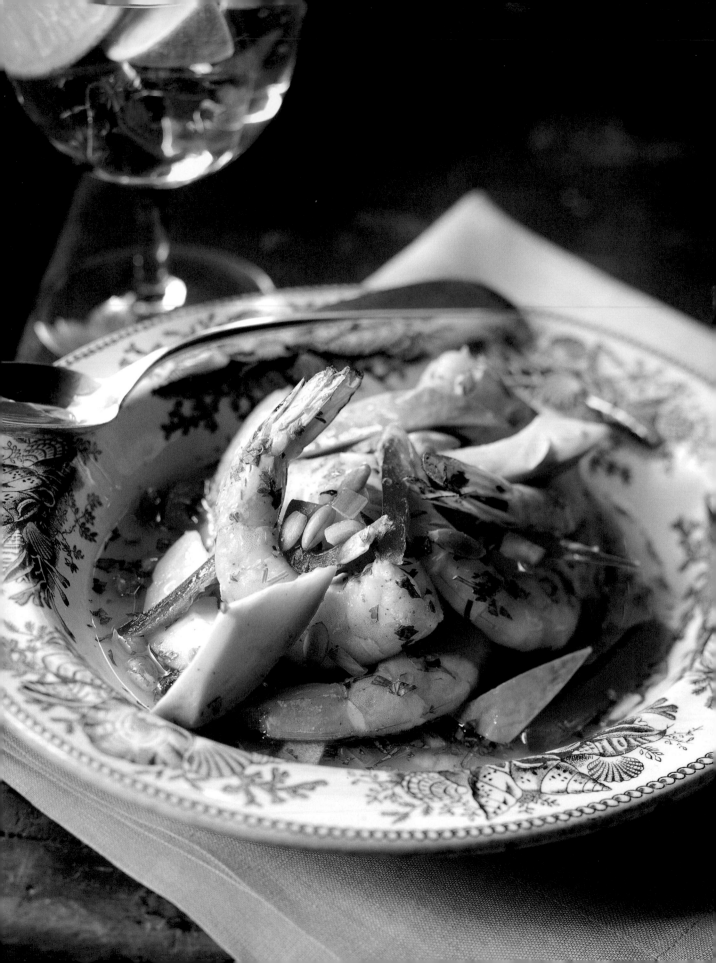

shrimp seviche with avocado & pumpkin seeds

This atypical seviche (the shrimp are cooked) is flavorful, colorful, and—because the citrus juices aren't subjected to heat—high in vitamin C.

1½	TEASPOONS GROUND CORIANDER
¾	TEASPOON SALT
1½	POUNDS MEDIUM SHRIMP, SHELLED AND DEVEINED
2	TEASPOONS GRATED ORANGE ZEST
2	CUPS ORANGE JUICE
3	TABLESPOONS FRESH LIME JUICE
¼	TEASPOON CAYENNE PEPPER
1	RED BELL PEPPER, CUT INTO MATCHSTICKS
¼	CUP DICED RED ONION
½	CUP CHOPPED CILANTRO
1	HASS AVOCADO, PEELED AND CUT INTO ½-INCH CHUNKS
3	TABLESPOONS (1½ OUNCES) HULLED ROASTED PUMPKIN SEEDS

1 In a large bowl, combine 1 teaspoon of the coriander and ¼ teaspoon of the salt. Add the shrimp, tossing to coat.

2 In a separate bowl, stir together the orange zest, orange juice, lime juice, remaining ⅓ teaspoon salt, ½ teaspoon coriander, and the cayenne. Stir in the bell pepper, onion, and cilantro.

3 Preheat the broiler. Broil the shrimp 6 inches from the heat for 3 minutes, or until cooked through; turn them once halfway through. Transfer the shrimp to the bowl with the orange mixture, and toss to coat. Refrigerate for at least 2 hours, or until well chilled.

4 Serve the chilled seviche topped with the avocado and pumpkin seeds.

Makes 4 servings. Per serving: 335 calories, 13g total fat (17% saturated), 33g protein, 23g carbohydrate, 3g fiber, 211mg cholesterol, 650mg sodium

salmon cakes with mustard-dill sauce

Light and crisp salmon cakes—light on the inside from mashed potatoes and crisp on the outside from a breadcrumb coating—are an excellent source of omega-3s, selenium, and vitamin B_{12}.

1	BAKING POTATO (8 OUNCES), THINLY SLICED
6	TEASPOONS DIJON MUSTARD
3	TABLESPOONS CHOPPED FRESH DILL
2	TABLESPOONS CIDER VINEGAR
1	TEASPOON LIGHT BROWN SUGAR
2	TABLESPOONS LIGHT MAYONNAISE
1	TEASPOON GRATED LEMON ZEST
2	TABLESPOONS FRESH LEMON JUICE
1	CAN (14¾ OUNCES) PINK SALMON, DRAINED
2	TABLESPOONS CHOPPED PARSLEY
2	TABLESPOONS PLAIN DRY BREADCRUMBS
1	TABLESPOON OLIVE OIL

1 In a small pot of boiling water, cook the potato for 7 minutes, or until tender. Drain, transfer to a large bowl, and mash with a potato masher. Set aside to cool to room temperature.

2 Meanwhile, in a small bowl, stir together 4 teaspoons of the mustard, the dill, vinegar, brown sugar, and 2 tablespoons of water. Set the mustard-dill sauce aside.

3 To the mashed potato, add the mayonnaise, the remaining 2 teaspoons mustard, the lemon zest, and lemon juice. Add the salmon and mix. Shape the mixture into 4 cakes.

4 In a shallow bowl or on a sheet of wax paper, stir together the parsley and breadcrumbs. Dredge the cakes in the parsley-crumb mixture, patting it on.

5 In a large nonstick skillet, heat the oil over medium heat. Add the salmon cakes and cook for 4 minutes per side, or until piping hot and crusty. Serve the salmon cakes with the mustard-dill sauce on top.

Makes 4 servings. Per serving: 271 calories, 12g total fat (21% saturated), 22g protein, 15g carbohydrate, 1.3g fiber, 60mg cholesterol, 852mg sodium

◀ **shrimp seviche with avocado & pumpkin seeds**

thai-style mussels

Pomegranate molasses, a sweet and tangy Middle Eastern condiment, is available in some specialty food stores. If you can't find pomegranate molasses, substitute 2 tablespoons of currant or cranberry jelly and increase the lime juice to 3 tablespoons.

- 3 TABLESPOONS FLAKED COCONUT
- ¾ CUP BOILING WATER
- 2 TEASPOONS OLIVE OIL
- 5 SCALLIONS, THINLY SLICED
- 3 CLOVES GARLIC, MINCED
- 2 TABLESPOONS MINCED FRESH GINGER
- ½ CUP CANNED CRUSHED TOMATOES
- 1 TABLESPOON REDUCED-SODIUM SOY SAUCE
- 2 TABLESPOONS POMEGRANATE MOLASSES
- ½ CUP CHOPPED CILANTRO
- ½ TEASPOON SALT
- 3 POUNDS MUSSELS, SCRUBBED AND DEBEARDED
- 2 TABLESPOONS FRESH LIME JUICE

1 In a small bowl, combine the coconut and boiling water. Let stand for 30 minutes, or until the coconut flakes are very soft and the water tastes of coconut. Strain the liquid into a bowl, pushing on the coconut to extract as much liquid as possible. Discard the coconut solids.

2 In a large pot, heat the oil over low heat. Add the scallions, garlic, and ginger, and cook for 3 minutes, or until the ginger is tender. Add the coconut water, tomatoes, soy sauce, pomegranate molasses, cilantro, and salt; bring to a boil.

3 Add the mussels; cover and boil for 5 minutes, or until the mussels have steamed open (discard any that do not open). To serve, lift the mussels into 4 large bowls. Stir the lime juice into the broth and spoon the broth over the mussels.

Makes 4 servings. *Per serving: 167 calories, 6.5g total fat (37% saturated), 13g protein, 14g carbohydrate, 1.2g fiber, 28mg cholesterol, 777mg sodium*

cod & vegetable stew

This simple fish stew, made with chunks of white, firm-fleshed cod, is rich in beta-carotene, B vitamins, selenium, potassium, and magnesium.

- 2 TABLESPOONS OLIVE OIL
- 2 MEDIUM ONIONS, FINELY CHOPPED
- 3 CLOVES GARLIC, THINLY SLICED
- 1 LARGE RED BELL PEPPER, CUT INTO MATCHSTICKS
- 1 POUND SWEET POTATOES, PEELED AND CUT INTO ½-INCH CHUNKS
- ¾ TEASPOON SALT
- ½ TEASPOON DRIED THYME
- 1½ CUPS FROZEN PEAS
- 1 CUP FROZEN CORN KERNELS
- 1½ POUNDS SKINLESS, BONELESS COD FILLET, CUT INTO BITE-SIZE PIECES

1 In a large skillet or Dutch oven, heat the oil over medium heat. Add the onions and garlic, and cook, stirring frequently for 5 minutes, or until the onion is light golden.

2 Add the bell pepper and sweet potatoes; cover and cook for 5 minutes, or until the sweet potatoes begin to soften. Stir in 1⅓ cups of water, the salt, and thyme; bring to a boil.

3 Reduce to a simmer; cover and cook for 5 minutes, or until the sweet potatoes are tender. Stir in the peas and corn.

4 Place the cod on top of the vegetables; cover and cook for 7 minutes, or until the fish is cooked through but still tender.

Makes 4 servings. *Per serving: 396 calories, 8.8g total fat (14% saturated), 37g protein, 43g carbohydrate, 6.8g fiber, 73mg cholesterol, 603mg sodium*

cod & vegetable stew ▶

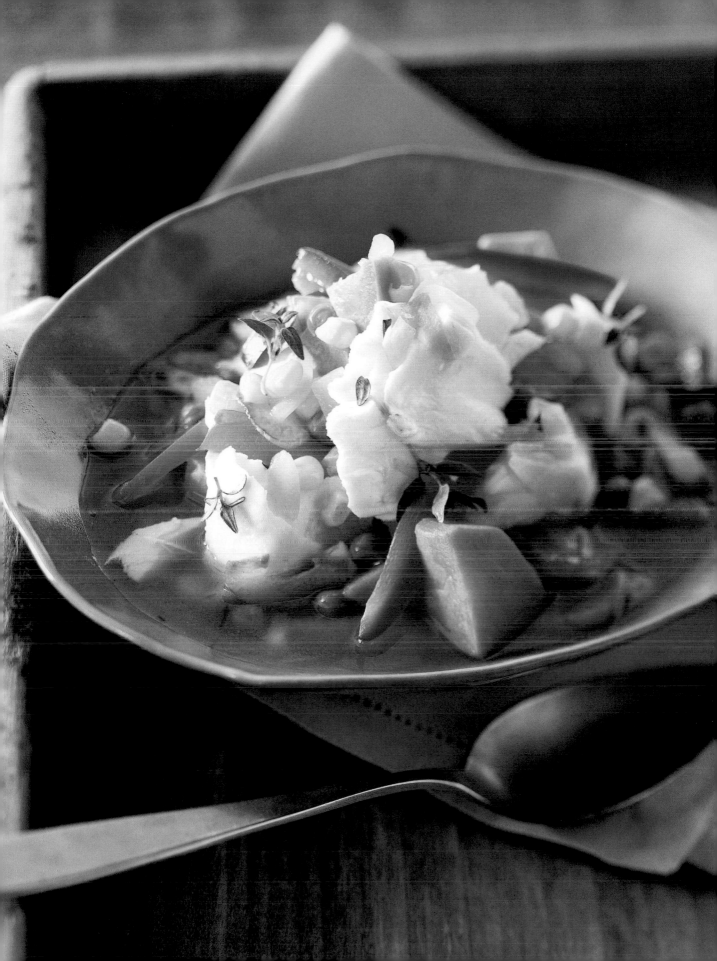

pasta with tuna-basil sauce

It's a common kitchen trick to use some of the pasta cooking water to help blend pasta sauce ingredients. For this sauce, the heat of the cooking water is also helpful in melting the Parmesan.

- 10 OUNCES PASTA SHELLS
- 1 TABLESPOON OLIVE OIL
- 1 LARGE RED ONION, FINELY CHOPPED
- 6 CLOVES GARLIC, MINCED
- 2 CUPS CANNED CRUSHED TOMATOES
- 2 TABLESPOONS TOMATO PASTE
- ½ TEASPOON CRUSHED RED PEPPER FLAKES
- ¼ TEASPOON SALT
- 4 CUPS SMALL BROCCOLI FLORETS
- 2 CANS (6½ OUNCES EACH) LIGHT TUNA PACKED IN OLIVE OIL, DRAINED
- 1 CUP CHOPPED FRESH BASIL
- ¼ CUP GRATED PARMESAN CHEESE

1 In a large pot of boiling water, cook the pasta according to package directions. Drain, reserving ½ cup of the pasta cooking water.

2 Meanwhile, in a large skillet, heat the oil over medium heat. Add the onion and garlic, and cook, stirring frequently for 7 minutes, or until the onion is tender.

3 Add the crushed tomatoes, tomato paste, red pepper flakes, and salt; bring to a boil. Reduce to a simmer; cover and cook for 5 minutes.

4 Stir in the broccoli; cook, uncovered, for 5 minutes, or until the broccoli is crisp-tender. Transfer the sauce to a large bowl. Add the tuna, basil, drained pasta, reserved liquid, and the Parmesan. Toss well to combine.

Makes 4 servings. Per serving: *565 calories, 14g total fat (15% saturated), 38g protein, 73g carbohydrate, 8.2g fiber, 37mg cholesterol, 975mg sodium*

crab cakes with melon relish

Crabmeat is sweet and delicate and doesn't require much fiddling with. Here it's combined with scallions, mustard, and stiffly beaten egg whites to make light crab cakes. The refreshing relish of cantaloupe, green pepper, and tomato provides a counterpoint to the richness of the cakes.

- ¼ CUP FRESH LIME JUICE
- 2 TABLESPOONS HONEY
- 1 TABLESPOON PLUS 2 TEASPOONS DIJON MUSTARD
- 2 CUPS CANTALOUPE CHUNKS (½-INCH)
- 1 GREEN BELL PEPPER, DICED
- 1 CUP CHERRY TOMATOES, QUARTERED
- 1 POUND LUMP CRABMEAT, PICKED OVER TO REMOVE ANY CARTILAGE
- 4 SCALLIONS, THINLY SLICED
- ½ TEASPOON SALT
- 2 EGG WHITES
- ½ CUP PLAIN DRY BREADCRUMBS
- 2 TABLESPOONS OLIVE OIL

1 In a medium bowl, whisk together the lime juice, honey, and 1 tablespoon of the mustard. Add the cantaloupe, bell pepper, and tomatoes; toss to combine. Refrigerate until ready to serve.

2 In a separate bowl, combine the crabmeat, scallions, remaining 2 teaspoons mustard, and the salt. Beat the egg whites until stiff peaks form and gently fold into the crabmeat mixture. Gently shape into 8 patties.

3 Dip the patties in the breadcrumbs. In a large non-stick skillet, heat 1 tablespoon of the oil over medium heat. Add 4 of the crab cakes to the pan, and cook for 2 to 3 minutes per side, or until hot and cooked through. Transfer the crab cakes to a plate. Repeat with the remaining 1 tablespoon oil and 4 crab cakes. Serve the crab cakes with the relish alongside.

Makes 4 servings. Per serving: *323 calories, 9.8g total fat (14% saturated), 28g protein, 30g carbohydrate, 2.2g fiber, 114mg cholesterol, 913mg sodium*

crab cakes with melon relish ▶

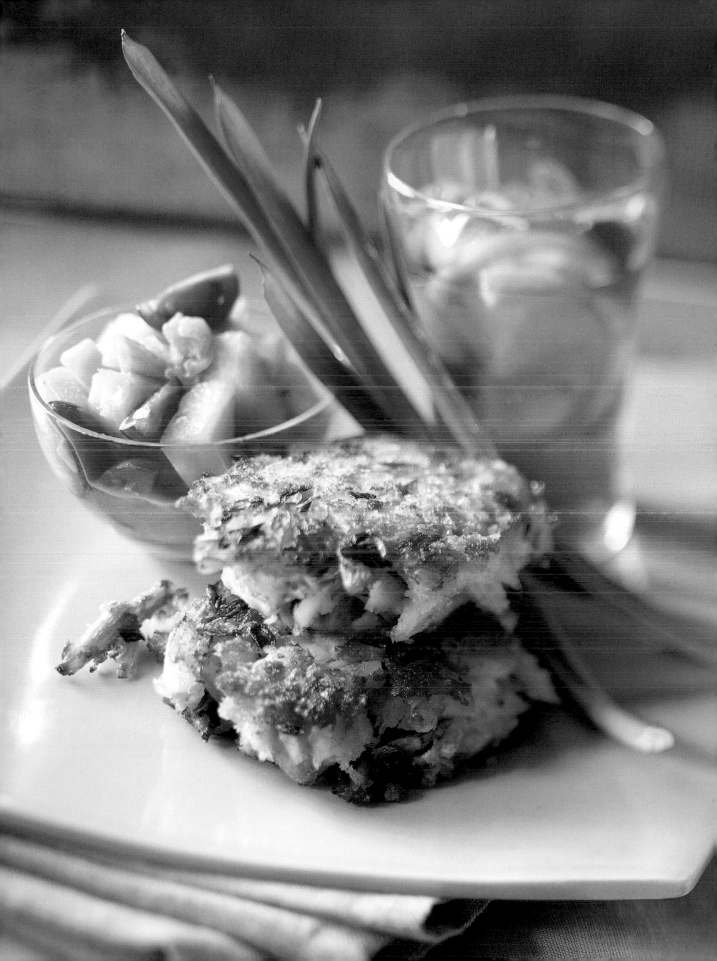

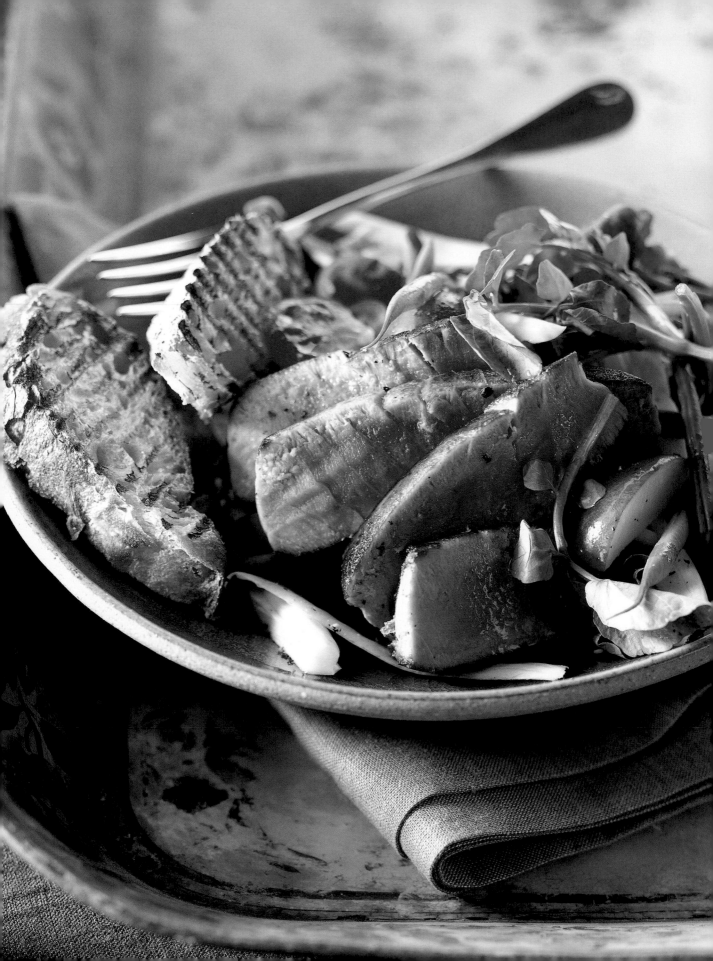

tossed tuna salad niçoise

Although the components for this classic French salad are usually arranged in separate piles on a plate, we've decided to toss the vegetables together in a lemon vinaigrette. Thick, fresh tuna steaks, brimming with omega-3s and vitamin B$_{12}$, are cooked to medium-rare, sliced, and placed on top of the tossed salad.

- 1 POUND SMALL RED-SKINNED POTATOES, CUT INTO EIGHTHS
- ⅓ CUP FRESH LEMON JUICE
- 2 TABLESPOONS OLIVE OIL
- 2 TABLESPOONS DIJON MUSTARD
- ½ TEASPOON SALT
- 12 OUNCES GREEN BEANS, CUT INTO 2-INCH LENGTHS
- 2 TUNA STEAKS (1 INCH THICK, 1½ POUNDS TOTAL)
- ½ TEASPOON PEPPER
- 1 PINT CHERRY TOMATOES, HALVED
- 1 BUNCH WATERCRESS, TOUGH STEMS TRIMMED
- 1 BELGIAN ENDIVE, CUT CROSSWISE INTO ½-INCH SLICES

1 In a large pot of boiling water, cook the potatoes for 10 minutes, or until tender. Drain.

2 Meanwhile, in a large bowl, whisk together the lemon juice, oil, mustard, and ¼ teaspoon of the salt. Add the potatoes while still warm, tossing to coat.

3 In a vegetable steamer, steam the green beans for 4 minutes, or until crisp-tender. Add to the bowl with the potatoes, and toss to combine.

4 Meanwhile, preheat the broiler. Place the tuna on a broiler pan and sprinkle with the remaining ¼ teaspoon salt and the pepper. Broil 6 inches from the heat for 3 minutes per side for medium-rare.

5 Add the tomatoes, watercress, and endive to the bowl, tossing well. To serve, slice the tuna and place on top of the salad mixture.

Makes 4 servings. Per serving: 427 calories, 15g total fat (20% saturated), 41g protein, 32g carbohydrate, 5.5g fiber, 58mg cholesterol, 566mg sodium

poached salmon with green sauce

The puree of spinach, parsley, cilantro, lemon juice, and olive oil may be made several hours ahead and refrigerated until serving time. The brief steaming of the spinach sets its color, giving the sauce a bright emerald hue.

- 2 CUPS PACKED FRESH SPINACH LEAVES (ABOUT 4 OUNCES)
- ½ CUP PACKED FLAT-LEAF PARSLEY LEAVES
- ½ CUP PACKED CILANTRO LEAVES AND TENDER STEMS
- 2 TABLESPOONS FRESH LEMON JUICE
- 1 PICKLED JALAPEÑO PEPPER
- 1 TABLESPOON OLIVE OIL
- ½ TEASPOON SALT
- ½ TEASPOON CELERY SEEDS
- 1 BAY LEAF
- 6 STRIPS (3 x ½ INCH EACH) LEMON ZEST
- 4 SALMON STEAKS (1 INCH THICK, 6 OUNCES EACH)

1 Steam the spinach over boiling water for 30 seconds, or until just wilted. Transfer the spinach to a food processor along with the parsley, cilantro, lemon juice, jalapeño, oil, and ¼ teaspoon of the salt; puree until thick and smooth.

2 In a large skillet, combine the celery seeds, bay leaf, lemon zest, and the remaining ¼ teaspoon salt. Add enough water to come halfway up the sides of the pan. Add the salmon; cover with wax paper and bring to a simmer over medium heat. Cook for 7 to 10 minutes, or until the salmon is just cooked through; turn the salmon over midway through the cooking. With a slotted spatula, remove the salmon from the skillet.

3 Serve the salmon warm, at room temperature, or chilled, with the green sauce spooned over it.

Makes 4 servings. Per serving: 321 calories, 20g total fat (19% saturated), 31g protein, 3g carbohydrate, 1.7g fiber, 88mg cholesterol, 463mg sodium

mackerel tandoori style

Mackerel, in addition to being rich in omega-3 fatty acids, has a rich flavor that stands up well to this traditional Indian spiced-yogurt marinade.

1 TEASPOON GROUND CUMIN

¼ CUP PLAIN LOW-FAT YOGURT

1 TABLESPOON FRESH LEMON JUICE

2 TEASPOONS MINCED FRESH GINGER

1 CLOVE GARLIC, PEELED

2 TEASPOONS PAPRIKA

½ TEASPOON SALT

¼ TEASPOON GROUND CARDAMOM

¼ TEASPOON CAYENNE PEPPER

4 MACKEREL FILLETS (ABOUT 6 OUNCES EACH), SKIN ON, EACH CUT CROSSWISE IN HALF

1 TABLESPOON PLUS 2 TEASPOONS OLIVE OIL

2 LARGE ONIONS, HALVED AND THINLY SLICED

1½ TEASPOONS SUGAR

1 LARGE RED BELL PEPPER, CUT INTO MATCHSTICKS

1 In a small skillet, toast the cumin over low heat for 2 minutes, or until fragrant. Transfer to a blender along with the yogurt, lemon juice, ginger, garlic, paprika, salt, cardamom, and cayenne; puree.

2 Place the mackerel pieces skin-side down in a shallow ovenproof pan and make several diagonal slashes in the mackerel flesh. Spread the yogurt mixture over the fish. Refrigerate for 2 hours or up to overnight.

3 About 30 minutes before serving time, remove the fish from the refrigerator. In a large skillet, heat 1 tablespoon of the oil over medium heat. Add the onions and sugar; cook, stirring frequently for 20 minutes, or until the onions are lightly browned. Add the bell pepper, and cook for 5 minutes, or until the pepper is crisp-tender; set aside.

4 Meanwhile, preheat the oven to 450°F. Sprinkle the mackerel with the remaining 2 teaspoons oil, and bake for 12 minutes, or until the mackerel is cooked through. Serve the mackerel topped with the caramelized onion mixture.

Makes 4 servings. Per serving: 414 calories, 26g total fat (21% saturated), 29g protein, 16g carbohydrate, 2.3g fiber, 100mg cholesterol, 432mg sodium

linguine with clams

The carrot juice adds a golden color and a substantial amount of beta-carotene to this pasta dish. A single serving provides more than 8mg of this phytonutrient, which is 102% of the daily recommended intake.

2 TEASPOONS OLIVE OIL

1 SMALL ONION, FINELY CHOPPED

3 CARROTS, QUARTERED LENGTHWISE AND THINLY SLICED CROSSWISE

4 CLOVES GARLIC, MINCED

1 CUP CARROT JUICE

2 DOZEN LITTLENECK CLAMS, WELL SCRUBBED

8 OUNCES LINGUINE

¼ TEASPOON SALT

¼ CUP CHOPPED PARSLEY

2 TEASPOONS UNSALTED BUTTER

1 In a large skillet, heat the oil over low heat. Add the onion, carrots, and garlic; cook, stirring frequently for 5 minutes, or until the onion is tender.

2 Add the carrot juice and bring to a boil. Add the clams; cover and cook for 5 minutes, or until the clams open (check after 3 minutes as some will open before others). Remove the clams as they open (discard any that do not open). Set the skillet with the carrot mixture aside. When the clams are cool enough to handle, remove the clam meat and discard the shells.

3 Meanwhile, in a large pot of boiling water, cook the linguine according to package directions. Drain.

4 Return the carrot mixture to a boil, and boil for 3 minutes. Stir in the salt. Transfer to a large bowl, add the drained pasta, clams, parsley, and butter; toss well.

Makes 4 servings. Per serving: 374 calories, 6.1g total fat (28% saturated), 20g protein, 59g carbohydrate, 3.8g fiber, 34mg cholesterol, 234mg sodium

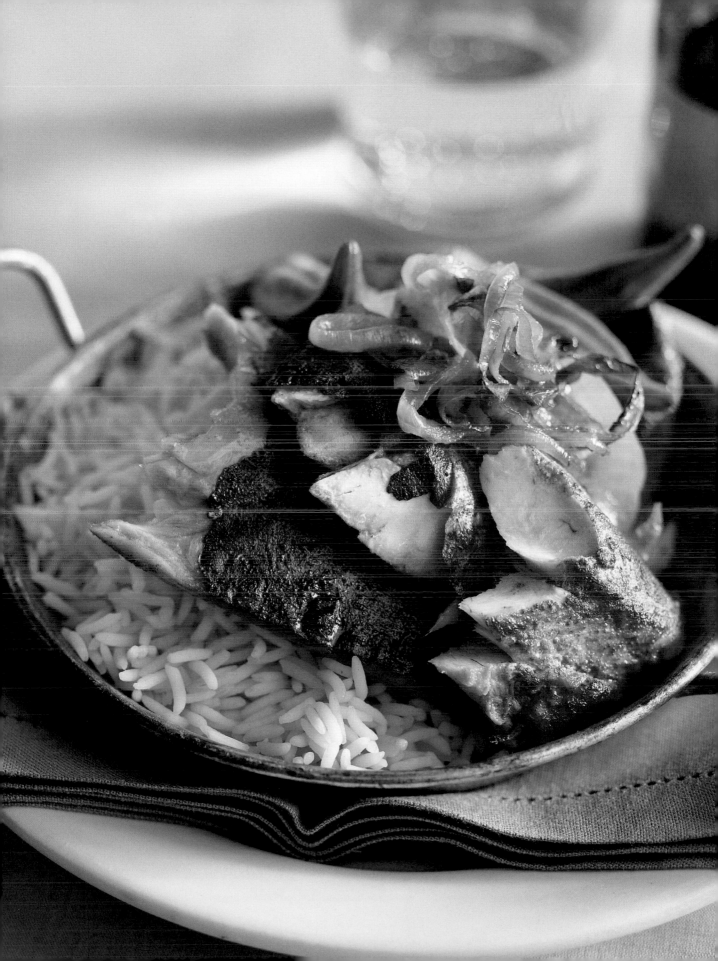

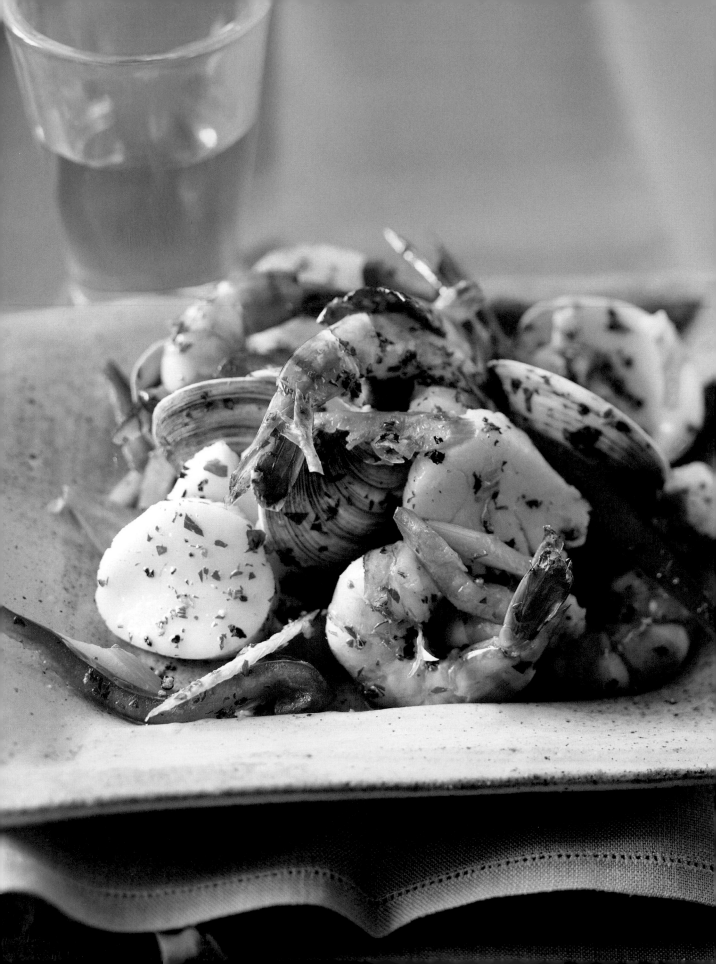

shellfish salad with herbed lemon dressing

Using some of the shellfish cooking liquid to make the salad dressing serves a dual purpose: The flavors are richer and some of the B vitamins that dissolved into the cooking liquid are retained.

- 1 CUP DRY WHITE WINE
- 1 TEASPOON DRIED TARRAGON
- ½ TEASPOON DRIED OREGANO
- 1 DOZEN LITTLENECK CLAMS, WELL SCRUBBED
- 12 OUNCES LARGE SHRIMP, SHELLED AND DEVEINED
- 8 OUNCES SEA SCALLOPS, HALVED HORIZONTALLY
- ¼ CUP FRESH LEMON JUICE
- 1 TABLESPOON OLIVE OIL
- 1½ TEASPOONS DIJON MUSTARD
- 2 CELERY STALKS, HALVED LENGTHWISE AND CUT CROSSWISE INTO ¼-INCH SLICES
- 2 RED BELL PEPPERS, DICED
- ⅓ CUP CHOPPED PARSLEY

1 In a large saucepan, combine the white wine, tarragon, and oregano; bring to a boil over high heat. Add the clams; cover and cook for 4 to 5 minutes, or until the clams open (check after 3 minutes as some will open before others). Remove the clams as they open (discard any that do not open); reserve the liquid in the pan. When the clams are cool enough to handle, remove the clam meat and place in a large bowl; discard the shells.

2 Heat the liquid in the pan over medium-low heat. Add the shrimp, and cook for 3 to 4 minutes, or until cooked through. With a slotted spoon, remove the shrimp, reserving the liquid in the pan. When the shrimp are cool enough to handle, halve them horizontally and add to the bowl with the clams.

3 Heat the liquid in the pan over medium-low heat. Add the scallops, and cook for 2 minutes, or until cooked through. With a slotted spoon, transfer the scallops to the bowl, reserving the liquid in the pan. Cool the shellfish cooking liquid to room temperature and measure out ½ cup.

4 In a medium bowl, whisk together the ½ cup reserved cooking liquid, the lemon juice, oil, and mustard. Pour the dressing over the shellfish. Add the celery, bell peppers, and parsley; toss to combine. Chill the salad until serving time.

Makes 4 servings. Per serving: 208 calories, 5.5g total fat (13% saturated), 30g protein, 9g carbohydrate, 1.2g fiber, 138mg cholesterol, 285mg sodium

sautéed scallops with fennel & tomatoes

To preserve as much of the vitamin C as possible, the orange juice is added at the end of the recipe and heated for only a brief time.

- 4 TEASPOONS OLIVE OIL
- 1 POUND SEA SCALLOPS, HALVED HORIZONTALLY
- 2 TABLESPOONS CORNSTARCH
- 1 BULB FENNEL, STALKS REMOVED, BULB HALVED LENGTHWISE AND THINLY SLICED CROSSWISE
- 1 MEDIUM ZUCCHINI (ABOUT 6 OUNCES), HALVED LENGTHWISE AND THINLY SLICED CROSSWISE
- 4 CLOVES GARLIC, SLIVERED
- 1 CUP CHERRY TOMATOES, HALVED
- 1 CAN (5½ OUNCES) TOMATO-VEGETABLE JUICE
- ½ TEASPOON SALT
- ½ TEASPOON DRIED TARRAGON
- ⅓ CUP FRESH ORANGE JUICE

1 In a large nonstick skillet, heat the oil over medium heat. Dredge the scallops in the cornstarch. Add the scallops to the skillet, and sauté for 1 minute per side, or until golden brown. With a slotted spoon, transfer the scallops to a plate.

2 Add the fennel, zucchini, and garlic to the pan; cook, stirring frequently for 5 minutes, or until the fennel is golden brown. Add the tomatoes, tomato-vegetable juice, salt, and tarragon; cook for 3 minutes, or until the tomatoes begin to collapse.

3 Return the scallops to the pan and add the orange juice; cook, stirring for 1 to 2 minutes, or until the scallops are heated through.

Makes 4 servings. Per serving: 207 calories, 5.7g total fat (13% saturated), 21g protein, 18g carbohydrate, 2.5g fiber, 38mg cholesterol, 637mg sodium

◀ **shellfish salad with herbed lemon dressing**

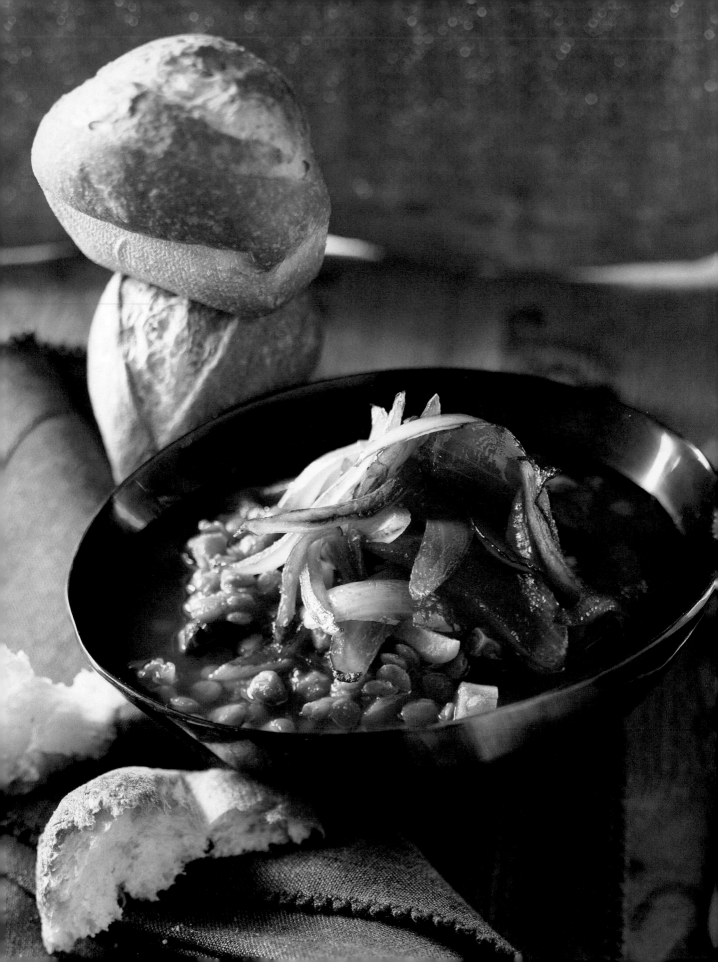

lentil-tomato stew with browned onions

This hearty vegetarian main course is rich in dietary fiber and also offers more than 300% of the daily recommended intake for beta-carotene. Nonvegans might want to serve the soup topped with some crumbled goat cheese or feta.

- 1 CUP DRIED SHIITAKE MUSHROOMS
- 1 CUP BOILING WATER
- 4 TEASPOONS OLIVE OIL
- 3 CARROTS, QUARTERED LENGTHWISE AND THINLY SLICED CROSSWISE
- 8 CLOVES GARLIC, THINLY SLICED
- ¾ CUP LENTILS, RINSED AND PICKED OVER
- 1 CUP CANNED CRUSHED TOMATOES
- ¾ TEASPOON SALT
- ¾ TEASPOON GROUND CUMIN
- ¾ TEASPOON GROUND GINGER
- ½ TEASPOON RUBBED SAGE
- 1 LARGE ONION, HALVED AND THINLY SLICED
- 2 TEASPOONS SUGAR
- 1 CUP FROZEN PEAS

1 In a small bowl, combine the shiitake mushrooms and boiling water. Let stand for 20 minutes, or until softened. With your fingers, remove the mushrooms from the soaking liquid, reserving the liquid. Trim any stems from the mushrooms and thinly slice the caps. Strain the reserved liquid through a fine-meshed sieve or coffee filter; set aside.

2 In a large saucepan, heat 3 teaspoons of the oil over medium heat. Add the carrots and garlic, and cook for 5 minutes, or until softened.

3 Stir in the lentils, tomatoes, salt, cumin, ginger, sage, mushrooms, and reserved liquid. Add 3 cups of water, and bring to a boil. Reduce to a simmer; cover and cook for 35 minutes, or until the lentils are tender.

4 Meanwhile, in a large skillet, heat the remaining 1 teaspoon oil over medium heat. Add the onion and sugar; cook, stirring frequently for 5 minutes, or until the onion is lightly browned.

5 Add the peas to the stew, and cook for 2 minutes to heat through. Serve the stew topped with the browned onions.

Makes 4 servings. Per serving: 290 calories, 5.5g total fat (13% saturated), 15g protein, 49g carbohydrate, 10g fiber, 0mg cholesterol, 601mg sodium

brown rice & chickpea pilaf

Although intended as a main course, this fiber- and folate-rich pilaf could just as easily serve 6 to 8 people as a side dish.

- 1 TABLESPOON OLIVE OIL
- 1 LARGE RED ONION, FINELY CHOPPED
- 5 CLOVES GARLIC, THINLY SLICED
- 12 OUNCES GREEN CABBAGE, CUT INTO 1-INCH CHUNKS (ABOUT 6 CUPS)
- ¾ CUP BROWN RICE
- ¾ TEASPOON SALT
- 1 CAN (19 OUNCES) CHICKPEAS, DRAINED AND RINSED
- 1 CUP CANNED TOMATOES, CHOPPED WITH THEIR JUICE
- ¾ CUP RAISINS

1 In a large saucepan, heat the oil over medium heat. Add the onion and garlic; cook, stirring frequently for 7 minutes, or until the onion is tender.

2 Stir in the cabbage; cover and cook for 5 minutes, or until the cabbage begins to wilt.

3 Stir in the brown rice, 2 cups of water, and the salt; bring to a boil. Reduce to a simmer; cover and cook for 25 minutes, or until the rice is almost done.

4 Stir in the chickpeas, tomatoes, and raisins; bring to a boil. Reduce to a simmer; cover and cook for 10 minutes, or until the rice is tender.

Makes 4 servings. Per serving: 392 calories, 7g total fat (12% saturated), 11g protein, 75g carbohydrate, 9.8g fiber, 0mg cholesterol, 710mg sodium

◄ **lentil-tomato stew with browned onions**

bulgur salad with tangerine-pomegranate dressing

Pomegranate molasses—a sweet-sour pomegranate concentrate—is available in Middle Eastern and some specialty food stores. If you can't find pomegranate molasses, substitute a mixture of currant jelly (2 tablespoons) and fresh lemon or lime juice (1 tablespoon).

- 1   CUP MEDIUM-GRAIN BULGUR
- 2½ CUPS BOILING WATER
- 1   TEASPOON GRATED TANGERINE OR ORANGE ZEST
- 1   CUP FRESH TANGERINE OR ORANGE JUICE
- 2   TABLESPOONS TOMATO PASTE
- 2   TABLESPOONS POMEGRANATE MOLASSES
- 2   TABLESPOONS OLIVE OIL
- ¾   TEASPOON SALT
- 1½ CUPS CORN KERNELS
- ⅔   CUP DRIED CHERRIES (3 OUNCES)
- ⅔   CUP THINLY SLICED SCALLIONS
- ⅓   CUP ROASTED PEANUTS, COARSELY CHOPPED

1 In a large bowl, combine the bulgur and the boiling water. Let stand for 30 minutes at room temperature. Drain well.

2 While the bulgur soaks, in a large bowl, whisk together the tangerine zest, tangerine juice, tomato paste, pomegranate molasses, oil, and salt.

3 Add the drained bulgur to the dressing, and fluff with a fork. Add the corn, cherries, scallions, and peanuts, tossing to combine. Serve at room temperature or chilled.

Makes 4 servings. Per serving: 414 calories, 14g total fat (14% saturated), 10g protein, 69g carbohydrate, 10g fiber, 0mg cholesterol, 520mg sodium

three-bean salad with manchego cheese

Chipotle peppers, which are smoked jalapeños, are sold in cans, packed in adobo sauce (a spicy, chili- and vinegar-based sauce). Although the chipotles add depth of flavor and heat to the dish, you could make this dressing with 1 teaspoon of regular chili powder instead.

- ¼   CUP RED WINE VINEGAR
- 2   TABLESPOONS OLIVE OIL
- 1   TABLESPOON HONEY
- 1   CHIPOTLE PEPPER IN ADOBO, FINELY CHOPPED (2 TEASPOONS)
- ¼   TEASPOON SALT
- 12 OUNCES GREEN BEANS, HALVED
- 1   CUP FROZEN CORN KERNELS
- 1   CAN (15 OUNCES) BLACK BEANS, DRAINED AND RINSED
- 1   CAN (15 OUNCES) RED KIDNEY BEANS, DRAINED AND RINSED
- 1   CELERY STALK, DICED
- ⅓   CUP FINELY CHOPPED RED ONION
- 4   OUNCES MANCHEGO OR MONTEREY JACK CHEESE, CUT INTO ¼-INCH-WIDE MATCHSTICKS

1 In a large bowl, whisk together the vinegar, oil, honey, chipotle, and salt.

2 Meanwhile, in a large vegetable steamer, steam the green beans for 5 minutes, or until crisp-tender. Add the corn during the final minute of steaming. Transfer the hot vegetables to the bowl with the dressing, and toss to coat.

3 Add the black beans, kidney beans, celery, onion, and cheese; toss to combine. Serve at room temperature or chilled.

Makes 4 servings. Per serving: 404 calories, 18g total fat (44% saturated), 20g protein, 43g carbohydrate, 10g fiber, 30mg cholesterol, 655mg sodium

three-bean salad with manchego cheese ▶

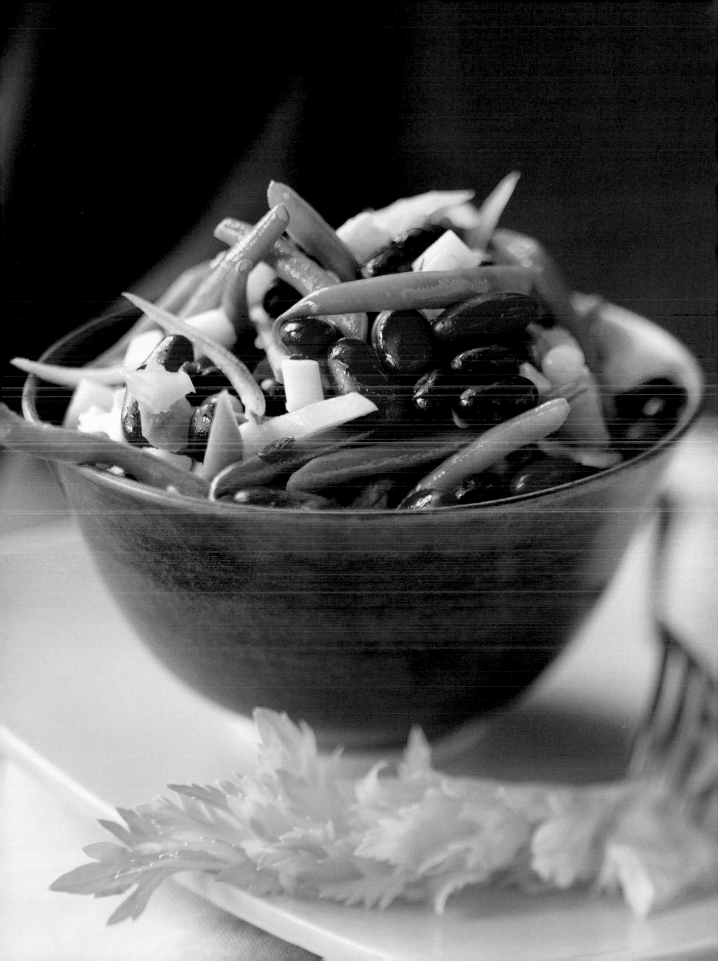

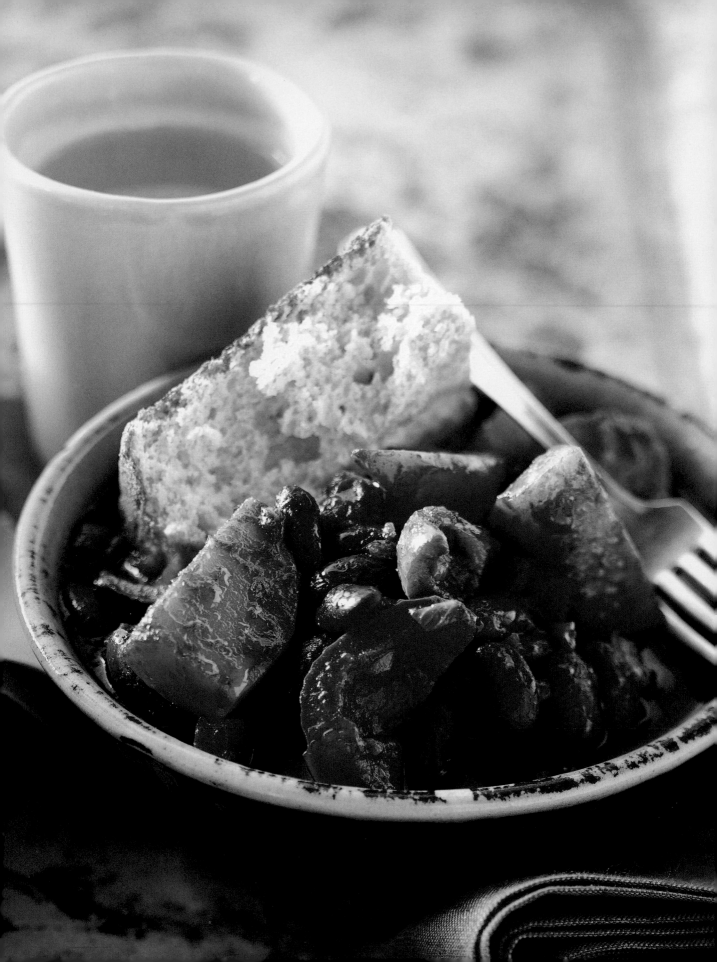

vegetarian chili

If you don't have the time to soak and cook dried beans, substitute 2½ cups of rinsed and drained canned beans. If you can't find chipotle peppers in adobo sauce (they're sold in cans and can be found in the international section of many supermarkets), substitute 1 teaspoon of hot chili powder.

1   CUP DRIED RED KIDNEY BEANS

1   TABLESPOON OLIVE OIL

1   LARGE ONION, FINELY CHOPPED

3   CLOVES GARLIC, MINCED

1   LARGE RED BELL PEPPER, CUT INTO
    ½-INCH CHUNKS

1   LARGE GREEN BELL PEPPER, CUT INTO
    ½-INCH CHUNKS

2   CUPS CHUNKS (1-INCH) BUTTERNUT SQUASH

2   TABLESPOONS UNSWEETENED COCOA POWDER

1   TABLESPOON LIGHT BROWN SUGAR

1   TEASPOON DRIED MARJORAM

½   TEASPOON SALT

1½ CUPS CANNED CRUSHED TOMATOES

1   CHIPOTLE PEPPER IN ADOBO, MINCED
    (2 TEASPOONS)

1 In a large saucepan, combine the kidney beans with water to cover by 3 inches; bring to a boil. Reduce to a simmer; cover and cook for 2¼ to 2½ hours, or until the beans are tender. Drain, reserving 1 cup of the liquid.

2 In a Dutch oven or flameproof casserole, heat the oil over medium heat. Add the onion and garlic, and cook for 7 minutes, or until tender. Stir in the bell peppers and butternut squash, and cook for 4 minutes, or until the peppers are crisp-tender. Add the cocoa powder, brown sugar, marjoram, and salt, stirring to coat.

3 Stir in the drained beans, the reserved liquid, the tomatoes, and chipotle pepper; bring to a boil. Reduce to a simmer; cover and cook for 30 minutes to blend the flavors.

Makes 4 servings. *Per serving: 293 calories, 4.7g total fat (16% saturated), 14g protein, 54g carbohydrate, 9.4g fiber, 0mg cholesterol, 477mg sodium*

pasta with cabbage, apples & leeks

For a calcium boost, add a cup of plain low-fat yogurt to the cabbage mixture before tossing it with the pasta.

2   TABLESPOONS OLIVE OIL

2   LEEKS, HALVED LENGTHWISE, THINLY SLICED
    CROSSWISE, AND WELL WASHED

3   CUPS PACKED SHREDDED GREEN CABBAGE (ABOUT
    12 OUNCES)

3   CLOVES GARLIC, MINCED

2   LARGE RED APPLES (UNPEELED), CUT INTO
    ½-INCH CHUNKS

½   TEASPOON SALT

½   TEASPOON PEPPER

2   TABLESPOONS CIDER VINEGAR

1   TABLESPOON DIJON MUSTARD

8   OUNCES FARFALLE (BOW-TIE) PASTA

1 In a large skillet, heat the oil over medium heat. Add the leeks, and cook, stirring frequently for 5 minutes, or until tender. Add the cabbage and garlic, and increase the heat to high; cook, stirring frequently for 5 minutes, or until the cabbage is golden brown.

2 Add the apples, salt, and pepper; cook for 2 minutes, or until the apple is crisp-tender. Stir in the vinegar and mustard, and cook for 30 seconds to blend the flavors.

3 In a large pot of boiling water, cook the pasta according to package directions. Drain, reserving ½ cup of the pasta cooking water. Transfer the drained pasta to a large bowl. Add the cabbage-apple mixture and the reserved pasta cooking water; toss to combine.

Makes 4 servings. *Per serving: 385 calories, 8.3g total fat (14% saturated), 9g protein, 70g carbohydrate, 6.1g fiber, 0mg cholesterol, 411mg sodium*

artichokes with lentils & lima beans

A wonderful combination of textures and flavors, this vegetarian dish is also a nutritional powerhouse: One serving provides more than 50% of the recommended daily intake of fiber and potassium, and more than 500% of beta-carotene.

4 LARGE ARTICHOKES

3 TABLESPOONS FRESH LEMON JUICE

1 TABLESPOON OLIVE OIL

1 SMALL ONION, FINELY CHOPPED

3 CLOVES GARLIC, MINCED

1 LARGE CARROT, DICED

¾ CUP LENTILS, PICKED OVER AND RINSED

1½ CUPS CARROT JUICE

¾ TEASPOON SALT

½ TEASPOON DRIED THYME

1 PACKAGE (10 OUNCES) FROZEN LIMA BEANS

3 OUNCES FETA CHEESE

1 To trim the artichokes: Remove the tough outer leaves. Trim the tough end of the stem; then, with a paring knife, peel the tough skin off the remaining stem. Cut off the top of the artichoke to just about 1 inch above the base. Halve the artichokes lengthwise, then scoop out and discard the chokes. Halve the artichokes again. Place the cleaned artichokes in a bowl with cold water to cover. Add 1 tablespoon of the lemon juice; set aside.

2 In a Dutch oven, heat the oil over medium heat. Add the onion and garlic; cook, stirring frequently for 5 minutes, or until the onion is golden brown. Stir in the carrot, and cook for 4 minutes.

3 Remove the artichokes from the water and place them in the Dutch oven. Stir in the lentils, the remaining 2 tablespoons lemon juice, the carrot juice, salt, thyme, and 1 cup of water; bring to a boil. Reduce to a simmer; cover and cook for 25 minutes.

4 Stir in the lima beans, and cook for 10 minutes, or until the artichokes, lima beans, and lentils are tender. Serve topped with crumbled feta cheese.

Makes 4 servings. Per serving: 423 calories, 8.9g total fat (43% saturated), 25g protein, 68g carbohydrate, 18g fiber, 19mg cholesterol, 907mg sodium

broiled marinated tofu

These marinated tofu "steaks" can be served hot, cold, or at room temperature. Serve 4 tofu triangles as a main course (perhaps on a bed of shredded spinach), or serve 2 to 3 as a first course or as part of a buffet. If you can find pressed tofu, skip step 1.

2 BLOCKS (19 OUNCES EACH) FIRM TOFU

¼ CUP REDUCED-SODIUM SOY SAUCE

2 TABLESPOONS FRESH LEMON JUICE

4 TEASPOONS DARK BROWN SUGAR

2 TEASPOONS DARK SESAME OIL

4 TEASPOONS SESAME SEEDS

4 SCALLIONS, THINLY SLICED

1 Slice each block of tofu in half horizontally. Lay the 4 pieces of tofu on a cutting board and place a can or small bowl under one end of the board to tilt it slightly. Set the board so that the low end hangs over the sink. Cover the tofu with paper towels, place another cutting board on top and weight it with a heavy pan or a couple of cans. Let drain for 2 hours.

2 In a shallow container (like a gratin dish or lasagna pan) large enough to hold the tofu in a single layer, whisk together the soy sauce, lemon juice, brown sugar, and sesame oil. Place the pressed tofu in the pan and let stand for 3 hours, or until the marinade has been absorbed about halfway up the tofu (there should still be some marinade in the container).

3 Preheat the broiler. Remove the tofu from the marinade, reserving any leftover. Place the tofu on a broiler pan, and broil 6 inches from the heat for 5 minutes per side, or until richly browned.

4 Meanwhile, in a small skillet, toast the sesame seeds over low heat for 3 minutes, or until golden.

5 To serve, cut each piece of tofu into 4 triangles and sprinkle with the scallions, sesame seeds, and any leftover marinade.

Makes 4 servings. Per serving: 461 calories, 27g total fat (14% saturated), 44g protein, 20g carbohydrate, 0.7g fiber, 0mg cholesterol, 642mg sodium

broiled marinated tofu ▶

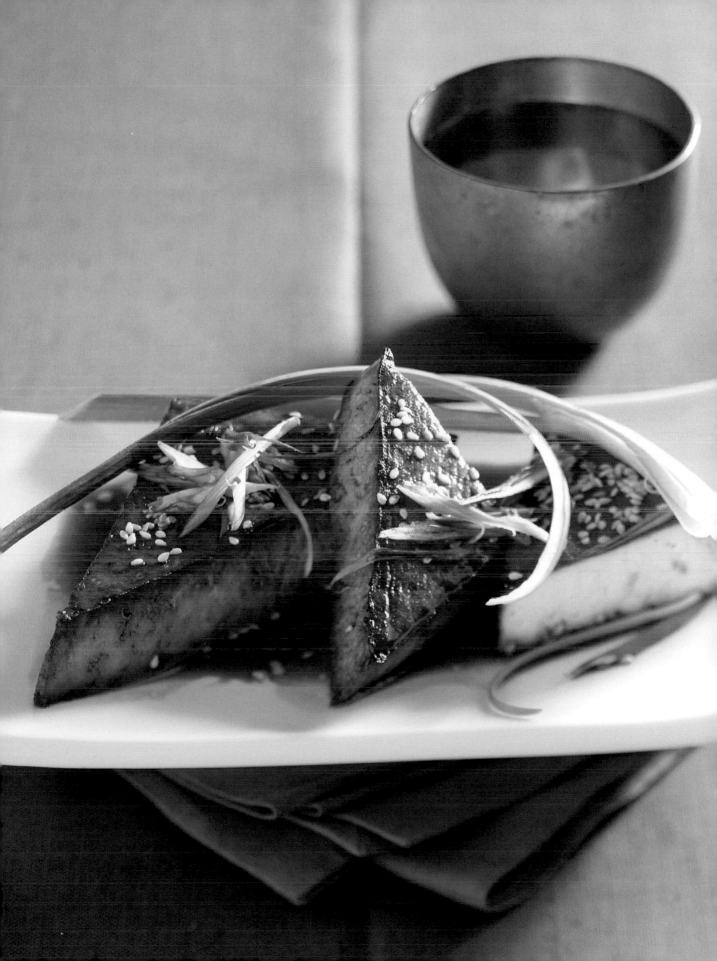

southwestern pizza

The secret ingredient in this pizza crust is carrot juice. It imparts a lovely golden color to the dough and also contributes a fair measure of beta-carotene.

- 1 PACKAGE (¼ OUNCE) ACTIVE DRY YEAST
- ¼ CUP WARM (105°F TO 115°F) WATER
- 3½ CUPS FLOUR
- ½ CUP YELLOW CORNMEAL
- 2 TABLESPOONS CHILI POWDER
- 1 TABLESPOON GROUND CUMIN
- 2 TEASPOONS SALT
- 1 CUP CARROT JUICE
- 3 TABLESPOONS OLIVE OIL
- 1 LARGE RED BELL PEPPER, THINLY SLICED
- 1 LARGE GREEN BELL PEPPER, THINLY SLICED
- 1 LARGE ONION, HALVED AND THINLY SLICED
- 1 CUP CORN KERNELS
- 2 TEASPOONS DRIED OREGANO
- 8 OUNCES MONTEREY JACK CHEESE, SHREDDED

1 In a measuring cup, sprinkle the yeast over the warm water. Let stand for 5 minutes to dissolve.

2 In a large bowl, combine the flour, cornmeal, chili powder, cumin, and salt. Stir in the yeast mixture, carrot juice, and 2 tablespoons of the oil. Transfer to a lightly floured surface, and knead for 7 to 10 minutes, or until the dough is smooth and elastic.

3 Transfer the dough to a large oiled bowl, cover with a dampened cloth, and let stand for 1½ hours in a warm draft-free spot, or until doubled in volume. Punch the dough down and divide in half. Cover and let rest for 15 minutes.

4 In a medium bowl, toss the peppers, onion, corn, and oregano with the remaining 1 tablespoon oil.

5 Roll each portion of dough to a 10-inch round, and place each on an ungreased baking sheet. Top each with cheese and the vegetable mixture; let stand for 20 minutes. Meanwhile, preheat the oven to 450°F.

6 Bake for 20 to 25 minutes, reversing the top and bottom pizzas midway, until the crust is crisp.

Makes 8 servings. Per serving: 440 calories, 15g total fat (38% saturated), 16g protein, 61g carbohydrate, 4.3g fiber, 30mg cholesterol, 770mg sodium

asparagus & potato frittata

A frittata (an Italian omelet) is usually made with whole eggs, but this lightened version is made with fewer egg yolks and more whites to reduce fat and cholesterol.

- 3 TEASPOONS OLIVE OIL
- 8 OUNCES RED-SKINNED POTATOES, CUT INTO ¼-INCH DICE
- 1 POUND ASPARAGUS, CUT INTO 1-INCH LENGTHS
- ¾ TEASPOON SALT
- ½ TEASPOON DRIED TARRAGON
- ½ TEASPOON DRIED MARJORAM
- 3 LARGE EGGS
- 4 LARGE EGG WHITES
- 3 TABLESPOONS GRATED PARMESAN CHEESE

1 In a large nonstick skillet, heat 2 teaspoons of the oil over medium heat. Add the potatoes, and cook, tossing occasionally for 7 minutes.

2 Add the asparagus, salt, tarragon, and marjoram; stir to combine. Cover and cook, stirring occasionally for 7 minutes, or until the asparagus and potatoes are tender.

3 Meanwhile, in a large bowl, whisk together the whole eggs, egg whites, and Parmesan. Reduce the heat under the skillet to low. Spoon the remaining 1 teaspoon oil around the inside edge of the pan. Add the egg mixture; cover and cook for 20 minutes, or until the eggs are set.

4 With a spatula, release the frittata from the pan and slide it onto a serving platter. Cut into wedges and serve hot, at room temperature, or chilled.

Makes 4 servings. Per serving: 191 calories, 8.6g total fat (28% saturated), 14g protein, 15g carbohydrate, 2g fiber, 162mg cholesterol, 615mg sodium

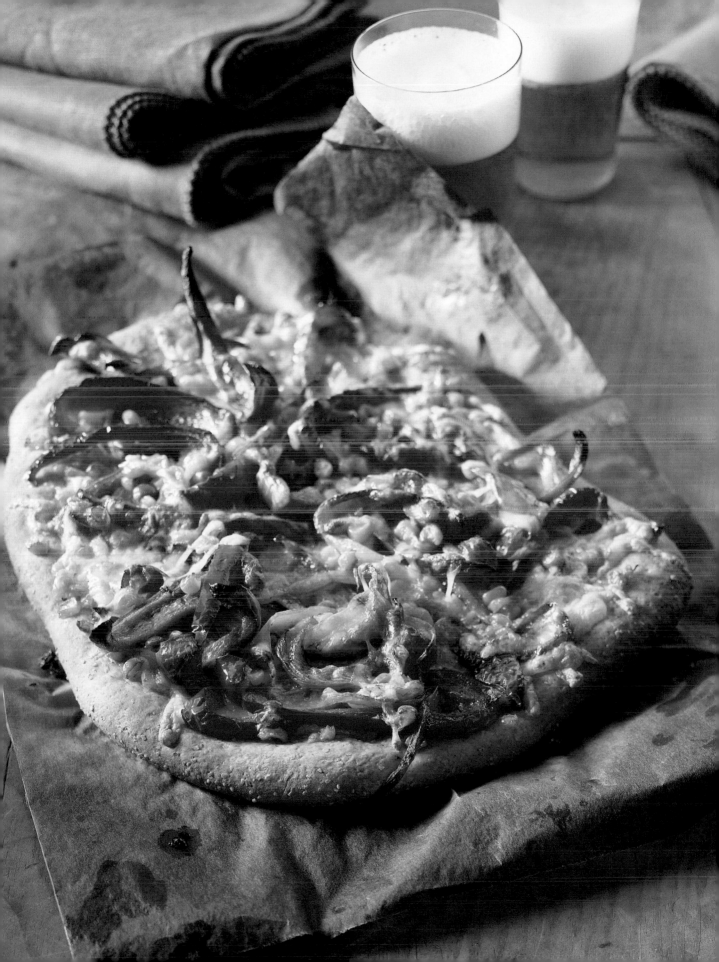

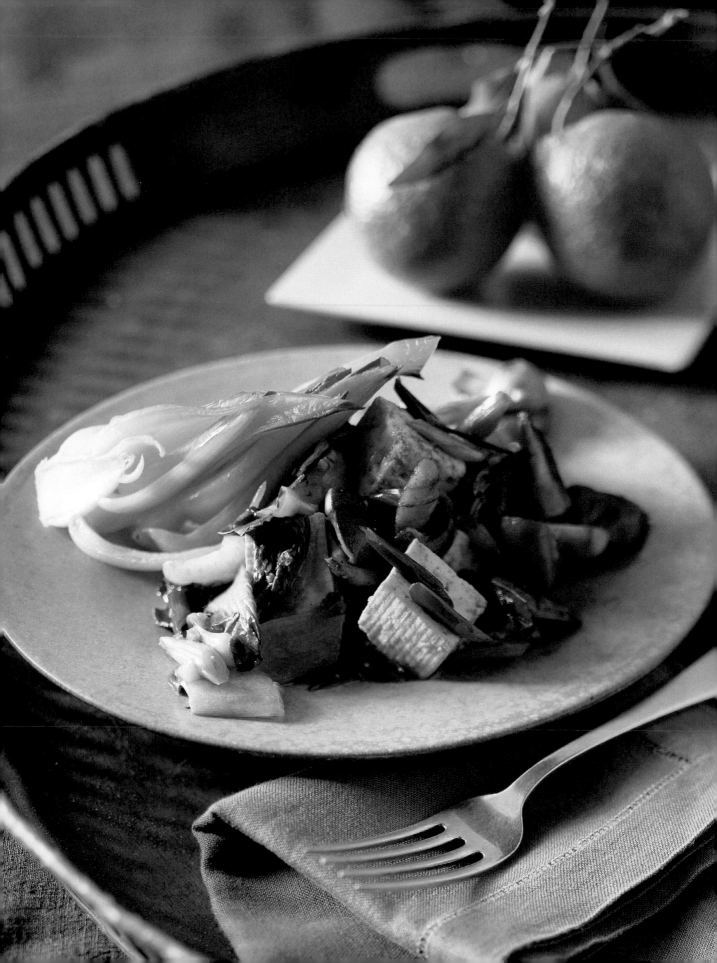

bok choy, tofu & mushroom stir-fry

In addition to the phytoestrogens from the tofu, this stir-fry is also rich in calcium, selenium, beta-carotene, and vitamin C.

- 1 PACKAGE (15 OUNCES) EXTRA-FIRM TOFU
- 3 TABLESPOONS REDUCED-SODIUM SOY SAUCE
- 4 TEASPOONS DARK BROWN SUGAR
- 1½ TEASPOONS CORNSTARCH
- 4 TEASPOONS OLIVE OIL
- 4 SCALLIONS, THINLY SLICED
- 2 TABLESPOONS MINCED FRESH GINGER
- 3 CLOVES GARLIC, MINCED
- 8 OUNCES FRESH SHIITAKE MUSHROOMS, STEMS REMOVED AND CAPS QUARTERED
- 8 OUNCES BUTTON MUSHROOMS, HALVED
- ¼ TEASPOON SALT
- 1 LARGE HEAD BOK CHOY, SLICED CROSSWISE INTO 1-INCH-WIDE STRIPS

1 Halve the block of tofu horizontally, then cut each piece into 12 squares or triangles; set aside. In a small bowl, stir together the soy sauce, brown sugar, cornstarch, and ½ cup of water; set the soy sauce mixture aside.

2 In a large nonstick skillet, heat 2 teaspoons of the oil over medium heat. Add the scallions, ginger, and garlic, and cook for 1 minute, or until tender.

3 Stir in the shiitakes and button mushrooms. Add ½ cup of water and the salt; cover and cook, stirring occasionally for 5 minutes, or until the mushrooms are tender. Transfer to a bowl.

4 Add the remaining 2 teaspoons oil and the bok choy to the pan; cook, stirring frequently for 5 minutes, or until the bok choy is tender.

5 Return the mushroom-scallion mixture to the pan and add the tofu. Stir the soy sauce mixture to recombine, and add it to the pan. Cook for 2 minutes, or until the tofu is heated through and the vegetables are coated with the sauce.

Makes 4 servings. Per serving: 240 calories, 11g total fat (11% saturated), 20g protein, 20g carbohydrate, 4g fiber, 0mg cholesterol, 760mg sodium

corn, cheese & tortilla strata

A strata—a layered casserole with an exotic Italian name but humble American roots—is most commonly made with bread. We've given it a twist by using corn tortillas instead. Corn tortillas have no fat and considerably less sodium than bread.

- 1 TABLESPOON OLIVE OIL
- 3 CLOVES GARLIC, MINCED
- 8 OUNCES FRESH SHIITAKE MUSHROOMS, STEMS REMOVED AND CAPS THINLY SLICED
- 1 PACKAGE (10 OUNCES) FROZEN CHOPPED COLLARD GREENS, THAWED AND SQUEEZED DRY
- 3 CUPS LOW-FAT (1%) MILK
- ¾ TEASPOON SALT
- ¼ TEASPOON CAYENNE PEPPER
- 3 TABLESPOONS FLOUR
- 1½ CUPS FROZEN CORN KERNELS
- 4 OUNCES MANCHEGO CHEESE, SHREDDED
- 5 CORN TORTILLAS (6-INCH DIAMETER), HALVED

1 Preheat the oven to 375°F. In a large saucepan, heat the oil over medium heat. Add the garlic, and cook for 10 seconds. Stir in the mushrooms, and cook, stirring frequently for 3 minutes, or until firm-tender. Stir in the collards, and cook, stirring for 5 minutes, or until the collards are tender.

2 In a small bowl, whisk the milk, salt, and cayenne into the flour until smooth.

3 Whisk the milk mixture into the collards, cook, stirring frequently for 3 to 5 minutes, or until the sauce is creamy and lightly thickened. Stir in the corn. Remove from the heat, and stir in the cheese until melted.

4 Arrange 5 tortilla halves over the bottom of a 9-inch-square glass baking dish. Top with half of the collard mixture. Place the remaining tortillas on top and spoon the remaining collard mixture over the tortillas. Bake for 25 minutes, or until the strata is bubbling hot.

Makes 4 servings. Per serving: 410 calories, 17g total fat (52% saturated), 5.1g fiber, 20g protein, 48g carbohydrate, 37mg cholesterol, 784mg sodium

◀ **bok choy, tofu & mushroom stir-fry**

vegetarian stuffed peppers with goat cheese

The bean mixture used to stuff these peppers has seasonings (cocoa, cinnamon, oregano, and raisins) that are reminiscent of a Latin American meat dish called picadillo.

1   LARGE RED BELL PEPPER, HALVED LENGTHWISE AND SEEDED

1   LARGE GREEN BELL PEPPER, HALVED LENGTHWISE AND SEEDED

1   TABLESPOON OLIVE OIL

1   LARGE RED ONION, FINELY CHOPPED

5   CLOVES GARLIC, MINCED

1   CAN (**19** OUNCES) CANNELLINI BEANS, DRAINED AND RINSED

2   TABLESPOONS TOMATO PASTE

2   TEASPOONS SESAME SEEDS

1½   TEASPOONS UNSWEETENED COCOA POWDER

½   TEASPOON DRIED OREGANO

½   TEASPOON CINNAMON

½   TEASPOON SALT

1½   CUPS CANNED CRUSHED TOMATOES

⅓   CUP RAISINS

3   OUNCES SOFT GOAT CHEESE, CRUMBLED

1 In a vegetable steamer, cook the pepper halves, cut-side down, for 10 minutes, or until crisp-tender.

2 Meanwhile, in a medium nonstick skillet, heat the oil over low heat. Add the onion and garlic, and cook for 5 minutes, or until the onion is golden brown. Measure out ¼ cup of the onion mixture and transfer it to a bowl. Add the beans and tomato paste to the bowl, and mash with a potato masher or a spoon.

3 To the onion mixture remaining in the skillet, add the sesame seeds, cocoa powder, oregano, cinnamon, and salt; cook for 1 minute. Stir in the crushed tomatoes and raisins; bring to a boil. Reduce to a simmer; cover and cook for 5 minutes to blend the flavors. Transfer to a food processor or blender and puree.

4 Return the puree to the skillet and stir in ⅓ cup of water. Add the steamed peppers, cut-side up. Spoon the bean mixture into the peppers; cover and cook for 5 minutes, or until the bean mixture is heated through. Spoon a little of the sauce over the beans and sprinkle with cheese; cover and cook for 2 minutes to melt the cheese.

5 To serve, spoon some of the sauce onto each plate, top with a pepper half and a little more sauce.

Makes 4 servings. Per serving: 295 calories, 10g total fat (38% saturated), 14g protein, 41g carbohydrate, 9.2g fiber, 10mg cholesterol, 752mg sodium

corn pasta with roasted asparagus

Corn pasta is a delicious gluten-free alternative to wheat-based pastas.

¼   CUP WALNUTS

1½   POUNDS ASPARAGUS, CUT INTO **1**-INCH LENGTHS

1½   CUPS FROZEN CORN KERNELS

1   TABLESPOON OLIVE OIL

8   OUNCES CORN PASTA

¼   CUP GRATED PARMESAN CHEESE

2   OUNCES SOFT GOAT CHEESE, CRUMBLED

2   TABLESPOONS CHOPPED PARSLEY

½   TEASPOON SALT

¼   TEASPOON PEPPER

1 Preheat the oven to 350°F. Toast the walnuts for 7 minutes, or until crisp and fragrant. Increase the oven temperature to 450°F. When the walnuts are cool enough to handle, coarsely chop.

2 In a 9 x 13-inch baking dish, toss the asparagus with the corn and oil. Bake for 10 minutes, or until the asparagus is tender and lightly browned.

3 Meanwhile, in a large pot of boiling water, cook the pasta according to package directions. Drain, reserving ¾ cup of the cooking liquid. Transfer the pasta to a large bowl.

4 To the pasta in the bowl, add the asparagus and corn, the reserved cooking liquid, Parmesan, goat cheese, parsley, salt, and pepper; toss well to combine. Serve the pasta sprinkled with the walnuts.

Makes 4 servings. Per serving: 438 calories, 15g total fat (33% saturated), 17g protein, 66g carbohydrate, 9.6g fiber, 15mg cholesterol, 464mg sodium

corn pasta with roasted asparagus ▶

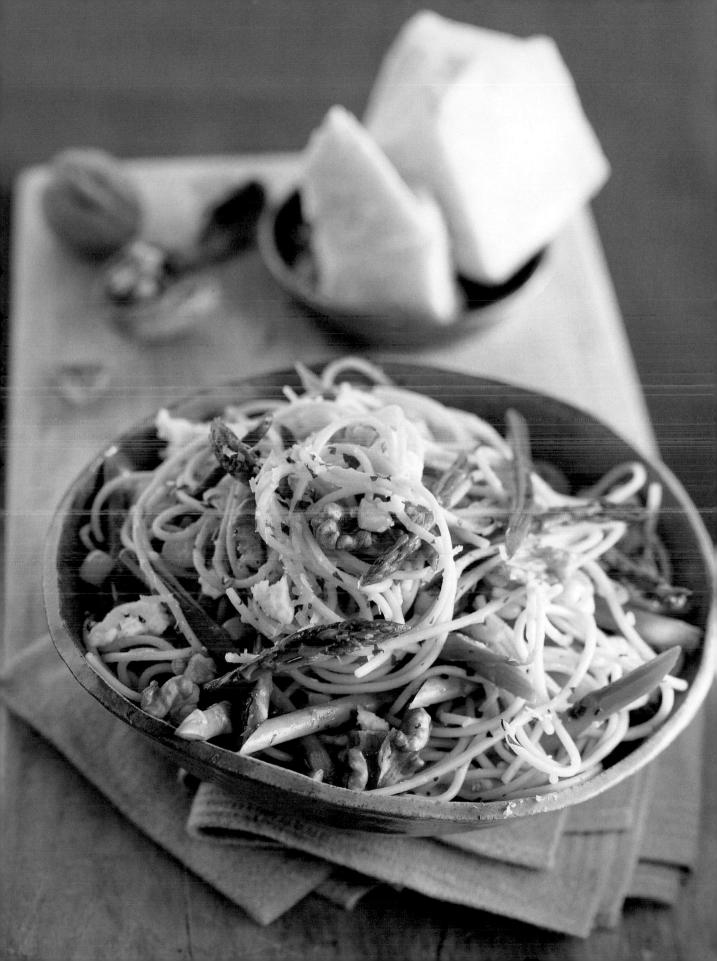

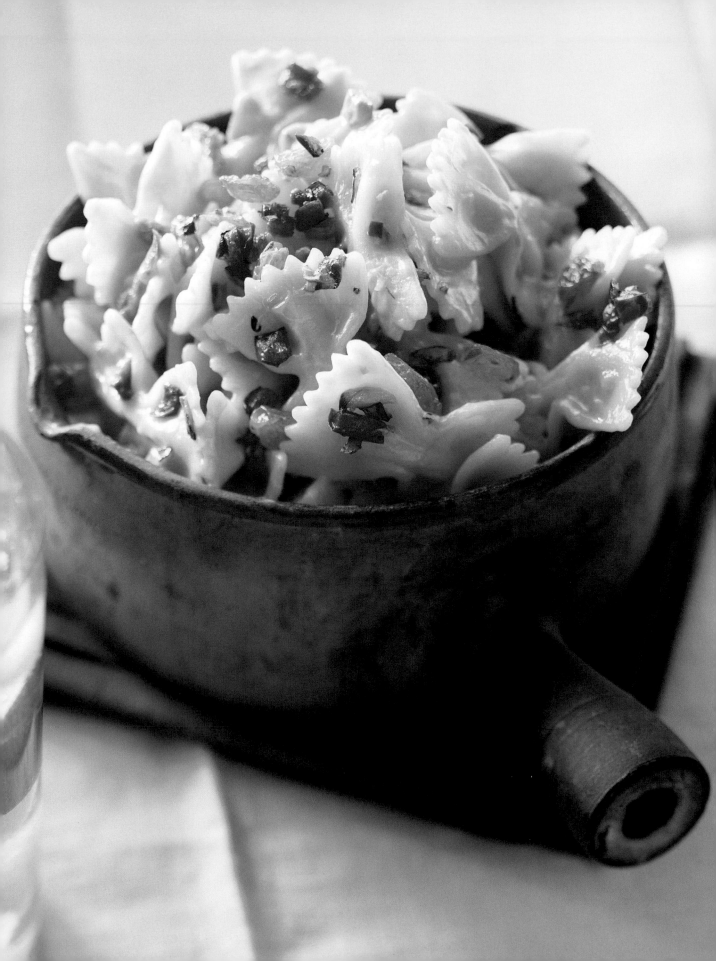

farfalle with winter squash sauce

Creamy, sweet butternut squash puree, enriched with Parmesan cheese and flecked with red bell pepper and raisins, makes a delicious and unusual pasta sauce. This dish provides ample amounts of beta-carotene, and also vitamin C, folate, selenium, and several B vitamins.

⅓	CUP RAISINS
1	CUP BOILING WATER
8	OUNCES FARFALLE (BOW-TIE) PASTA
1	TABLESPOON OLIVE OIL
1	LARGE RED BELL PEPPER, DICED
4	CLOVES GARLIC, MINCED
2	PACKAGES (9 OUNCES EACH) WINTER SQUASH PUREE, THAWED
1	TEASPOON RUBBED SAGE
1	TEASPOON SALT
½	TEASPOON BLACK PEPPER
3	TABLESPOONS REDUCED-FAT CREAM CHEESE (NEUFCHÂTEL)
⅓	CUP GRATED PARMESAN CHEESE

1 In a small bowl, soak the raisins in boiling water for 5 minutes, or until plump. In a large pot of boiling water, cook the pasta according to package directions. Drain, reserving ⅓ cup of the cooking liquid.

2 While the pasta cooks, in a large skillet, heat the oil over medium heat. Add the bell pepper and garlic; cook, stirring frequently for 5 minutes, or until the pepper is tender. Add the squash puree, sage, salt, and black pepper; cook until heated through.

3 Stir in the raisins and their soaking liquid and the cream cheese, and cook until the cream cheese has melted. Transfer to a large bowl. Add the pasta, the reserved cooking liquid, and the Parmesan; toss to combine.

Makes 4 servings. Per serving: 418 calories, 8.7g total fat (39% saturated), 14g protein, 73g carbohydrate, 7.4g fiber, 13mg cholesterol, 760mg sodium

basil & red pepper terrine

To achieve the proper texture for this colorful terrine, it's important to use "silken" tofu, which is much smoother than the regular variety. The dish serves 4 as a vegetarian main course, or 8 as a first course.

3	CLOVES GARLIC, PEELED
1	PACKAGE (19 OUNCES) SOFT SILKEN TOFU
1	PACKAGE (8 OUNCES) NONFAT CREAM CHEESE
½	CUP GRATED PARMESAN CHEESE
2	TABLESPOONS FLOUR
1	LARGE EGG
2	LARGE EGG WHITES
½	TEASPOON SALT
2	CUPS PACKED FRESH BASIL LEAVES
1	CUP JARRED ROASTED RED PEPPERS, DRAINED AND RINSED
3	TABLESPOONS TOMATO PASTE
¼	TEASPOON CAYENNE PEPPER

1 Preheat the oven to 350°F. Coat an 8½ x 4½-inch loaf pan with nonstick cooking spray. In a small pot of boiling water, cook the garlic for 2 minutes to blanch. Drain.

2 In a food processor, combine the blanched garlic, tofu, cream cheese, Parmesan, flour, whole egg, egg whites, and salt; process until smooth. Pour half of the tofu mixture into a bowl.

3 To the tofu mixture remaining in the food processor, add the basil and puree until smooth. Pour the basil-tofu mixture into the prepared pan.

4 Return the tofu mixture in the bowl to the food processor (no need to rinse). Add the roasted peppers, tomato paste, and cayenne; puree until smooth. Spoon the red pepper-tofu mixture on top of the basil mixture. With a small knife, make several cuts through the 2 layers.

5 Bake for 1 hour, or until set. Cool in the pan on a wire rack, then refrigerate for at least 4 hours. To serve, invert onto a serving platter and cut into 8 slices.

Makes 4 servings. Per serving: 260 calories, 9.2g total fat (31% saturated), 25g protein, 21g carbohydrate, 4.3g fiber, 67mg cholesterol, 964mg sodium

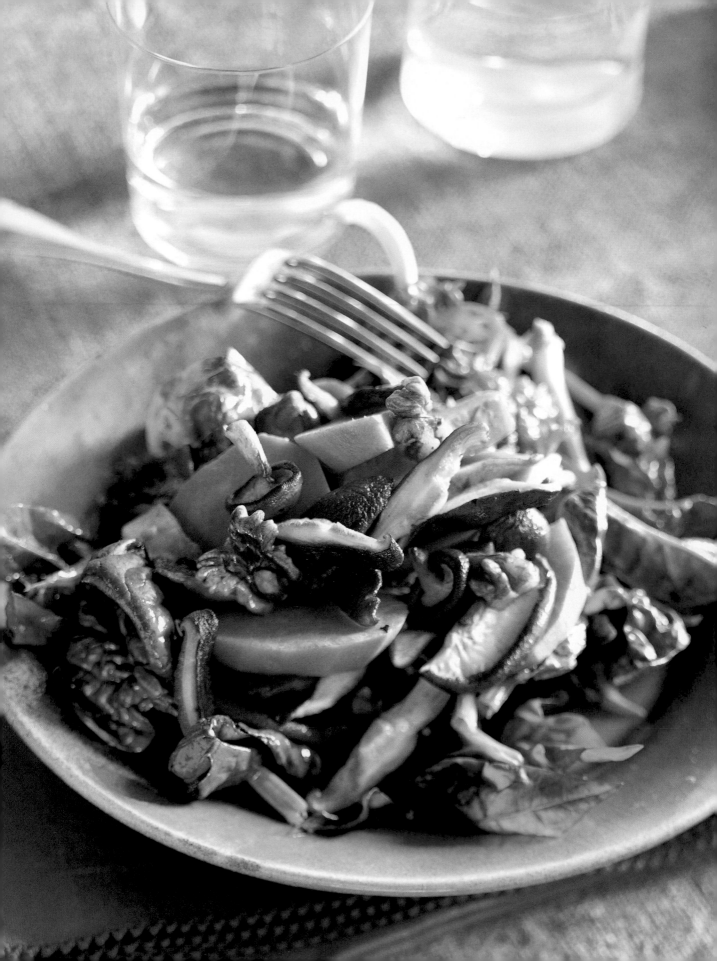

spinach, sweet potato & shiitake salad

To save some time, instead of baking sliced sweet potatoes, you can microwave whole, unpeeled potatoes and then peel and slice them after cooking.

- 1 POUND SWEET POTATOES, PEELED, HALVED LENGTHWISE, AND CUT CROSSWISE INTO ½-INCH SLICES
- ⅓ CUP WALNUTS
- 1 TABLESPOON PLUS 4 TEASPOONS OLIVE OIL
- 2 CLOVES GARLIC, SLIVERED
- 12 OUNCES FRESH SHIITAKE MUSHROOMS, STEMS DISCARDED AND CAPS THICKLY SLICED
- ½ TEASPOON SALT
- 12 CUPS SPINACH LEAVES
- ½ CUP RED WINE VINEGAR
- 1 TABLESPOON DIJON MUSTARD

1 Preheat the oven to 400°F. Place the sweet potatoes on a lightly oiled baking sheet, and bake for 15 to 20 minutes, or until tender. Toast the walnuts in a separate pan in the oven for 5 to 7 minutes, or until crisp. When cool enough to handle, coarsely chop the nuts.

2 In a large skillet, heat 1 tablespoon of the oil over medium heat. Add the garlic, and cook for 30 seconds, or until fragrant.

3 Add half the mushrooms, sprinkle them with ¼ teaspoon of the salt, and cook for 4 minutes, or until they begin to soften. Add the remaining mushrooms and ¼ teaspoon salt, and cook for 5 minutes, or until all the mushrooms are tender.

4 Place the spinach in a large bowl. Add the sweet potatoes and walnuts. Remove the mushrooms from the skillet with a slotted spoon, and add them to the bowl with the spinach.

5 Add the vinegar, mustard, and remaining 4 teaspoons oil to the skillet, and whisk over high heat until warm. Pour the dressing over the salad, and toss to combine.

Makes 4 servings. Per serving: 283 calories, 15g total fat (12% saturated), 9g protein, 32g carbohydrate, 8.1g fiber, 0mg cholesterol, 524mg sodium

garlic mashed potatoes & peas

Here's comfort food at its best. Buttermilk adds a slight tang to these mashed potatoes, while tarragon underscores the sweetness of the peas. Lots of garlic and sautéed scallions round out the flavors.

- 1½ POUNDS BAKING POTATOES, PEELED AND CUT INTO LARGE CHUNKS
- 8 CLOVES GARLIC, PEELED AND CRUSHED
- 1 TEASPOON SALT
- 1½ CUPS FROZEN PEAS
- ½ CUP BUTTERMILK
- 1 TEASPOON DRIED TARRAGON
- 1 TABLESPOON OLIVE OIL
- 8 SCALLIONS, THINLY SLICED

1 In a large saucepan, combine the potatoes, garlic, ¼ teaspoon of the salt, and water to cover by 1 inch; bring to a boil. Reduce to a simmer and cook for 20 minutes, or until the potatoes are tender. Add the peas, and cook for 1 minute. Drain.

2 Return the potatoes, peas, and garlic to the saucepan. Add the remaining ¾ teaspoon salt, the buttermilk, and tarragon. With a potato masher, mash the potatoes until creamy.

3 In a small skillet, heat the oil over medium heat. Add the scallions, and cook for 3 minutes, or until very soft. Stir the scallions into the mashed potato mixture, and cook over low heat until the potatoes are heated through.

Makes 4 servings. Per serving: 205 calories, 4g total fat (17% saturated), 8g protein, 36g carbohydrate, 4.9g fiber, 1mg cholesterol, 609mg sodium

stir-fried broccoli, shiitakes & new potatoes

Broccoli stalks are full of flavor (and nutrients). To use them, first separate them from the florets. Then trim the tough end of the stalks and peel off the tough outer layer. Thinly slice the peeled stalks crosswise and cook them along with the florets.

- 2 TABLESPOONS OLIVE OIL
- 12 OUNCES SMALL RED-SKINNED POTATOES, CUT INTO ½-INCH CHUNKS
- ¾ TEASPOON SALT
- 8 OUNCES FRESH SHIITAKE MUSHROOMS, STEMS DISCARDED AND CAPS QUARTERED
- 4 CUPS BROCCOLI FLORETS AND SLICED STALKS
- 3 SCALLIONS, THINLY SLICED
- 4 CLOVES GARLIC, MINCED

1 In a large skillet, heat the oil over medium heat. Add the potatoes and ¼ teaspoon of the salt; cook, stirring frequently for 10 minutes, or until the potatoes are golden brown.

2 Add the mushrooms. Reduce the heat to low; cover and cook for 4 minutes, or until the mushrooms have softened.

3 Add the broccoli, scallions, and garlic; cook, stirring frequently for 2 minutes, or until the scallions are tender. Add ¾ cup of water and the remaining ½ teaspoon salt, and cook, uncovered, for 5 minutes, or until the broccoli is crisp-tender.

Makes 4 servings. Per serving: 170 calories, 7.2g total fat (13% saturated), 6g protein, 24g carbohydrate, 4.6g fiber, 0mg cholesterol, 467mg sodium

roasted harvest vegetables

Fall and winter vegetables stand up well to roasting, and you can easily mix and match. You could make this with parsnips or carrots instead of brussels sprouts, or throw in some small onions. This particular combination is rich in fiber, potassium, beta-carotene, and calcium (most of which comes from the squash and brussels sprouts, not the cheese!).

- 3 TABLESPOONS OLIVE OIL
- 6 CLOVES GARLIC, SLICED
- 3 CUPS CHUNKS (1-INCH) BUTTERNUT SQUASH
- 10 OUNCES BRUSSELS SPROUTS, TRIMMED AND HALVED LENGTHWISE
- 8 OUNCES FRESH SHIITAKE MUSHROOMS, STEMS DISCARDED AND CAPS THICKLY SLICED
- 2 LARGE RED APPLES (UNPEELED), CUT INTO 1-INCH CHUNKS
- ¼ CUP OIL-PACKED SUN-DRIED TOMATOES, DRAINED AND THINLY SLICED
- 1 TEASPOON DRIED ROSEMARY, MINCED
- ½ TEASPOON SALT
- ¼ CUP GRATED PARMESAN CHEESE

1 Preheat the oven to 400°F. In a large roasting pan, combine the olive oil and garlic. Heat for 3 minutes in the oven. Add the squash, brussels sprouts, mushrooms, apples, sun-dried tomatoes, rosemary, and salt; toss to combine.

2 Roast for 35 minutes, or until the vegetables are tender; toss the vegetables every 10 minutes. Sprinkle the Parmesan over the vegetables, and roast for 5 minutes longer.

Makes 4 servings. Per serving: 292 calories, 14g total fat (17% saturated), 8g protein, 39g carbohydrate, 9.3g fiber, 4mg cholesterol, 464mg sodium

roasted harvest vegetables ▶

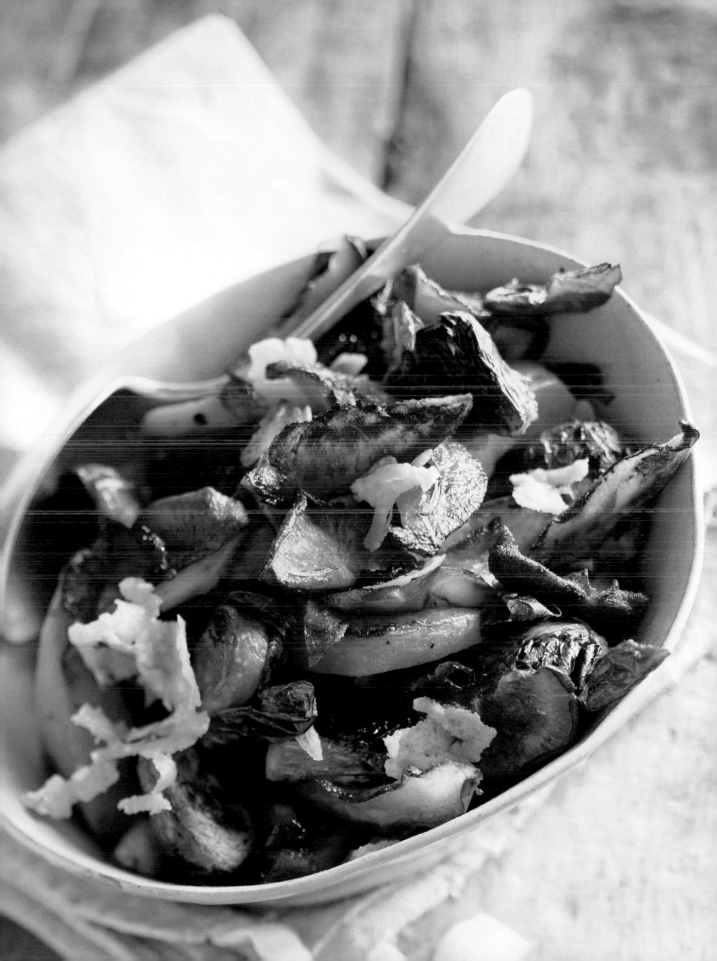

roasted jerusalem artichokes & garlic

Also known as sunchokes, Jerusalem artichokes have a creamy consistency and nutty flavor when roasted. They are a rich source of inulin, which may prove helpful in maintaining the balance between good and bad bacteria in the intestines.

- 2 TABLESPOONS OLIVE OIL
- 12 CLOVES GARLIC, UNPEELED
- 1 TABLESPOON DRIED ROSEMARY, CRUMBLED
- 2 POUNDS JERUSALEM ARTICHOKES, WELL SCRUBBED AND SLICED ½ INCH THICK
- ½ TEASPOON SALT

1 Preheat the oven to 400°F. In a roasting pan large enough to hold the Jerusalem artichokes in a single layer, combine the oil, garlic, and rosemary. Heat the pan in the oven for 3 to 5 minutes, or until the oil begins to sizzle.

2 Add the Jerusalem artichokes, and toss well to coat with the oil. Roast the artichokes, shaking the pan occasionally, for 35 to 40 minutes, or until the artichokes are tender. Sprinkle the salt over the artichokes and serve.

Makes 4 servings. Per serving: 248 calories, 6.9g total fat (14% saturated), 5g protein, 43g carbohydrate, 4.2g fiber, 0mg cholesterol, 301mg sodium

toasted buckwheat pilaf with dried fruit

Toasting brings out the flavors of many ingredients, especially nuts and grains. This pilaf calls for whole grains of buckwheat (called groats) that have been preroasted. This form of buckwheat is sold in most supermarkets as "kasha" and comes in both whole-grain and cracked versions.

- ½ CUP WALNUTS
- 1 TABLESPOON OLIVE OIL
- 1 RED BELL PEPPER, DICED
- 4 CLOVES GARLIC, MINCED
- 1 CUP WHOLE-GRAIN ROASTED BUCKWHEAT GROATS (KASHA)
- ½ CUP RED LENTILS
- 3 CUPS BOILING WATER
- ¾ TEASPOON DRIED ROSEMARY, MINCED
- ¾ TEASPOON SALT
- ½ TEASPOON BLACK PEPPER
- ⅔ CUP DRIED APRICOTS, DICED
- ⅔ CUP DRIED FIGS, DICED
- ¼ CUP CHOPPED PARSLEY

1 Preheat the oven to 350°F. Toast the walnuts for 7 minutes, or until crisp and fragrant. When cool enough to handle, coarsely chop.

2 In a large skillet, heat the oil over medium heat. Add the bell pepper and garlic, and cook for 4 minutes, or until the pepper is tender.

3 Stir in the buckwheat and red lentils, and cook for 3 minutes, or until the buckwheat is well coated.

4 Add the boiling water, rosemary, salt, and black pepper; bring to a boil. Reduce to a simmer; cover and cook for 15 minutes, or until the buckwheat is tender. Stir in the walnuts, apricots, figs, and parsley.

Makes 4 servings. Per serving: 482 calories, 13g total fat (12% saturated), 16g protein, 85g carbohydrate, 13g fiber, 0mg cholesterol, 453mg sodium

toasted buckwheat pilaf with dried fruit ▶

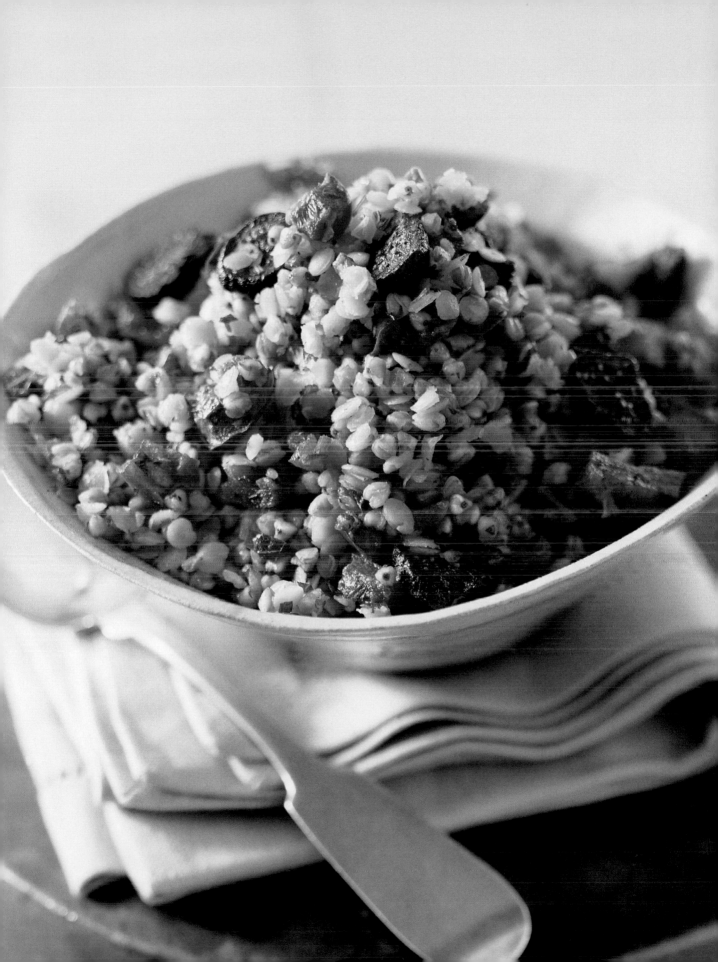

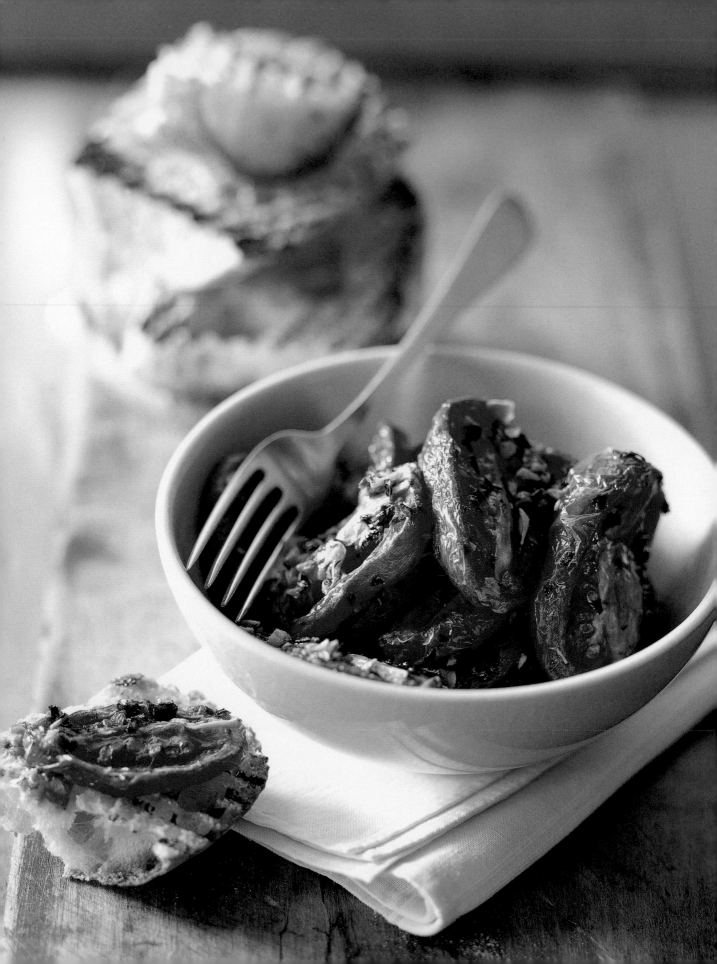

roasted tomatoes with garlic & herbs

Even in the winter months, when plum tomatoes are not at their best, these taste like a burst of summer. Although they do bake a long time, they require very little attention. Once baked, they'll keep for several days in the refrigerator. Eat them as is or use them in pasta sauces and salads.

3 POUNDS PLUM TOMATOES, HALVED LENGTHWISE

2 TABLESPOONS OLIVE OIL

5 CLOVES GARLIC, MINCED

½ CUP FINELY CHOPPED FRESH BASIL

2 TABLESPOONS MINCED FRESH ROSEMARY

1 TEASPOON SUGAR

¾ TEASPOON SALT

1 Preheat the oven to 250°F. Line a jelly-roll pan with foil.

2 In a large bowl, toss the tomatoes with the oil, garlic, basil, rosemary, sugar, and salt. Place the tomatoes cut-side up in the prepared pan, and bake for 3 hours, or until the tomatoes have collapsed and their skins have wrinkled.

3 Serve at room temperature or chilled.

Makes 4 servings. Per serving: 148 calories, 8g total fat (13% saturated), 4g protein, 19g carbohydrate, 5.4g fiber, 0mg cholesterol, 468mg sodium

braised artichokes, potatoes & peas

In order to preserve the most fiber and phytonutrients in the artichokes, they are not trimmed all the way down to their hearts: A good inch of the leaves is left on.

4 LARGE ARTICHOKES

4 TABLESPOONS FRESH LEMON JUICE

2 TABLESPOONS OLIVE OIL

1 SMALL RED ONION, FINELY CHOPPED

3 CLOVES GARLIC, MINCED

¾ TEASPOON DRIED MARJORAM

¾ TEASPOON SALT

1 POUND SMALL RED-SKINNED POTATOES, CUT INTO ½-INCH CUBES

1½ CUPS FROZEN PEAS

½ CUP CHOPPED PARSLEY

1 To trim the artichokes: Remove the tough outer leaves. Trim the tough end of the stem; then, with a paring knife, peel off the tough skin of the remaining stem. Cut off the top of the artichoke to just about 1 inch above the base. Halve the artichokes, scoop out and discard the chokes. Halve the artichokes again. Place the cleaned artichokes in a bowl with cold water to cover. Add 1 tablespoon of the lemon juice and set aside.

2 In a large skillet, heat the oil over medium heat. Add the onion and garlic, and cook, stirring frequently for 5 minutes, or until the onion is light golden.

3 Lift the artichokes from the water and add them to the skillet, stirring to coat. Add 1½ cups of water, the remaining 3 tablespoons lemon juice, the marjoram, and ¼ teaspoon of the salt; bring to a boil. Reduce to a simmer; cover and cook for 10 minutes.

4 Stir in the potatoes and remaining ½ teaspoon salt; cover and cook for 15 to 20 minutes, or until the potatoes and artichokes are tender.

5 Stir in the peas and parsley; cover and cook for 5 minutes, or until the peas are heated through.

Makes 4 servings. Per serving: 289 calories, 7.5g total fat (13% saturated), 11g protein, 50g carbohydrate, 13g fiber, 0mg cholesterol, 662mg sodium

◀ **roasted tomatoes with garlic & herbs**

toasted oat & bran tea bread

Flaxseeds add a nutty flavor to this tea bread. Look for them in health-food stores, but do not buy preground flaxseed meal, which loses much of its nutrient value due to exposure to air and light. If you cannot easily find whole flaxseeds, use unhulled sesame seeds instead.

- 1½ CUPS OLD-FASHIONED ROLLED OATS
- ½ CUP FLAXSEEDS
- ½ CUP WHEAT BRAN
- 1 CUP FLOUR
- ½ CUP FIRMLY PACKED LIGHT BROWN SUGAR
- 2 TEASPOONS BAKING POWDER
- ¾ TEASPOON SALT
- 1½ CUPS PLAIN LOW-FAT YOGURT
- ⅔ CUP HONEY
- 1 LARGE EGG
- 1 CUP (6 OUNCES) DARK RAISINS

1 Preheat the oven to 350°F. Lightly grease a 9 x 5-inch metal loaf pan.

2 Place the oats, flaxseeds, and wheat bran on a baking sheet, and bake for 7 to 9 minutes, or until the oats are golden brown. Transfer to a food processor and process until finely ground.

3 Transfer the oat mixture to a large bowl. Stir in the flour, brown sugar, baking powder, and salt.

4 In a separate bowl, whisk together the yogurt, honey, and egg. Make a well in the center of the dry ingredients and fold in the yogurt mixture until just combined. Fold in the raisins.

5 Spoon the batter into the prepared pan, smoothing the top. Bake for 1 hour, 20 minutes, or until a cake tester inserted in the center of the loaf comes out clean. Cool for 5 minutes in the pan, then invert the loaf onto a wire rack to cool completely.

Makes 12 servings. Per serving: 276 calories, 4.3g total fat (20% saturated), 7g protein, 57g carbohydrate, 4.9g fiber, 20mg cholesterol, 261mg sodium

whole wheat-parmesan flatties

These flat biscuits get lots of flavor (and a good amount of calcium) from the Parmesan and the yogurt. The walnuts add richness and healthful fats.

- ½ CUP WALNUTS
- 1¼ CUPS WHOLE-WHEAT FLOUR
- ½ CUP GRATED PARMESAN CHEESE
- 1 TABLESPOON SUGAR
- 2 TEASPOONS BAKING POWDER
- 1 TEASPOON SALT
- ½ TEASPOON BAKING SODA
- 1 CUP PLAIN LOW-FAT YOGURT
- 1 LARGE EGG

1 Preheat the oven to 400°F. Toast the walnuts for 5 minutes, or until golden brown and crisp. Leave the oven on. Transfer the toasted walnuts to a food processor along with ¼ cup of the flour, and process until the nuts are finely ground.

2 Transfer the walnut mixture to a large bowl. Add the remaining 1 cup flour, the Parmesan, sugar, baking powder, salt, and baking soda.

3 In a separate bowl, whisk together the yogurt and egg. Make a well in the center of the dry ingredients and stir in the yogurt mixture until just combined.

4 Turn out the dough onto a lightly floured surface. Pat out the dough to a ¾-inch thickness. Cut the dough with a 2-inch-round biscuit cutter, gathering up the scraps each time and patting it out again; you should end up with about 24 rounds.

5 Place the rounds 1 inch apart on an ungreased baking sheet, and bake for 15 to 17 minutes, or until golden brown and baked through.

Makes 24 flatties. Per flattie: 55 calories, 2.3g total fat (27% saturated), 3g protein, 7g carbohydrate, 1g fiber, 11mg cholesterol, 205mg sodium

toasted oat & bran tea bread ▶

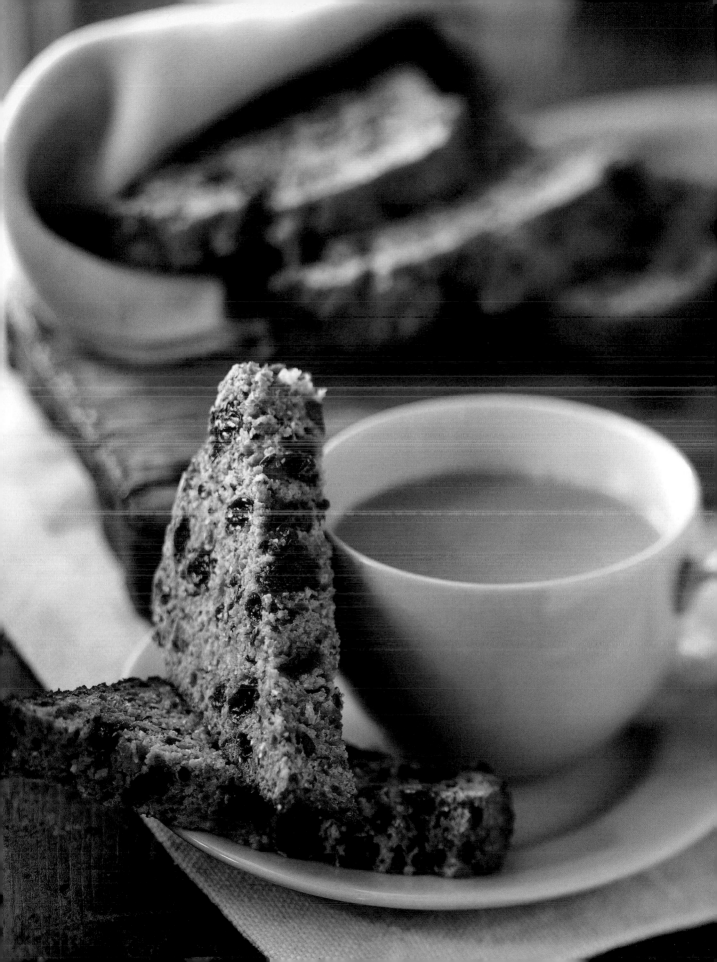

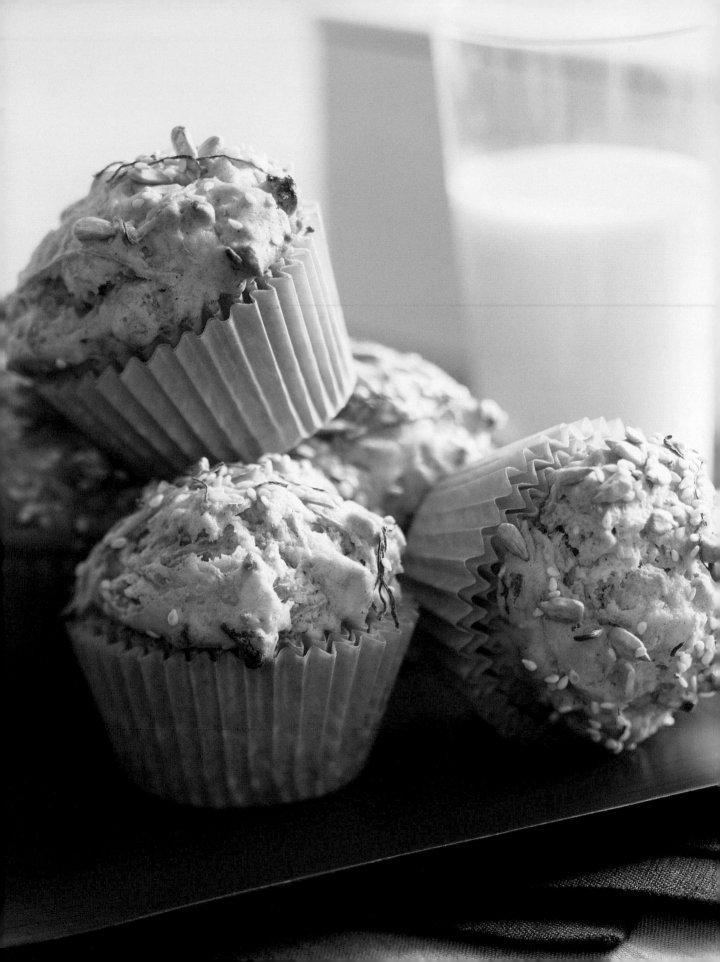

carrot-apricot muffins

Bursting with good-for-you ingredients—carrots, sunflower seeds, and apricots—these muffins make a substantial breakfast.

⅔ CUP SUNFLOWER SEEDS

3 TABLESPOONS SESAME SEEDS

1¾ CUPS FLOUR

2 TEASPOONS BAKING POWDER

½ TEASPOON BAKING SODA

½ TEASPOON SALT

¾ TEASPOON CINNAMON

¾ TEASPOON GROUND CARDAMOM

¾ TEASPOON GROUND GINGER

1 CUP BUTTERMILK

½ CUP FIRMLY PACKED LIGHT BROWN SUGAR

¼ CUP LIGHT OLIVE OIL

1 LARGE EGG

3 LARGE CARROTS, SHREDDED (1½ CUPS)

½ CUP DRIED APRICOTS, FINELY CHOPPED

1 Preheat the oven to 375°F. Line twelve 2½-inch muffin pan cups with paper liners. In a baking pan, toast the sunflower seeds and sesame seeds for 4 minutes, or until the sesame seeds are light golden, cool. Leave the oven on.

2 In a large bowl, combine the flour, baking powder, baking soda, salt, cinnamon, cardamom, and ginger.

3 In a separate bowl, whisk together the buttermilk, brown sugar, oil, and egg until well combined. Make a well in the center of the dry ingredients, pour in the egg mixture, and stir until just combined.

4 Fold in the sunflower seeds, sesame seeds, carrots, and apricots.

5 Spoon the batter into the prepared muffin cups, and bake for 30 minutes, or until a toothpick inserted in the center of a muffin comes out clean. Remove the muffins from the pan and cool on a wire rack.

Makes 12 muffins. Per muffin: 234 calories, 10g total fat (14% saturated), 6g protein, 31g carbohydrate, 1.6g fiber, 19mg cholesterol, 267mg sodium

creamy cornmeal & rice bread

A treat for anyone with gluten intolerance or wheat allergies, this cornmeal- and rice-based side dish has a wonderfully creamy center—much like southern spoonbread (which is more like corn pudding or soufflé than a bread).

⅓ CUP YELLOW CORNMEAL

⅓ CUP GRATED PARMESAN CHEESE

1 TABLESPOON PACKED LIGHT BROWN SUGAR

¾ TEASPOON BAKING POWDER

¾ TEASPOON SALT

½ TEASPOON CHILI POWDER

¾ CUP LOW-FAT (1%) MILK

⅔ CUP CANNED CREAMED CORN

2 TABLESPOONS OLIVE OIL

1 LARGE EGG, SEPARATED

¾ CUP COOKED RICE

2 LARGE EGG WHITES

1 Preheat the oven to 375°F. Lightly grease an 8-inch-square metal baking pan.

2 In a large bowl, stir together the cornmeal, Parmesan cheese, brown sugar, baking powder, salt, and chili powder.

3 In a separate bowl, stir together the milk, creamed corn, oil, and egg yolk. Make a well in the center of the dry ingredients and stir in the milk mixture. Fold in the cooked rice.

4 In a medium bowl, beat the 3 egg whites until stiff peaks form. Fold the whites into the batter.

5 Spoon the batter into the prepared pan. Bake for 30 minutes, or until the top is puffed and richly browned, and the bread is set. Serve warm.

Makes 4 servings. Per serving: 271 calories, 12g total fat (26% saturated), 10g protein, 31g carbohydrate, 1.3g fiber, 60mg cholesterol, 844mg sodium

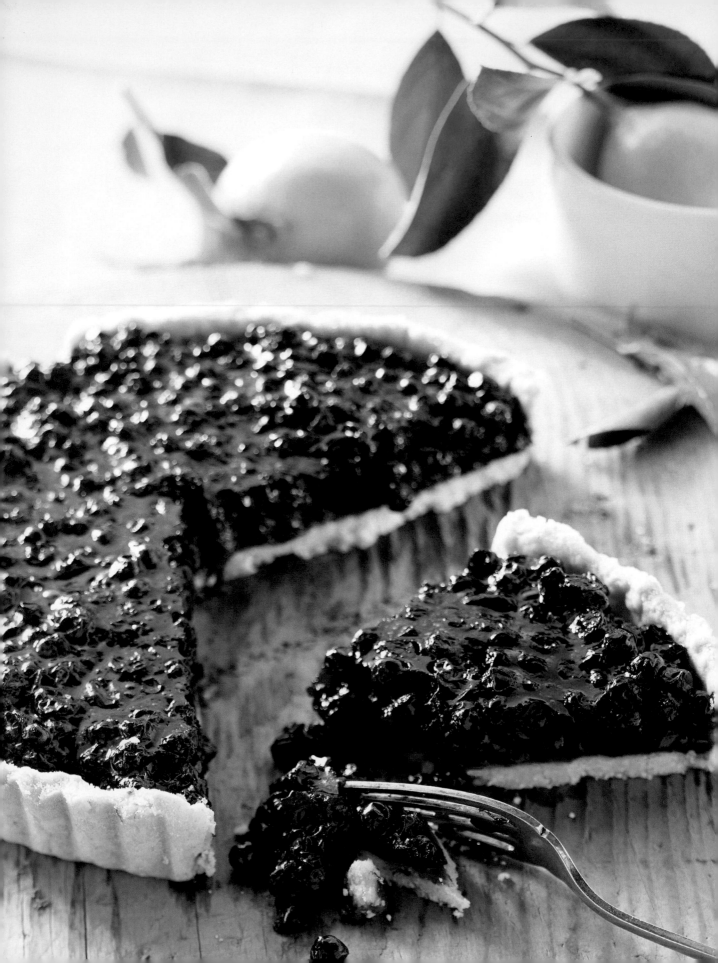

blueberry-orange tart

Don't be surprised by the small amount of pepper in the filling—it heightens the blueberry flavor. The dough for the tart shell is made with monounsaturated olive oil instead of butter.

- 1½ CUPS FLOUR
- ⅓ CUP CONFECTIONERS' SUGAR
- 2 TEASPOONS GRATED ORANGE ZEST
- ½ TEASPOON BAKING POWDER
- ½ TEASPOON SALT
- ¼ CUP PLUS 3 TABLESPOONS OLIVE OIL
- 2 TABLESPOONS PLUS ¼ CUP ORANGE JUICE
- 2 BAGS (12 OUNCES EACH) FROZEN UNSWEETENED BLUEBERRIES
- 8 TABLESPOONS GRANULATED SUGAR
- ½ TEASPOON PEPPER
- ⅛ TEASPOON NUTMEG
- 3 TABLESPOONS CORNSTARCH

1 In a large bowl, stir together the flour, confectioners' sugar, orange zest, baking powder, and salt. Add the oil and 2 tablespoons of the orange juice, and stir until the mixture comes together. Transfer the dough to a lightly floured work surface and knead 10 times, or until the dough forms a ball. Flatten into a disk, wrap in plastic wrap, and let stand for 30 minutes at room temperature.

2 Preheat the oven to 350°F. With your fingertips, gently press the dough onto the bottom and sides of a 9-inch tart pan with a removable bottom. Prick the bottom of the shell with a fork and line the pan with foil. Fill the foil with pie weights or dried beans, and bake the shell for 15 minutes. Remove the foil and weights, and bake the shell for 10 minutes, or until golden brown. Cool on a wire rack.

3 Meanwhile, in a saucepan, combine the blueberries, the remaining ¼ cup orange juice, 6 tablespoons of the granulated sugar, the pepper, and nutmeg; bring to a boil. Reduce to a simmer and cook for 5 minutes.

4 In a small bowl, stir together the remaining 2 tablespoons granulated sugar and the cornstarch. Stir the cornstarch mixture into the berries, and cook for 2 minutes, or until the berry mixture is thick.

5 Cool the blueberry mixture to room temperature, then spoon into the baked shell. Chill the tart for 1 hour before serving.

Makes 8 servings. Per serving: 319 calories, 13g total fat (13% saturated), 3g protein, 50g carbohydrate, 3.4g fiber, 0mg cholesterol, 177mg sodium

mint-chocolate chip pudding

The soy milk used in this recipe is the type most commonly found in supermarkets, and is slightly sweetened with malted corn and barley extract. If you use a completely unsweetened soy milk (such as the type often found in Chinese markets), increase the brown sugar to taste.

- ½ CUP FIRMLY PACKED DARK BROWN SUGAR
- ⅓ CUP CORNSTARCH
- 3 TABLESPOONS UNSWEETENED COCOA POWDER
- ½ TEASPOON SALT
- 3 CUPS SOY MILK
- ½ TEASPOON PURE MINT EXTRACT
- ½ TEASPOON VANILLA EXTRACT
- ¼ CUP MINI CHOCOLATE CHIPS (1 OUNCE)

1 In a large saucepan, stir together the brown sugar, cornstarch, cocoa powder, and salt. Gradually whisk in the soy milk until smooth.

2 Bring to a boil over medium heat, stirring constantly. Boil for 1 minute, or until the pudding is thick. Remove from the heat and stir in the mint and vanilla extracts. Cool to room temperature and stir in the chocolate chips.

3 Spoon into 4 dessert dishes. Cover and refrigerate for 2 hours, or until chilled.

Makes 4 servings. Per serving: 291 calories, 5.3g total fat (27% saturated), 8g protein, 53g carbohydrate, 1.3g fiber, 0mg cholesterol, 387mg sodium

fruit & nut-studded amaranth pudding

Cultivated since ancient times, amaranth is rich in magnesium, iron, fiber, and the amino acid lysine (which is rare in plant sources). You'll find amaranth in health-food stores. In this homey pudding, the amaranth remains somewhat crunchy and has a nutty flavor, which is emphasized by the addition of pine nuts.

- 2 TABLESPOONS PINE NUTS
- 3 CUPS LOW-FAT (1%) MILK
- 1 CUP WHOLE-GRAIN AMARANTH
- ¼ CUP MAPLE SUGAR
- 2 TEASPOONS GRATED ORANGE ZEST
- 2 TEASPOONS GRATED LEMON ZEST
- ¼ TEASPOON GROUND CARDAMOM
- ¼ TEASPOON SALT
- ⅓ CUP RAISINS
- ½ TEASPOON VANILLA EXTRACT

1 Preheat the oven to 350°F. Toast the pine nuts for 3 minutes, or until golden brown.

2 In a large saucepan, combine the milk, amaranth, maple sugar, orange zest, lemon zest, cardamom, and salt; bring to a boil. Reduce to a simmer; cover and cook, stirring occasionally for 35 minutes, or until the amaranth is tender.

3 Remove from the heat and stir in the pine nuts, raisins, and vanilla. Serve the pudding at room temperature or chilled.

Makes 4 servings. Per serving: 354 calories, 7.4g total fat (32% saturated), 15g protein, 60g carbohydrate, 8.6g fiber, 7mg cholesterol, 248mg sodium

cherry crisp

For an even better-tasting crisp, use fresh cherries. To get the amount of pitted cherries you need here, buy 2 pounds of fresh cherries and pit them; this should yield the same quantity as the 24 ounces of frozen pitted cherries. Sour cherries (pie cherries)—fresh or frozen—can be substituted for the sweet cherries, but increase the granulated sugar in the cherry mixture to ⅓ or ½ cup, to taste.

- ¼ CUP GRANULATED SUGAR
- 2 TABLESPOONS CORNSTARCH
- 1 TEASPOON CINNAMON
- ½ TEASPOON PEPPER
- ½ TEASPOON SALT
- ⅛ TEASPOON ALLSPICE
- 2 TEASPOONS GRATED LIME ZEST
- 2 BAGS (12 OUNCES EACH) FROZEN PITTED SWEET CHERRIES, THAWED
- 1 TABLESPOON FRESH LIME JUICE
- ¾ CUP OLD-FASHIONED ROLLED OATS
- ⅓ CUP FLOUR
- ⅓ CUP FIRMLY PACKED LIGHT BROWN SUGAR
- 3 TABLESPOONS COLD UNSALTED BUTTER, CUT UP

1 Preheat the oven to 400°F. In a large bowl, stir together the granulated sugar, cornstarch, cinnamon, pepper, ¼ teaspoon of the salt, the allspice, and lime zest. Add the cherries and lime juice, tossing to coat. Transfer to a 9-inch-square glass baking dish; set aside.

2 In a medium bowl, stir together the remaining ¼ teaspoon salt, the oats, flour, and brown sugar. With a pastry blender or two knives, cut in the butter until the mixture resembles coarse crumbs. Sprinkle the mixture over the fruit.

3 Bake for 25 minutes, or until the fruit is bubbly and piping hot and the topping is golden brown and crisp.

Makes 6 servings. Per serving: 257 calories, 6.9g total fat (55% saturated), 4g protein, 48g carbohydrate, 1.4g fiber, 16mg cholesterol, 201mg sodium

cherry crisp ▶

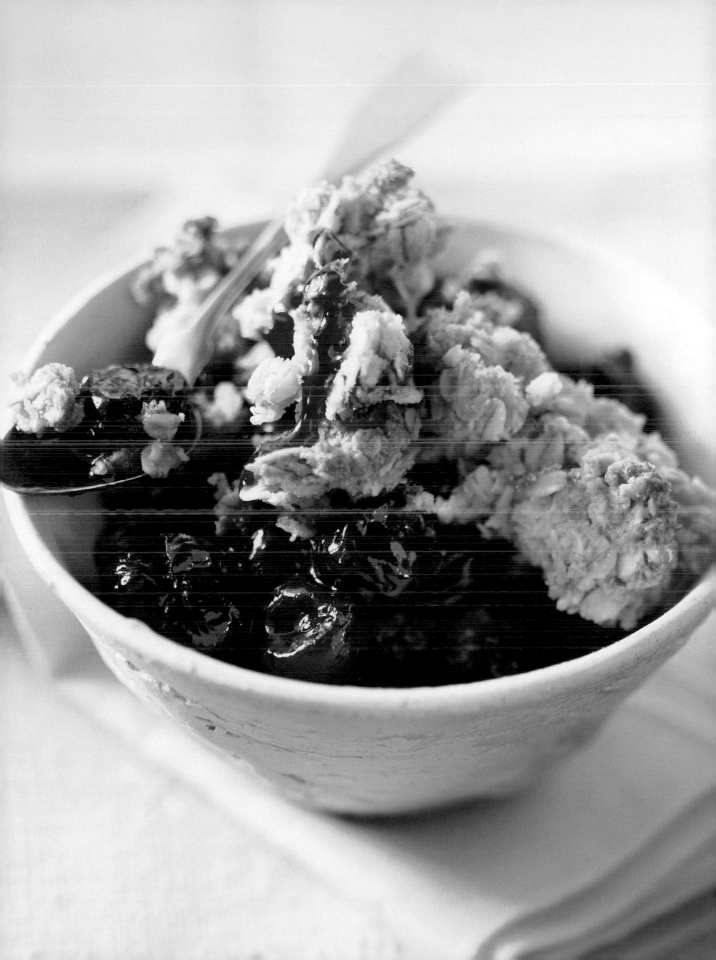

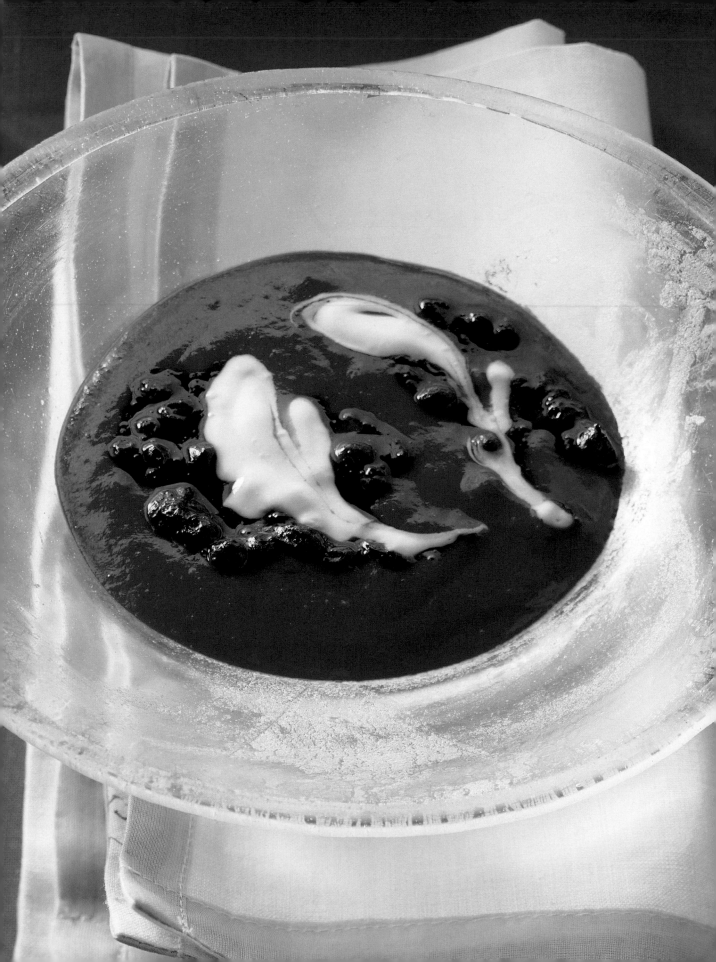

three-berry fool

Although many recipes call for straining out the seeds from raspberry purees and sauces, we have purposely left them in, because the seeds account for a goodly amount of the dietary fiber.

- 1   QUART PLAIN LOW-FAT YOGURT
- 1   PACKAGE (12 OUNCES) FROZEN UNSWEETENED RASPBERRIES, THAWED
- 2   CUPS FROZEN UNSWEETENED STRAWBERRIES, THAWED
- ½   CUP SUGAR
- 1½   TEASPOONS VANILLA EXTRACT
- 3   TEASPOONS CORNSTARCH BLENDED WITH 2 TABLESPOONS WATER
- 1   PACKAGE (12 OUNCES) FROZEN UNSWEETENED BLUEBERRIES
- 2   TABLESPOONS ORANGE JUICE
- ¼   TEASPOON PEPPER
- ¼   TEASPOON ALLSPICE
- 1   TABLESPOON FRESH LEMON JUICE

1 Spoon the yogurt into a fine-mesh strainer or a coffee filter set over a bowl to catch the drips. Let the yogurt stand for 4 hours at room temperature.

2 In a food processor, combine the raspberries, strawberries, ¼ cup of the sugar, and ½ teaspoon of the vanilla; puree. Transfer the puree to a small saucepan and bring to a boil over medium heat. Stir in half of the cornstarch mixture and bring to a boil. Boil, stirring constantly for 1 minute, until lightly thickened. Cool to room temperature, transfer to a bowl, cover, and refrigerate.

3 In a small saucepan, combine 2 tablespoons of the sugar, the blueberries, orange juice, pepper, and allspice; bring to a simmer over low heat. Cook, stirring frequently for 5 minutes, or until the blueberries are tender. Stir in the remaining cornstarch mixture and bring to a boil; cook, stirring constantly, for 1 minute, or until thickened. Transfer to a bowl and stir in the lemon juice; cover and refrigerate.

4 In a medium bowl, combine the drained yogurt, the remaining 2 tablespoons sugar, and the remaining 1 teaspoon vanilla.

5 To serve, spoon the raspberry-strawberry mixture into 4 bowls. Spoon the blueberry mixture into the center and top with the yogurt. Gently swirl the mixture to lightly marble the yogurt with fruit puree.

Makes 4 servings. Per serving: 331 calories, 4.5g total fat (0% saturated), 13g protein, 63g carbohydrate, 2.8g fiber, 6mg cholesterol, 75mg sodium

creamy citrus & vanilla rice pudding

Rice milk (available in many supermarkets) is used here instead of cow's milk for a creamy, lactose-free pudding. The basmati rice is used for extra flavor, but regular long-grain rice would be fine.

- 4   CUPS RICE MILK
- 3   STRIPS (3 x ½ INCH EACH) ORANGE ZEST
- 3   STRIPS (3 x ½ INCH EACH) LIME ZEST
- 1   CINNAMON STICK, SPLIT LENGTHWISE
- ½   TEASPOON SALT
- ½   CUP BASMATI, JASMINE, OR TEXMATI RICE
- ¼   CUP SUGAR
- 2   LARGE EGG YOLKS
- ½   TEASPOON VANILLA EXTRACT

1 In a large saucepan, stir together the rice milk, orange and lime zests, cinnamon, and salt. Add the rice, and bring to a simmer over medium-low heat. Cover and cook for 15 minutes, stirring occasionally.

2 Meanwhile, in a medium bowl, whisk together the sugar and egg yolks.

3 Uncover the rice and cook, stirring frequently for 15 minutes, or until the rice is very tender. Whisk some of the hot rice mixture into the egg mixture to warm it, then whisk the egg mixture into the saucepan. Cook, stirring constantly, for 2 minutes, or until the pudding is slightly thickened.

4 Transfer the pudding to a bowl and stir in the vanilla. When cool, remove the orange zest, lime zest, and cinnamon stick. Cool to room temperature, then cover and refrigerate until serving time.

Makes 4 servings. Per serving: 279 calories, 5g total fat (16% saturated), 5g protein, 56g carbohydrate, 0.3g fiber, 106mg cholesterol, 394mg sodium

panforte cluster cookies

A true panforte is a dense, nearly flourless, nut cake from Siena, Italy. Here is a cookie-size adaptation made with nutrient-rich dried fruits and crystallized ginger in place of some of the nuts.

- 1 CUP NATURAL (UNBLANCHED) ALMONDS
- ½ CUP DICED DRIED PINEAPPLE (3½ OUNCES)
- ½ CUP DICED DRIED MANGO (3 OUNCES)
- ⅓ CUP DRIED CRANBERRIES, FINELY CHOPPED
- ¼ CUP CHOPPED CRYSTALLIZED GINGER (1½ OUNCES)
- ½ CUP FLOUR
- ¾ TEASPOON CINNAMON
- ¼ TEASPOON GROUND CORIANDER
- ¼ TEASPOON ALLSPICE
- ¼ TEASPOON NUTMEG
- ¼ TEASPOON SALT
- ⅓ CUP HONEY
- ⅓ CUP SUGAR

1 Preheat the oven to 350°F. Toast the almonds for 7 minutes, or until crisp and fragrant. Leave the oven on. When the almonds are cool enough to handle, finely chop them.

2 Line a large baking sheet with parchment paper or lightly greased aluminum foil.

3 In a large bowl, combine the pineapple, mango, cranberries, ginger, and almonds. On a sheet of wax paper, stir together the flour, cinnamon, coriander, allspice, nutmeg, and salt.

4 In a small saucepan, stir together the honey and sugar; bring to a boil over medium heat. Boil for 2 minutes. Pour the hot honey mixture over the fruit mixture, and stir to combine. Add the flour mixture and stir until combined.

5 With dampened hands, shape the dough into walnut-size pieces. Place 1 inch apart on the prepared baking sheet, then flatten each to ¼-inch thickness. Bake for 10 minutes, or until just set. Let cool on the pan for 5 minutes before transferring to a wire rack to cool completely.

Make 32 cookies. Per cookie: 75 calories, 2.2g total fat (0% saturated), 1g protein, 14g carbohydrate, 0.8g fiber, 0mg cholesterol, 23mg sodium

ginger pancake with banana-walnut topping

Serve this oversized pancake for dessert or as the main attraction at a Sunday brunch.

- ⅓ CUP WALNUTS
- ½ CUP FLOUR
- ½ CUP LOW-FAT (1%) MILK
- 1 LARGE EGG
- 1 LARGE EGG WHITE
- 1 TABLESPOON LIGHT OLIVE OIL
- 1 TABLESPOON BUTTER, MELTED
- 2 TEASPOONS GRANULATED SUGAR
- 1 TEASPOON VANILLA EXTRACT
- ¼ TEASPOON SALT
- ⅓ CUP FINELY CHOPPED CRYSTALLIZED GINGER (2 OUNCES)
- ¼ CUP FRESH LIME JUICE
- 2 TABLESPOONS PACKED LIGHT BROWN SUGAR
- 3 BANANAS, THINLY SLICED

1 Preheat the oven to 350°F. Toast the walnuts for 5 minutes, or until crisp and fragrant. When the walnuts are cool enough to handle, coarsely chop.

2 Increase the oven temperature to 425°F. Lightly oil a 10-inch nonstick skillet and place it in the oven.

3 In a large bowl, stir together the flour, milk, whole egg, egg white, oil, butter, granulated sugar, vanilla, and salt until well combined. Stir in the ginger.

4 Pour the batter into the hot pan, return the pan to the oven, and bake for 12 to 15 minutes, or until the pancake has puffed and is golden brown.

5 Meanwhile, in a large skillet, combine the lime juice and brown sugar, and cook over medium heat until the sugar has melted. Add the sliced bananas and cook for 3 minutes, or until the bananas have softened. Stir in the walnuts.

6 To serve, cut the pancake into wedges and top with the banana-walnut mixture.

Makes 4 servings. Per serving: 402 calories, 15g total fat (24% saturated), 7g protein, 63g carbohydrate, 2.9g fiber, 62mg cholesterol, 238mg sodium

ginger pancake with banana-walnut topping ▶

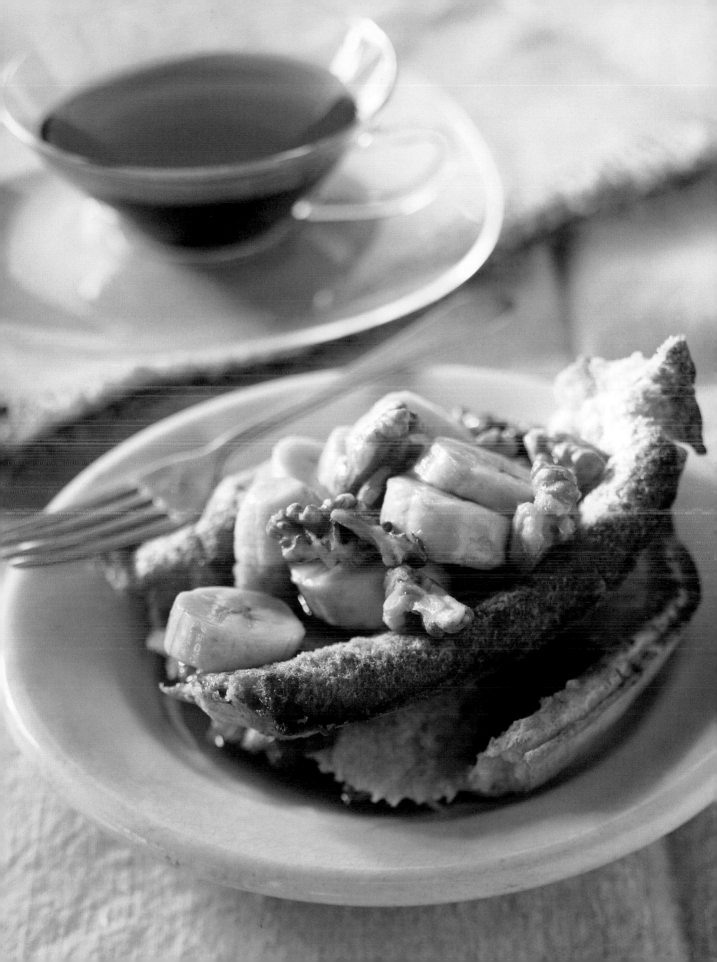

cheese blintzes with strawberry sauce

Blintzes are simply crêpe-like pancakes folded around a filling. The pancakes can be cooked in advance and frozen; thaw them before filling and baking. In addition to tasting great, these cheese blintzes are high in calcium, iron, vitamin C, and the B vitamins thiamin, riboflavin, niacin, and B_{12}.

- 1 PACKAGE (20 OUNCES) FROZEN UNSWEETENED STRAWBERRIES, THAWED
- ½ CUP PLUS 1 TEASPOON SUGAR
- 3 TABLESPOONS RASPBERRY ALL-FRUIT SPREAD
- 2 LARGE EGGS
- 2 LARGE EGG WHITES
- 1 CUP LOW-FAT (1%) MILK
- 1 TABLESPOON LIGHT OLIVE OIL
- ¼ TEASPOON SALT
- 1 CUP PLUS 3 TABLESPOONS FLOUR
- 1 CONTAINER (16 OUNCES) LOW-FAT (1%) COTTAGE CHEESE, DRAINED
- 1½ TEASPOONS VANILLA EXTRACT

1 In a food processor, combine the strawberries, ¼ cup of the sugar, and the raspberry fruit spread; puree until smooth.

2 In a blender, combine the whole eggs, egg whites, milk, oil, 1 teaspoon of the sugar, and the salt; blend until combined. Add 1 cup of the flour and blend until smooth. Let stand for 30 minutes.

3 Brush a 10-inch nonstick skillet with oil and place over medium heat. Pour a scant ¼ cup of batter into the pan, and swirl to cover the bottom. Cook for 10 seconds, or until the bottom is light golden. Turn the blintz over and cook for 5 seconds longer on the other side. Transfer the blintz to a plate lined with wax paper. Repeat with the remaining batter, separating the cooked blintzes with sheets of wax paper.

4 Preheat the oven to 400°F. Lightly oil a 9 x 13-inch baking dish.

5 In a medium bowl, stir together the remaining ¼ cup sugar, 3 tablespoons flour, the cottage cheese, and vanilla. One at a time, lay a blintz on a work surface and spoon 2 tablespoons of filling into the center. Fold the sides over the filling, then roll up the blintz. Place the blintzes seam-side down in the prepared baking dish. Bake for 10 to 15 minutes, or until the pancake is lightly crisped.

6 To serve, spoon the strawberry sauce onto 4 serving plates; place 2 blintzes on each plate and serve.

Makes 4 servings. Per serving: 524 calories, 10g total fat (26% saturated), 25g protein, 82g carbohydrate, 1g fiber, 113mg cholesterol, 697mg sodium

blushing applesauce

Making your own applesauce is a cinch, and when the apples are combined with grape juice, cinnamon, and a hint of black pepper, the sauce is much more interesting than the store-bought variety. In addition to adding some sweetness and the "blush" color, the purple grape juice provides the heart-healthy phytochemical resveratrol.

- 4 LARGE GRANNY SMITH APPLES, PEELED, CORED, AND HALVED
- 2 CUPS UNSWEETENED CONCORD GRAPE JUICE
- 2 TABLESPOONS HONEY
- ½ TEASPOON CINNAMON
- ¼ TEASPOON BLACK PEPPER
- 1 TEASPOON VANILLA EXTRACT

1 In a medium saucepan, combine the apples, grape juice, honey, cinnamon, and pepper; bring to a boil over medium heat. Reduce to a gentle boil and cook for 30 minutes, or until the apples are slightly chunky and the mixture has become thick.

2 Remove from the heat and stir in the vanilla. If you prefer a smoother applesauce, mash with a potato masher. Serve the applesauce chilled or at room temperature.

Makes 4 servings. Per serving: 200 calories, 0.5g total fat (15% saturated), 0g protein, 51g carbohydrate, 2.8g fiber, 0mg cholesterol, 1mg sodium

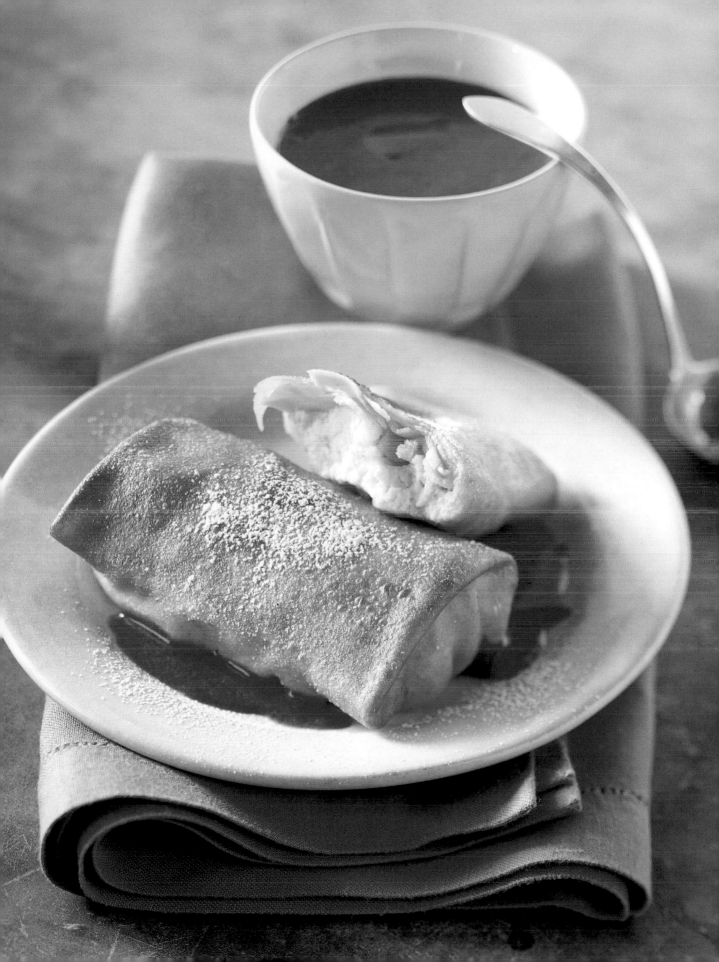

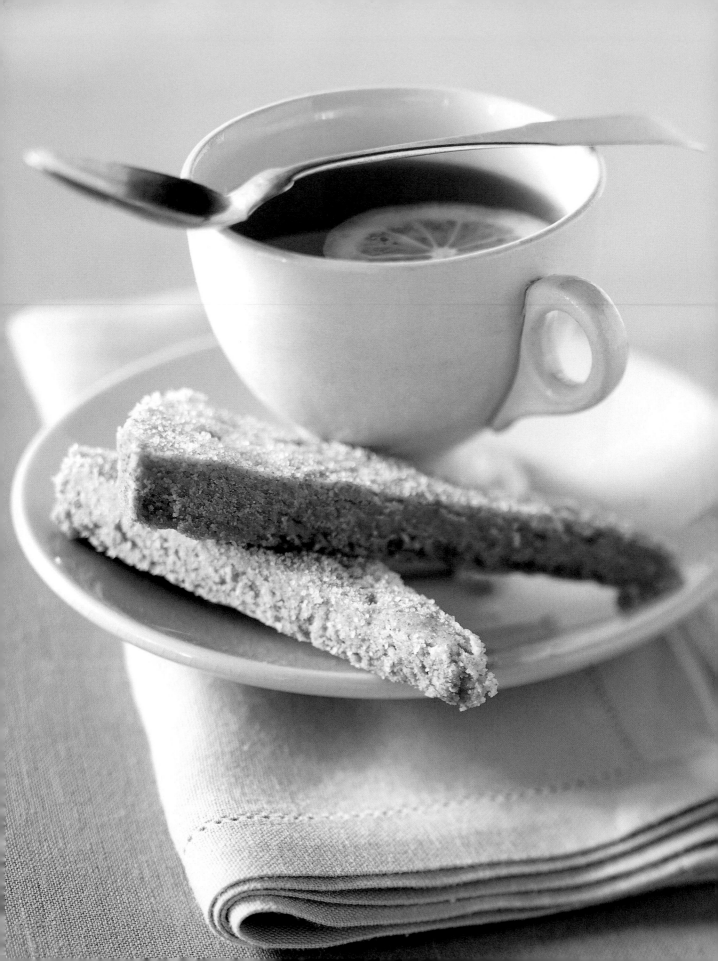

walnut shortbread

Although shortbread is usually made with butter, we've found that replacing it with ground walnuts, olive oil, and walnut oil works beautifully. The result is a rich-tasting cookie with no cholesterol and healthful monounsaturated fats instead of saturated fats. Walnuts and walnut oil also have ellagic acid, a potent antioxidant.

- ⅔ CUP WALNUTS
- ¾ CUP ALL-PURPOSE FLOUR
- ½ CUP WHOLE-WHEAT FLOUR
- ½ CUP CONFECTIONERS' SUGAR
- ¼ TEASPOON SALT
- ¼ CUP WALNUT OIL
- ¼ CUP LIGHT OLIVE OIL
- 1½ TEASPOONS GRATED LEMON ZEST
- 1 TEASPOON VANILLA EXTRACT

1 Preheat the oven to 325°F. Toast the walnuts for 7 minutes, or until crisp and fragrant. Leave on the oven. Cool the walnuts, then transfer to a food processor with the all-purpose flour, and process until the nuts are finely ground.

2 Transfer the flour-walnut mixture to a large bowl. Stir in the whole-wheat flour, confectioners' sugar, and salt. Add the walnut oil, olive oil, lemon zest, and vanilla, and stir until well combined.

3 Press the dough onto the bottom of a 9-inch tart pan with a removable bottom. With the tines of a fork, prick the dough. With a sharp knife, score the dough into 16 wedges, cutting almost, but not quite through, to the bottom.

4 Bake for 30 minutes, or until crisp and light golden. Check the shortbread after 20 minutes; if it is over-browning, decrease the oven temperature to 300°F. Remove from the oven and, while the shortbread is still warm, cut the wedges through to the bottom. Cool in the pan on a wire rack.

Makes 8 servings. Per serving: 273 calories, 19g total fat (11% saturated), 3g protein, 24g carbohydrate, 1.7g fiber, 0mg cholesterol, 73mg sodium

kiwi-mango salad

While the avocado may come as a surprise in this dessert salad, its smooth, silky texture and rich flavor are a nice counterpoint to the other fruits. Prepare this shortly before serving, or the fruit—especially the banana—will become mushy as the acid in the lime juice starts to break it down.

- ¼ CUP FRESH LIME JUICE
- 2 TABLESPOONS SUGAR
- ¼ CUP FRESH MINT LEAVES, MINCED (2 TABLESPOONS)
- 6 KIWIFRUIT, PEELED, QUARTERED LENGTHWISE, AND CUT CROSSWISE INTO THIRDS
- 2 BANANAS, HALVED LENGTHWISE AND THICKLY SLICED
- 1 MANGO, PEELED AND CUT INTO 1-INCH CHUNKS
- 1 AVOCADO, PEELED AND CUT INTO 1-INCH CHUNKS

In a large bowl, whisk together the lime juice, sugar, and mint. Add the kiwifruit, bananas, mango, and avocado; toss well. Refrigerate for up to 1 hour before serving.

Makes 4 servings. Per serving: 267 calories, 8.6g total fat (16% saturated), 3g protein, 51g carbohydrate, 6.7g fiber, 0mg cholesterol, 14mg sodium

banana bread pudding

Made with rice milk instead of cow's milk, and egg whites instead of whole eggs, this sweet, mildly spiced banana bread pudding is rich tasting without being high in fat. Soothing to both the body and spirit, the pudding is a good source of B vitamins, potassium, folate, and selenium.

- 6 OUNCES ITALIAN SEMOLINA BREAD, CUT INTO 1-INCH PIECES
- 1 POUND VERY RIPE BANANAS
- ¼ CUP FIRMLY PACKED DARK BROWN SUGAR
- 2½ CUPS RICE MILK
- 3 LARGE EGG WHITES
- ½ TEASPOON VANILLA EXTRACT
- ¼ TEASPOON GRATED NUTMEG
- ¼ TEASPOON SALT

1 Preheat the oven to 400°F. Toast the bread cubes for 7 minutes, or until crisp. Remove from the oven and reduce the oven temperature to 350°F.

2 In a large bowl, mash the bananas with a potato masher or a fork. Stir in the brown sugar until combined. Whisk in the rice milk, egg whites, vanilla, nutmeg, and salt.

3 Place the toasted bread cubes in a 9-inch-square glass baking dish. Pour the banana mixture over the bread.

4 Bake for 35 minutes, or until the pudding is puffed and set. Cool to room temperature before serving.

Makes 4 servings. Per serving: 325 calories, 3.1g total fat (17% saturated), 8g protein, 68g carbohydrate, 2.5g fiber, 0mg cholesterol, 495mg sodium

pumpkin-ginger cheesecake

Bake this creamy cake the day before you plan to serve it, because it has to sit overnight to firm up. In addition to being a good source of calcium, each serving provides 140% of the daily recommended intake of beta-carotene.

- 9 OUNCES GINGERSNAPS (ABOUT **36** COOKIES)
- 2 TABLESPOONS OLIVE OIL
- 3 PACKAGES (8 OUNCES EACH) REDUCED-FAT CREAM CHEESE (NEUFCHÂTEL)
- 1 CUP REDUCED-FAT SOUR CREAM
- 1 CAN (**15** OUNCES) SOLID-PACK PUMPKIN PUREE
- 1 CUP FIRMLY PACKED DARK BROWN SUGAR
- 2 LARGE EGGS
- 2 LARGE EGG WHITES
- 1½ TEASPOONS VANILLA EXTRACT
- 2 TEASPOONS CINNAMON
- 1½ TEASPOONS GROUND GINGER
- 1½ TEASPOONS GROUND CARDAMOM
- 1 TEASPOON ALLSPICE
- ½ TEASPOON SALT
- 1 CUP WALNUTS, COARSELY CHOPPED

1 Preheat the oven to 350°F. In a food processor, combine the gingersnaps and oil, and process until finely ground. Press the mixture onto the bottom of a 9-inch springform pan. Bake for 10 minutes, or until set and crisp. Leave the oven on.

2 In the same food processor bowl (no need to rinse), combine the cream cheese, sour cream, pumpkin puree, brown sugar, whole eggs, egg whites, vanilla, cinnamon, ginger, cardamom, allspice, and salt; process until smooth.

3 Pour the batter into the prepared pan. Sprinkle the walnuts over the batter. Bake for 1 hour.

4 Turn off the oven, prop open the oven door slightly, and let the cheesecake stand for 45 minutes in the turned-off oven. Cool to room temperature, then cover and refrigerate overnight.

Makes 12 servings. Per serving: 447 calories, 26g total fat (42% saturated), 12g protein, 41g carbohydrate, 1.6g fiber, 82mg cholesterol, 516mg sodium

pumpkin-ginger cheesecake ▶

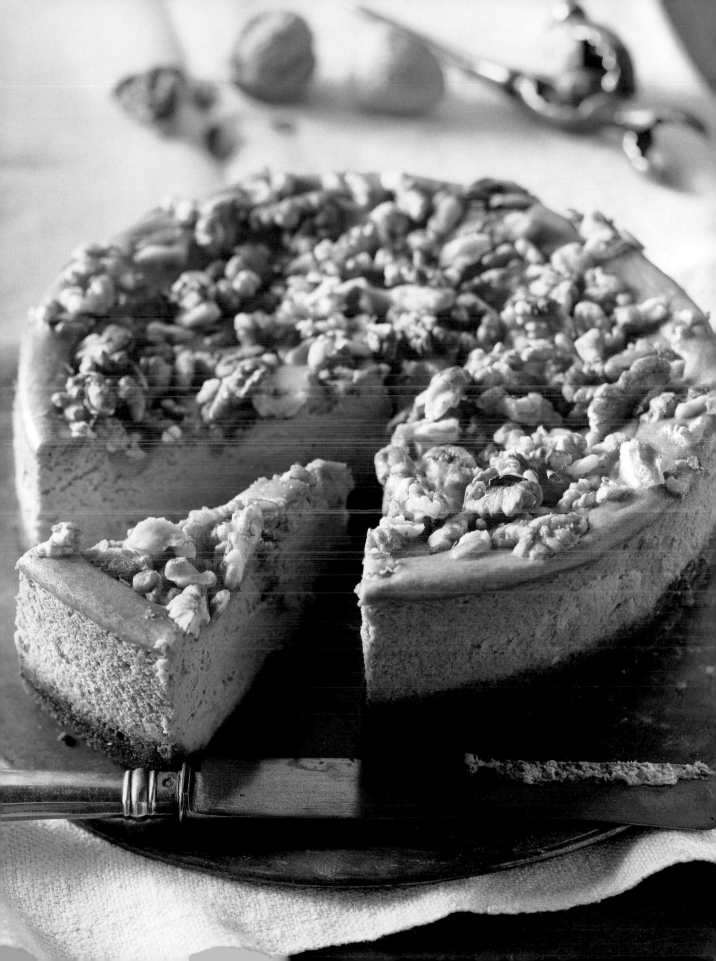

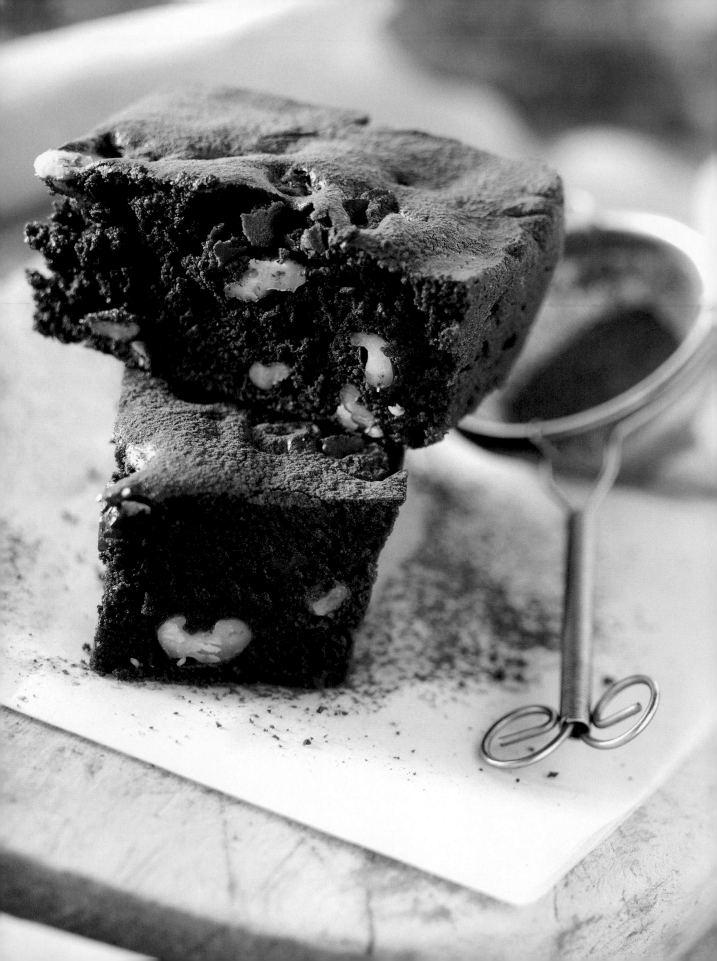

fig bars with sesame crust

Shredded carrots are added to the filling of these bar cookies both to lighten the mixture and to add a subtle sweetness (as well as soluble fiber).

- ½ CUP NATURAL (UNBLANCHED) ALMONDS
- 1 TABLESPOON SESAME SEEDS
- 1 CUP FLOUR
- ⅓ CUP CONFECTIONERS' SUGAR
- ½ TEASPOON SALT
- ⅓ CUP DARK SESAME OIL
- 1½ TEASPOONS GRATED ORANGE ZEST
- 1 CUP DRIED FIGS, COARSELY CHOPPED
- 2 CARROTS, VERY THINLY SLICED
- ¾ CUP ORANGE JUICE
- 2 TABLESPOONS FRESH LEMON JUICE
- ¾ TEASPOON GROUND CARDAMOM
- 1 TEASPOON VANILLA EXTRACT

1 Preheat the oven to 350°F. Toast the almonds and sesame seeds for 5 to 7 minutes, or until the almonds are fragrant and the seeds are golden.

2 Transfer the almonds and sesame seeds to a food processor. Add the flour, confectioners' sugar, and salt; process until powdery. Add the sesame oil and orange zest, and process until evenly moistened.

3 Press the crust mixture into a 9-inch-square metal baking pan. With the tines of a fork, prick the dough all over and bake for 20 minutes. Cool on a wire rack.

4 While the crust bakes, in a medium saucepan, combine the figs, carrots, orange juice, lemon juice, and cardamom; bring to a boil over medium heat. Reduce to a simmer; cover and cook 20 minutes, or until the figs and carrots are soft and most of the liquid has been absorbed. Cool to room temperature.

5 Transfer the fig-carrot mixture to a food processor. Add the vanilla, and process to a coarse puree. Spread the mixture over the crust, and bake for 20 minutes. Cool in the pan on a wire rack before slicing into 32 pieces.

Makes 32 cookies. Per cookie: 75 calories, 3.6g total fat (0% saturated), 1g protein, 10g carbohydrate, 1.1g fiber, 0mg cholesterol, 39mg sodium

peanut butter brownies with walnuts & cranberries

Peanut butter and olive oil replace the butter in these brownies, and walnuts and cranberries add some healthful phytochemicals.

- ⅔ CUP FLOUR
- ½ CUP UNSWEETENED COCOA POWDER
- 1 TEASPOON BAKING POWDER
- ¼ TEASPOON BAKING SODA
- ¼ TEASPOON SALT
- ¾ CUP FIRMLY PACKED LIGHT BROWN SUGAR
- ¼ CUP CREAMY PEANUT BUTTER
- 3 TABLESPOONS LIGHT OLIVE OIL
- 1 LARGE EGG
- 2 TEASPOONS VANILLA EXTRACT
- ½ CUP CHOPPED WALNUTS
- ⅓ CUP DRIED CRANBERRIES OR CHERRIES
- 1 OUNCE SEMISWEET CHOCOLATE, CHOPPED

1 Preheat the oven to 350°F. Lightly grease an 8-inch square metal baking pan. On a sheet of wax paper, combine the flour, cocoa powder, baking powder, baking soda, and salt.

2 In a medium bowl, with an electric mixer, beat together the brown sugar, peanut butter, oil, and egg until well combined. Beat in the vanilla. On low speed, add the flour mixture. Fold in the walnuts, cranberries, and chocolate.

3 Bake for 25 to 30 minutes, or until a toothpick inserted in the center comes out clean, but with some crumbs clinging to it. Cool in the pan on a wire rack before cutting into 8 brownies.

Makes 8 brownies. Per brownie: 318 calories, 17g total fat (19% saturated), 3.2g fiber, 6g protein, 40g carbohydrate, 27mg cholesterol, 228mg sodium

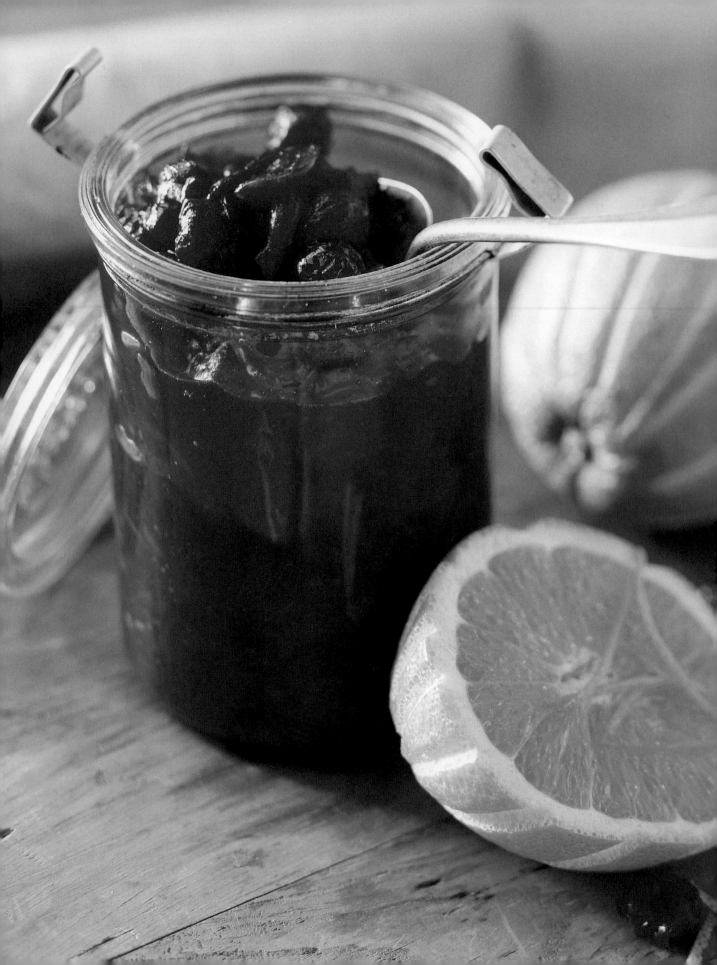

wasabi-miso dressing

Wasabi, a type of horseradish, can be found in paste form or as a powder in Asian food markets and in the international section of some supermarkets. Once opened, store the wasabi in the refrigerator—it will keep for several months. Serve this spicy dressing on mixed greens, sliced cucumbers, or in a chicken salad.

- 2 TABLESPOONS WASABI POWDER
- 2 TABLESPOONS YELLOW SHIRO MISO PASTE
- ¼ CUP FRESH LIME JUICE
- 1 TABLESPOON DARK SESAME OIL
- 1 TABLESPOON HONEY
- ½ TEASPOON SALT
- ½ TEASPOON GROUND GINGER

1 In a large bowl, stir together the wasabi powder and 2 tablespoons of water to form a paste. Stir in the miso.

2 Whisk in the lime juice, sesame oil, honey, salt, and ginger until smooth.

Makes 4 servings. Per serving: 74 calories, 4g total fat (14% saturated), 2g protein, 10g carbohydrate, 0.5g fiber, 0mg cholesterol, 603mg sodium

savory cranberry chutney

It's getting easier to make cranberry dishes year round now that many supermarkets have figured out that cranberries freeze well. If you're fond of cranberries, you can buy several bags of fresh cranberries when they're available in the late fall, and simply throw them into the freezer for later use.

- 2 TEASPOONS OLIVE OIL
- 1 LARGE RED ONION, FINELY CHOPPED
- 3 CLOVES GARLIC, MINCED
- 1 PACKAGE (12 OUNCES) FRESH OR FROZEN CRANBERRIES
- ½ CUP FIRMLY PACKED LIGHT BROWN SUGAR
- ½ CUP DRIED CHERRIES
- 2 TEASPOONS GRATED ORANGE ZEST
- ½ CUP ORANGE JUICE
- ½ TEASPOON PEPPER
- ¼ TEASPOON SALT
- ⅛ TEASPOON ALLSPICE

1 In a large saucepan, heat the oil over medium-low heat. Add the onion and garlic; cook, stirring frequently for 7 minutes, or until the onion is tender.

2 Stir in the cranberries, brown sugar, dried cherries, orange zest, orange juice, pepper, salt, and allspice. Cook, stirring occasionally for 10 minutes, or until the berries have popped. Cool to room temperature. Serve at room temperature or chilled.

Makes 6 servings. Per serving: 175 calories, 1.7g total fat (12% saturated), 1g protein, 42g carbohydrate, 2.8g fiber, 0mg cholesterol, 108mg sodium

roasted garlic-buttermilk ranch dressing

Use this as you would any creamy salad dressing. It can be made several days in advance and refrigerated until serving time.

- 1 BULB GARLIC (3 OUNCES)
- 2 TEASPOONS GRATED LEMON ZEST
- 1 TABLESPOON FRESH LEMON JUICE
- 1 TABLESPOON OLIVE OIL
- 1 TEASPOON ONION POWDER
- ½ TEASPOON SALT
- ⅛ TEASPOON CAYENNE PEPPER
- 1 CUP BUTTERMILK

1 Preheat the oven to 400°F. Wrap the garlic bulb in foil and roast for 45 minutes, or until the packet is soft to the touch.

2 Cut off the top of the garlic bulb and squeeze the garlic pulp into a medium bowl. Whisk in the lemon zest, lemon juice, oil, onion powder, salt, and cayenne until smooth. Whisk in the buttermilk. Keep refrigerated until serving time.

Makes 4 servings. Per serving: 85 calories, 4g total fat (20% saturated), 3g protein, 10g carbohydrate, 0.5g fiber, 2mg cholesterol, 357mg sodium

◀ savory cranberry chutney

general index

recipe index